AF904741

CARDIOTOXICITY OF ONCOLOGIC TREATMENTS

Edited by **Manuela Fiuza**

Cardiotoxicity of Oncologic Treatments
Edited by Manuela Fiuza

Published by InTech
Janeza Trdine 9, 51000 Rijeka, Croatia

Copyright © 2012 InTech
All chapters are distributed under the Creative Commons Attribution 3.0 license, which allows users to download, copy and build upon published articles even for commercial purposes, as long as the author and publisher are properly credited, which ensures maximum dissemination and a wider impact of our publications. After this work has been published by InTech, authors have the right to republish it, in whole or part, in any publication of which they are the author, and to make other personal use of the work. Any republication, referencing or personal use of the work must explicitly identify the original source.

As for readers, this license allows users to download, copy and build upon published chapters even for commercial purposes, as long as the author and publisher are properly credited, which ensures maximum dissemination and a wider impact of our publications.

Notice
Statements and opinions expressed in the chapters are these of the individual contributors and not necessarily those of the editors or publisher. No responsibility is accepted for the accuracy of information contained in the published chapters. The publisher assumes no responsibility for any damage or injury to persons or property arising out of the use of any materials, instructions, methods or ideas contained in the book.

Publishing Process Manager Sasa Leporic

Technical Editor Teodora Smiljanic

Cover Designer InTech Design Team

Additional hard copies can be obtained from orders@intechopen.com

Cardiotoxicity of Oncologic Treatments, Edited by Manuela Fiuza
p. cm.
ISBN 978-953-51-0273-1

We are IntechOpen, the world's leading publisher of Open Access books
Built by scientists, for scientists

4,200+
Open access books available

116,000+
International authors and editors

125M+
Downloads

151
Countries delivered to

Our authors are among the
Top 1%
most cited scientists

12.2%
Contributors from top 500 universities

WEB OF SCIENCE™

Selection of our books indexed in the Book Citation Index
in Web of Science™ Core Collection (BKCI)

Interested in publishing with us?
Contact book.department@intechopen.com

Numbers displayed above are based on latest data collected.
For more information visit www.intechopen.com

For EU product safety concerns:
IN TECH d.o.o., Prolaz Marije Krucifikse Kozulić 3, 51000 Rijeka, Croatia,
info@intechopen.com or visit our website at intechopen.com.

Meet the editor

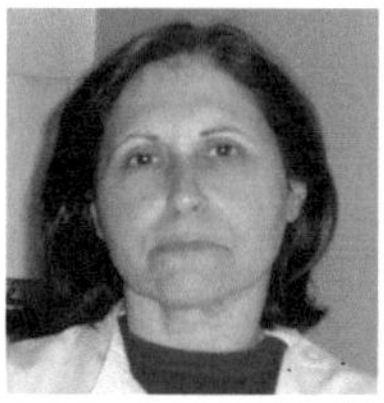

Manuela Fiuza was born in Lisbon, Portugal in 1956. She attended Lisbon Medical University and graduated in 1981. She did the fellowship of cardiology at the Hospital Santa Maria in Lisbon and graduated in 1991. During that time she developed special interest in echocardiography and intensive care. Dr. Fiuza is currently working at the Department of Cardiology of Hospital Santa Maria. Since 1999 she has been working as a senior cardiologist at the Echocardiography Laboratory. In 2000, she received her Ph.D. from Lisbon Medical University. While holding a position as a Professor of Cardiology, she also coordinated several pre- and post- graduated projects. She received several awards for scientific research. Her latest research interests are focused on cardio-oncology. Dr. Fiuza is a member of several scientific societies and is fellow of the European Society of Cardiology.

Contents

Preface

Many drugs, including those used in cancer patient treatments can cause injuries to human heart. As number of cured cancer patients continues to increase, the issue of cardiotoxicity is currently being subject of intensive research, since it can harmly influence long-term health condition of patients. This book reviews this subject over seven chapters which are briefly described below.

In Chapter 1 the authors address the issue of cardiac damage caused by natural toxins. This compressive review focuses on toxins affecting heart physiology through modulation of the ionic channels in plasma membrane, describing most of the toxins affecting heart function, their targets in the heart tissue, mode of action and the most important clinical effects of envenomation.

Chapter 2 revisits the issue of nitric acid as a protective mechanism involved in the recovery of myocardial ischaemia. The results of this study clearly show the action of NO in isoproterenol-induced myocardial infarction and suggest the importance to assess the role of NO in pre infarction and early post infarction stages in patients. It is possible that the therapeutic modulation of NO release might prevent the cytotoxic actions of the excessive NO release which facilitate the recovery of the patient at the post infarction stage.

Chapter 3 reviews in depth the problem of cardiotoxicity of cancer therapy. The authors review different most used drugs and their potential mechanisms responsible for cardiac injury and major cardiac manifestations. Authors also revised the issue of cardiac involvement in patients undergoing mediastinal radiotherapy.

Chapter 4 addresses the issue of Neureregulin1-Erb signaling in Doxorubicin-induced cardiotoxicity. In this chapter authors review several studies, from basic and clinical findings regarding the potential cardioprotective role of neureregulin in prevention and promising therapeutic approach to prevent or reverse myocardial dysfunction of doxorubicin-induced cardiotoxicity.

In Chapter 5 authors deal with cardiotoxicity related to doxorubicin therapy. The mechanisms underlying cardiotoxicity of doxorubicin are complex. No single drug is able to prevent cardiotoxicity therefore, more clinical studies are needed to elucidate the mechanism and develop strategies in prevention against doxorubicin-induced cardiotoxicity.

Chapter 6 deals with the question of trastuzumab cardiotoxicity in patients with breast cancer Her2+. The use of trastuzumab has changed the natural history of patients with HER-2 positive breast cancer, both in adjuvant and metastatic setting, and has become the standard of care for treatment of these patients. However, the occurrence of symptomatic and asymptomatic cardiac dysfunction is one of major concerns. Several methods are proposed to early identify at-risk patients.

Chapter 7 reviews the issue of critical importance - the detection and prediction of early cardiotoxicity using biomarkers and echocardiographic techniques that can provide the diagnosis of myocardial injury in real time which is one of the main goals for both cardiologists and oncologists.

Manuela Fiuza
Echocardiography Laboratory of the Cardiology
Department of University Hospital Santa Maria,
Lisbon Medical University,
Portugal

1

Cardiovascular Pathophysiology Produced by Natural Toxins and Their Possible Therapeutic Implications

Robert Frangež, Marjana Grandič and Milka Vrecl
University of Ljubljana, Veterinary Faculty, Slovenia

1. Introduction

Venoms are complex concentrates of biologically highly active molecules known as toxins, and they exist mainly as peptides and proteins. Several natural toxins are produced by plants, bacteria, phytoplanktonic dinoflagellates, sea anemones, insects, fungi and animals. In nature, toxins have two main functions: to capture their preferred prey (e.g. spiders, snakes, scorpions, etc.) or to serve as defence (e.g. bee sting, frog poison, etc.). Toxins produced by micro-organisms are important virulence factors. On the other hand they are also tools to combat diseases. Some of them are used in low quantities as drugs, to prepare vaccines and as important tools in biomedical research. Toxins affecting heart physiology are very effective in the sense of defence and especially in capturing prey. They can disturb electrical (producing arrhythmias) and mechanical activity of the heart affecting pumping or leading even to cardiac arrest. The aim of this chapter is to describe most of the toxins affecting heart function, their targets in the heart tissue, mode of action and the most important clinical effects of envenomation.

2. Main molecular targets of the toxins in the heart

2.1 Sodium channels

Voltage-gated sodium channels are an essential part of excitable membranes and enable fast depolarisation, which is responsible for action potential (AP) generation in cardiomyocytes and in the some parts of the conduction system of the heart. Their density is very low in some parts of the heart's conductive system, e.g. sinoatrial node and atrioventricular node cells, and the highest in Purkinje cells and cardiomyocytes (Fozzard, 1996). Hence, they are targeted by several neurotoxins from plants and animals that use these molecules for defence and protection.

2.2 Calcium channels

Different types of Ca^{2+}-permeable channels have been described in the plasma membrane of heart cells: the L- and T-type channels, both voltage activated, and a background channel (for a review see Carmeliet et al., 1999). Inward current through L-type high voltage-gated calcium channels is responsible for prolonged AP in cardiac muscle cells and cardiac muscle contraction. L-type voltage-gated Ca^{2+}-channels are especially target for some bacterial (saxitoxin) and animal toxins (atrotoxin, maitotoxin, ω-conotoxin, crotoxin).

2.3 Potassium channels

The role of potassium channels is to repolarize the membrane during the AP or to maintain hyperpolarizing potential. They are involved in the regulation of duration of the AP. Therefore, changes in the function of potassium channels may cause life-threatening arrhythmias (Carmeliet et al., 1999). Important potassium channels that can be the target of natural toxins are calcium-activated potassium channels (charybdotoxin, iberiotoxin, apamin) and voltage-gated potassium channels (some dendrotoxins).

3. Biologically active molecules from different sources

3.1 Biologically active molecules from plants

3.1.1 Aconitine

Aconitines are a group of very poisonous alkaloids derived from various aconite species. They are neurotoxins that open TTX-sensitive Na^+ channels in the heart and other tissues (Wang & Wang, 2003). Some of them can bind to the high affinity receptor site 2 of sodium channels (K_i ~1.2 μM) and some of them to a low affinity binding site (Ki ~11.5 μM). The compounds of the high affinity group, which increases synaptosomal sodium and calcium activity (EC_{50} 3 μM), are the most toxic and provoke tachyarrhythmia. Binding of aconitine to the site II of voltage-dependent Na^+ channels prolongs the open state responsible for Na^+ influx leading to the permanent depolarization. Now it is commonly accepted that aconitine produces arrhythmias by prolonging opening or delaying the inactivation of voltage-dependent Na^+ channels. Low affinity alkaloids from aconitum species are less-toxic, reduce intracellular calcium activity and induce bradycardia (Friese et al., 1997).

3.1.2 Grayanotoxins

At least four grayanotoxins (GTXs) have been isolated from the leaves of *Rhododendron decorum* (Ericaceae). These toxins are responsible for so called "mad honey" intoxication. Early in the 1980s it was published that GTXs produce cardiac tachyarrhythmias. The pathophysiological mechanism, underlying tachyarrhythmia, is the triggered activity in the form of oscillatory afterpotentials, as it was shown in feline cardiac Purkinje fibres (Brown et al., 1981). After intoxication, GTXs can produce bradyarrhythmias in man and livestock (Koca & Koca, 2007). It was shown that GTXs-induced cardiac toxicity in rats is a consequence of increased sodium channel permeability and activated vagus nerve (Onat et al., 1991). Intoxication is associated with the fatal bradyarrhythmias that include second degree atrio-ventricular block and circulatory collapse (Okuyan et al., 2010).

3.1.3 Veratridine

Veratrum species plants contain more than 200 different alkaloids, which are the principal toxins. The opening of voltage-gated sodium channels is probably one of the most relevant pathophysiological mechanisms of its toxicity. Veratridine injected intravenously in rats induced the Bezold-Jarisch-like effect (transient hypotension) accompanied by bradicardia (Chianca et al., 1985). It is well known that persistent sodium current, which can be enhanced during heart ischemia, is one of the major contributors to ischemic arrhythmias. Prolonged cardiac AP, which can also be induced by veratridine, favours the occurrence of early afterdepolarizations that is one of the pathophysiological mechanisms of tachyarrhythmias. Increased Na+ uptake activates the Na+/Ca2+ exchanger that leads to cardomyocytes' Ca2+ overload. The latter can trigger the late depolarization after-potentials (DAPs), which is another pathophysiological mechanism underlying arrhythmias. If the amplitude of the DAPs reaches the threshold potential, a new AP is triggered. Such large, late DAPs often occur in the case of oscillations of the cytosolic Ca2+ concentration (Pignier et al., 2010).

Name	Source (produced by)	Chemical structure	Target	Mode of action	Effects	Acute LD_{50} in mice	Reference
Cardiotoxic toxins from plants							
Aconitine	Plants from genus *Aconitum*	Alkaloid	Voltage-gated Na^+ channels	Depolarization, AP duration increase	Arrhythmias	0.1 mg/kg	Gutser, 1998
Grayanotoxins (GTX)	Species from genus *Rhododendron*	Polyhydroxylated cyclic diterpene	Increase Na^+ channel permeability and activate vagus nerve	Alteration of excitability	Fatal cardiac bradyarrhythmias	1.28 mg/kg *i.p.*	Brown et al., 1981; Okuyan et al., 2010 ; Scott et al., 1971
Veratridine	Plants in the family *Liliaceae*	Steroid-derived alkaloid	Binding to the activated Na^+ ion channels	Depolarization, AP duration increase	Arrhythmias	1.35 mg/kg *i.p.*	Chianca et al., 1985; Pignier et al., 2010; Swiss & Bauer, 1951

Table 1. Natural cardiotoxic toxins from plants: source, structure, receptors, mode of action, effects on heart and toxicity.

3.2 Cardiotoxic toxins derived from mushrooms

3.2.1 Ostreolysin

Ostreolysin (Oly) is an acidic, 15 kDa protein isolated from the edible oyster mushroom (Pleurotus ostreatus) (Berne et al., 2002). It is a toxic, pore-forming cytolysin (Sepčić et al., 2003). When administered intravenously (i.v.), Oly causes electrocardiographic, arterial blood pressure and respiratory changes. Oly produces changes such as transient increase of arterial blood pressure followed by a progressive fall to mid-circulatory pressure accompanied by bradicardia, myocardial ischaemia and ventricular extrasystoles. Oly also induces lysis of rat erythrocytes in vitro and in vivo, resulting in hyperkalemia. Although direct action of the protein on the cardiomyocytes or heart circulation cannot be excluded (Oly is pore-forming toxin), the hyperkalemia resulting from the haemolytic activity seems to play an important role in its cardiotoxicity (Žužek et al., 2006). Additionally, an important mechanism of the cardiotoxic effect may also be its concentration-dependent contractile effect on elastic blood vessels, such as aorta (Rebolj et al., 2009) and coronary vessels (Juntes et al., 2009).

Name	Source (produced by)	Chemical structure	Target	Mode of action	Effects	Acute LD_{50} in mice	Refer-ence
Cardiotoxic toxins derived from mushrooms							
Ostreolysin	Oyster mushroom (*Pleurotus ostreatus*)	Pore-forming protein	Cell membranes	Pore formation	Bradycardia; myocardial ischaemia; ventricular extrasystoles, hyperkalemia	1.17 mg/kg	Žužek et al., 2006

Table 2. Natural cardiotoxic toxins from mushrooms: source, structure, receptors, mode of action, effects on heart and toxicity.

3.3 Biologically active molecules produced by micro-organisms

3.3.1 Bacterial toxins

3.3.1.1 *Vibrio parahemolyticus* haemolysin (toxin)

Vibrio parahemolyticus toxin is lethal for rats when injected *i.v.* in a dose of 5 μg/kg or higher. It decreases intra-atrial and ventricular conductivity, and produces atrioventricular block. Before cardiac arrest occurs, ventricular flutter develops. The toxin is also toxic for cardiomyocytes in culture. Similar to the heart, the beating rhythm of cardiomyocytes exposed to the toxin increases and then abruptly stops (Honda et al., 1976).

3.3.1.2 Streptolysin O

Streptolisin O is a pore-forming toxin released in the extracellular medium by the majority of group A and some of group C and G *Streptococci*. It belongs to the sulphydryl- or thiol-activated toxins. It is a protein with a molecular weight of about 67 kDa. Streprolysin O is capable of forming cation permeable pores in cholesterol-rich membranes. Administered *i.v.* in high doses it produces sudden cardiac arrest, probably due to a non-specific binding to the lipid bilayers of cardiac cells (for a review see Harvey, 1990).

3.3.1.3 Saxitoxin

Saxitoxin (STX) is produced by certain marine species of dinoflagellates (*Alexandrium sp., Gymnodinium sp.*) and cyanobacteria species (*Anabaena sp.,* some *Aphanizomenon spp., Cylindrospermopsis sp.*). STX, usually administered through shellfish ingestion, is responsible for the human illness known as paralytic shellfish poisoning (PSP). STX acts primarily as a sodium channel blocker; it binds to the binding site 1 (Mebs & Hucho, 1990). Additionally it was found that STX also inhibits L-type Ca^{2+} currents in adult mouse ventricular myocytes (Su et al., 2003).

3.3.1.4 Tetrodotoxin

Tetrodotoxin (TTX) is a toxin of microbial origin. A number of marine bacteria probably produce TTX, especially members of the genus *Vibrio* (most common species is *Vibrio alginolyticus*). The link between this species and production of TTX in animals has not been definitely confirmed as it is not clear whether the source of TTX in animals is the above-mentioned bacteria. TTX has been isolated from many animal species (pufferfish, toads of the genus *Atelopus*, octopuses of the genus *Hapalochlaena*, etc. (Mebs & Hucho, 1990). It was shown that both high and low affinity receptors (sodium channels) for TTX exist on the rat cardiomyocytes. Only a low affinity binding site is functional on the cardiac cells, which has dissociation constant for TTX about three orders of magnitude higher compared to the reported dissociation constant for TTX receptors in muscle and nerve. The concentration needed to block cardiac sodium channels is very high (Renaud et al., 1983). The myocytes in the heart express fast voltage-gated sodium channel and therefore the generation of AP and

Name	Source (produced by)	Chemical structure	Target	Mode of action	Effects	Acute LD_{50} in mice	Reference
Microbial toxins							
Bacterial toxins							
Hemolysin TDH, TRH	*Vibrio parahaemolyticus*	Protein	Heart	Alteration in conductance of the conductive system	Arrhythmias, cardiac arrest	Between 2.5 and 5 μg/kg in rats	Honda et al., 1976
Streptolysin O	*Streptococci* group A, C and G	Protein	Nonspecific binding (membranes rich on cholesterol)	Pore formation	Bradycardia, atrio-ventricular conduction block	8 μg/kg *i.v.*	Gill, 1982; Harvey, 1990
Tetrodotoxin (TTX)	Bacteria: *Pseudoalteromo-nas tetraodonis*, certain species of *Pseudomonas* and *Vibrio*	heterocyclic, organic, water-soluble non-protein molecule	Voltage dependent Na^+ channels	Shorten the AP duration and decrease the initial depolarizing phase of the AP	Cardiac arrest	10.7 μg/kg *i.p.*; 12.5 μg/kg *s.c.*; 532 μg/kg *i.g.*	Mebs & Hucho, 1990; Xu et al., 2003
Saxitoxin	Marine dinoflagellates (*Alexandrium sp.*, *Gymnodinium sp.*) and cyanobacteria (*Anabaena sp.*, some *Aphanizomenon spp.*, *Cylindrospermopsis sp.*)	Heterocyclic guanidine	Voltage-gated Na^+ channels-block L-type Ca^{2+} channels-partial block	Shorten the AP duration and decrease the initial depolarizing phase of the AP	Prolongation of P-Q interval, first degree of atrio-ventricular block, ventricular fibrilation	3 – 10 μg/kg *i.p.*	Anderson, 2000; Su et al., 2003

Table 3. Natural cardiotoxic toxins from microbes: source, structure, receptors, mode of action, effects on heart and toxicity; *i.g.*- intra-gastric administration

electrical activity is blocked leading to blockade of myocardium excitability and cardiac arrest, although sodium channels are usually not affected in case of intoxication.

3.3.2 Algal toxins affecting heart physiology

Algae are ubiquitous micro-organisms in aqueous environments. Some of them will periodically form harmful "blooms." *Karenia brevis* is a dinoflagellate that can form harmful blooms known as "Florida red tides". Blooms are associated with the production of a group of powerful neurotoxins known as brevetoxins.

3.3.2.1 Brevetoxins

Brevetoxin (PbTx) is produced by marine dinoflagellates. It is polyether neurotoxin that targets the voltage-gated sodium channels present in all excitable membranes including heart tissues. Brevetoxins open voltage-gated sodium ion channels in cell membranes and cause uncontrolled sodium influx into the cell leading to the depolarization (Purkerson et al., 1999). Humans can be exposed to PbTx by ingesting brevetoxin-contaminated shellfish or through other environmental exposures. Its affinity for the rat heart tissue is much lower in contrast to the heart tissue of marine animals, but comparable with the skeletal muscle and brain (Dechraoui et al., 2006). At least 10 different brevetoxins have been isolated from seawater blooms and *K. brevis* cultures. PbTx in a dose higher than 25 μg/kg produces heart block, ventricular extrasystoles and idioventricular rhythms in conscious rats. It was concluded that brevetoxin causes changes in the cardiac conduction system and multiple changes in the function of the nervous system (Templeton et al., 1989). Systemic accumulation of the toxin in artificially respirated cats injected with PbTx leads to cardiovascular collapse and death (Borison et al., 1985).

3.3.2.2 Yessotoxins

Yessotoxins (YTXs) are polycyclic ether compounds produced by phytoplanktonic dinoflagellates (algal toxins). They can accumulate in shellfish which are a source of human intoxication through contaminated seafood ingestion. YTX, homoyessotoxin and 45-hydroxy-homoyessotoxin are lethal when administered intraperitonealy (*i.p.*) to mice. Although the mechanisms of the cardiotoxicity of YTX and homoyessotoxins are not well understood, some data from *in vitro* experiments, such as changes of intracellular calcium and cyclic AMP concentrations, alteration of cytoskeletal and adhesion molecules, caspases activation and opening of the permeability transition pore of mitochondria, support their cardiotoxic action (Dominguez et al., 2010; for a review see Tubaro et al., 2010). They induce microscopically visible ultrastructural changes in heart tissue after intraperitoneal and oral exposure. Noticeable intracytoplasmic oedema of cardiac muscle cells was observed within three hours after the *i.p.* administration of YTX at a dose of 300 μg/kg or higher (Terao et al., 1990). In mice YTX produces swelling of cardiomyocytes and separation of organelles in the area near capillaries after oral (10 mg/kg) and *i.p.* (1 mg/kg) toxin administration (Aune et al., 2002).

3.3.2.3 Ciguatoxin

Ciguatera caused by fish poisoning is a foodborne disease caused by eating certain fishes whose meat is contaminated with ciguatoxins produced by dinoflagellates such as *Gambierdiscus toxicus*. These toxins include ciguatoxin (CTX), maitotoxin, scaritoxin and palytoxin. Ciguatera fish poisoning is primarily endemic in tropical regions of the world. On neuroblastoma cells, CTX induces a membrane depolarization which is due to an action that increases Na^+ permeability and is prevented by voltage-gated sodium channel blocker TTX (Bidard et al., 1984). Intravenous injections of ciguatoxin evoke dose-dependent effects: bradycardia and atrioventricular conduction block at low doses, ventricular tachycardia at sublethal doses, and heart failure at high doses (up to 160 µg/kg) (Legrand et al., 1982). The Caribbean ciguatoxin (C-CTX-1) stimulates the release of *acetylcholin* (ACh) and produces muscarinic effect on frog atrial fibres (Sauviat, 1999; Sauviat et al., 2002).

Name	Source (produced by)	Chemical structure	Target	Mode of action	Effects	Acute LD_{50} in mice	Reference
Algal toxins							
Brevetoxin	Dinoflagellate *Karenia brevis*	Cyclic polyether	Voltage-gated Na^+ channels	Depolarization, AP duration increase	Heart block, ventricular extrasystoles and idioventricular rhythms	250 µg/kg *i.p.*	Purkerson et al., 1999; Templeton et al., 1989; Selwood et al., 2008
Yes-sotoxins	Algae	Polycyclic ether compounds	Voltage gated Ca^{2+} channels	Reduction of the firing and biting frequency of rat cardiac cells	Changes of intracellular Ca^{2+} and cyclic AMP concentrations, alteration of cytoskeletal and adhesion molecules, caspases activation and opening of the permeability transition pore of mitochondria	444-512 µg/kg *i.p.*	Tubaro et al., 2003; Dell'Ovo et al., 2008
Ciguatoxin	Dinoflagellate *Gambierdiscus toxicus*	Polyether toxins	Voltage-gated Na^+ channels	Depolarization, AP duration increase, arrhythmias	Biphasic inotropic and chronotropic excitatory, and inhibitory effects	0.3 – 10 µg/kg *i.p.*	Dechraoui et al., 1999
Maitotoxin	Dinoflagellate *Gambierdiscus toxicus*	N/A	Ca^{2+} channels	Agonist	AP amplitude increase	0.17 mg/kg *i.p.*	Igarashi et al., 1999; Mebs & Hucho, 1990

Table 4. Natural cardiotoxic toxins from algae: source, structure, receptors, mode of action, effects on heart and toxicity. (N/A - not applicable).

3.3.2.4 Maitotoxin

Maitotoxin (MTX) plays an important role in the syndrome named ciguatera poisoning. The toxin is derived from *Gambierdiscus toxicus*, a marine dinoflagellate species (for a review see

Mebs & Hucho, 1990). MTX causes dose-dependent effects on the heart. It has positive inotropic effects on heart preparations and causes irreversible contracture of isolated rat cardiomyocytes that can be prevented by specific voltage-dependent Ca^{2+} channel blocker verapamil (Kobayashi et al., 1986). MTX increases dose-dependent increase in Ca^{2+} activity in freshly dispersed cardiomyocytes. This effect of MTX may be inhibited by reducing Ca^{2+} concentration in the culture medium or by the calcium-channel blocker verapamil. Therefore, it has been concluded that MTX specifically activates voltage-dependent Ca^{2+} channels. This influx of Ca^{2+} into the cells is considered an important mechanism for cardiotoxicity of the MTX (Santostasi et al., 1990).

4. Biologically active molecules from animals affecting heart physiology

Animal venoms are usually a complex mixture of polypeptides, enzymes and molecules which can cause cell injury. Polypeptides exert their effect through action on ion channels and in a cell's plasma membrane. Enzymes can cause membrane lysis, pore formation, etc.

4.1 Palytoxin

Palytoxin (PTX) was first toxin isolated from the soft coral *Palythoa toxica*. PTX is one of the most powerful marine biotoxins of a high molecular weight (~ 3.3 kDa). It is the most potent non-proteinic and non-peptidic toxic substance known, with a lethal dose LD_{50} of 0.15 μg/kg in mice by the *i.v.* route (Moore & Scheuer, 1971).

4.2 Iberiotoxin

Iberiotoxin (IbTX) is derived from the venom of Eastern Indian red scorpion *Buthus tamulus*. IbTX selectively inhibits current through the calcium-activated potassium channels. IbTX in a 2 μM concentration increased the stimulation-induced ACh release (Kawada et al., 2010). It was reported that some patients who had been stung by a scorpion had signs such as hypertension and supraventricular tachycardia (Bawaskar & Bawaskar, 1992), to which may contribute also IbTX.

4.3 Batrachotoxins

Batrachotoxins (BTXs) are neurotoxic steroidal alkaloids first isolated from a Colombian poison-dart frog. BTXs are lipid-soluble toxins that bind with a high affinity to the type 2 receptor site of voltage-gated sodium channels in nerve and muscle membranes, keeping them in an open state (Albuquerque et al., 1971; Huang et al., 1984). This results in cell depolarization since BTXs inhibit inactivation of sodium channels. BTXs seem to play the most important role in cardiotoxicity. The cardiotoxic effects of BTXs accompanied by arrhythmia and cardiac arrest are connected to the activation of voltage-gated sodium channels in cardiac cells (Mebs & Hucho, 1990). It can evoke premature heart beat and fatal ventricular fibrillation associated with the haemodynamic arrest (Albuquerque et al., 1971).

4.4 Atrotoxin

Atrotoxin (ATX) is isolated from a venomous rattlesnake species *Crotalus atrox* found in the United States and Mexico. ATX binds reversibly to the voltage-gated calcium channels, leading to the increase of voltage-dependent calcium currents in single, dispersed guinea pig ventricular cells. ATX acts as a specific Ca^{2+} channel agonist (Hamilton et al., 1985).

4.5 Equinatoxins

Equinatoxins are pore-forming proteins isolated from the sea anemone *Actinia equine*. First evidence that equinatoxins are cardiotoxic was provided by Sket et al. (1974) by administration of tentacle extract of sea anemone *i.v.* into rats. Later, the isolation of three cardiotoxic proteins named Equinatoxin I, II and III with median lethal doses of 23, 35 and 83 μg/kg in mice, respectively (Macek & Lebez, 1988), was reported. EqT II is a pore forming toxin that through *de novo* formed pores evokes significant increase of intracellular Ca^{2+} activity, which cannot be blocked by conventional sodium and calcium channel blockers and probably plays an important role in direct (cytotoxic) or indirect cardiotoxicity through coronary vessel contraction and drop of the coronary perfusion rate (Frangež et al., 2000; Frangež et al., 2008; Zorec et al., 1990). All three equinatoxins are highly haemolytic and can cause a dose-dependent increase in potassium activity in blood plasma, leading to arrhythmias and cardiac arrest. Administered *i.v.* they produce dose-dependent disturbances in electrical activity of the heart accompanied by blood pressure changes. Additional information about direct dose-dependent cardiotoxic effects of EQT IIs were provided from the experiments on Langendorff's heart preparations. It causes a concentration-dependent drop of the perfusion rate, decreases left ventricular pressure and produces arrhythmias followed by cardiac arrest (Bunc et al., 1999).

4.6 Cardiotoxic-cytotoxic protein from cobra *Naja kaouthia*

A cytolytic protein was isolated from the Indian monocellate cobra (Naja kaouthia) venom. Intraperitoneal median lethal dose was estimated to be 2.5 mg/kg in Balb/C in male mice. *In vitro* the toxin produces auricular blockade as shown on isolated guinea pig auricle (Debnath et al., 2010).

4.7 Taicatoxin

Taicatoxin (TCX) is a snake toxin derived from the Australian taipan snake *Oxyuranus scutellatus scutellatus*. TCX reversibly and specifically blocks voltage-dependent L-type calcium channels in nanomolar concentrations (Brown et al., 1987). TCX decreases the plateau of AP in cardiomyocytes leading to a decrease in contractility. TCX has a negative chronotropic effect and evokes arrhythmias (Fantini et al., 1996). Electrocardiographic abnormalities were described in patients envenomed with a number of different species including *Oxyuranus spp.* Electrocardiographic changes include septal T wave inversion and bradycardia, and atrioventricular block. One of possible mechanisms which might be responsible for such clinical signs is a calcium channel blockade on cardiomyocytes (Lalloo et al., 1997).

4.8 Conotoxins

Conotoxins are peptides derived from the marine snail *Conus geographus* and consist of 10 to 30 amino acid residues. Many of these peptides modulate the activity of different ion channels. ω-conotoxin inhibits N-type voltage-dependent Ca^{2+} channels. It decreases the magnitude of cardiac AP and possesses a negative inotropic effect (Nielsen, 2000).

4.9 Crotoxin

Crotoxin (CTX) is derived from the venom of the South American rattlesnake, *Crotalus durissus terrificus*. *In vitro*, CTX decreases contractile force, increases the P-R interval and displaces the S-T segment. Arrhythmias are uncommon. The reduction of the contractile force and the increase in creatine kinase (CK) activity are ascribed to the release of free fatty acids and lysophospholipids, and to a cellular lesion (Santos et al., 1990; Zhang et al., 2010).

4.10 Sarafotoxin and bibrotoxin

Sarafotoxins (SRTs) and bibrotoxins are a group of extremely poisonous cardiotoxic snake venom peptides that show a striking structural similarity to endothelins (Becker et al., 1993; Kloog et al., 1988). SRTs are highly lethal peptides: in mice, the LD_{50} is 15 µg/kg body weight equalling the LD_{50} for endothelin (Bdolah et al., 1989), which is quite surprising for a peptide naturally occurring in the plasma of healthy humans. Sarafotoxin S6C, the most acidic endothelin-like peptide, shows reduced vasoconstrictive potency and is a highly selective natural ET_BR agonist (over 100 000 times higher affinity for the ET_BR vs. the ET_AR; [Williams et al., 1991]).

4.11 Anti-arrhytmic toxin from tarantula *Grammostola spatulata*

Gs-Mtx-4 is an amfipathic peptide toxin derived from the venom of the tarantula spider (*Grammostola spatulata*) with a molecular weight of 4 kDa (Hodgson & Isbister, 2009). It is the only toxin known that specifically affects cationic stretch activated ion channels and is therefore able to inhibit atrial fibrillation (Bowman et al., 2007).

5. Natural toxins as drugs

Some of the natural toxins acting on the cardiovascular system are very potent and highly specific for some receptors in cardiac and neuronal tissue. They can block, activate and even modulate the ion channels activity in excitable membranes. Although they are very stable molecules and possess high receptors specificity, they are seldom used as therapeutic drugs. Information about their three dimensional structure and data from structure-function studies of protein toxins may provide useful information for synthesis of smaller analogues with lower toxicity. Few natural toxins have potential in clinical use for treatment of cardiovascular dysfunction. Some of them have a positive inotropic effect, i.e. grayanotoxin, veratridine (Brill & Wasserstrom, 1986; Tirapelli et al., 2008). Due to their high toxicity, none of the described natural cardiotoxic substances are used as therapeutic drugs for treating cardiovascular diseases. Recently, sarafotoxins have been utilized to develop new, low molecular weight substances with metalloproteinase inhibitory activity. The modified molecule of the sarafotoxin 6b is used as a starting point, which has retained metalloproteinase inhibitory activity and removed vasoconstrictor activity. From this, the peptide (STX-S4-CT) was developed, which will hopefully provide a foundation for further development of improved candidate molecules (Hodgson & Isbister, 2009). Some promising

Name	Source (produced by)	Chemical structure	Target	Mode of action	Effects	Acute LD_{50} in mice	Source
Animal toxins							
Palytoxin	Soft coral: *Palythoa toxica*	Aliphatics carbon chain containing a series of heterocyclic rings	Na^+/K^+-ATPase; Hemolysin	Voltage-dependent K^+ channels	Haemolysis, arrhythmias	0.15 μg/kg	Sosa et al., 2009
Equinatoxin I, II, II	Sea anemone: *Actinia equina*	Proteins	Haemolysin	New cation non-selective pore formation	Dose-dependent arrhythmias, cardiac arrest, haemolysis	25,30 and 83 μg/kg *i.v.*	Maček & Lebez, 1988; Sket et al., 1974
Batrachotoxins (BTX)	Some frogs species (poison-dart frog), melyrid beetles and birds (*Ifrita kowaldi, Colluricincla megarhyncha*)	Steroidal alkaloids	Na^+ channels	Depolarize, lengthen the AP	Arrhythmias, extrasystoles, ventricular fibrillation	2 μg/kg *s.c.*	Albuquerque et al., 1971; Mebs & Hucho, 1990
Atrotoxin	Snake: *Crotalus atrox*	N/A	Ca^{2+} channels	Agonist, AP amplitude increase	Arrhythmias	89.4 - 137 μg *i.v.*	Hamilton et al., 1985; Barros et al., 1998
Cardiotoxic-cytotoxic protein (MW 6.76 kDa)	Indian monocellate cobra (*Naja kaouthia*)	Protein	Heart	Sinuauricular blockade	Arrhythmias	2.5 mg/kg *i.p.*	Debnath et al., 2010
Taicatoxin (TCX)	Australian taipan snake *Oxyuranus scutellatus*	N/A	Ca^{2+} channels	Antagonist	Bradycardia, atrioventricular block	N/A	Brown et al., 1987; Lalloo et al., 1997
Omega-conotoxin	Cone snail from genus *Conus*	Peptide	N-type voltage-dependent Ca^{2+} channels	Antagonist	Decreases the magnitude of AP plateau, negative inotropic effects	N/A	Nielsen, 2000
Crotoxin (CTX)	South American rattlesnake (*Crotalus durissus terrificus*)	Protein; crotapotin basic phospholipase A_2	L-type Ca^{2+} channels	Agonist	Elongation of AP duration, an increase of its amplitude	55.5 - 70.5 μg/kg *i.p.*	Rangel-Santos et al., 2004
Sarafotoxin (SRTs) and bibrotoxin	Snake: *Atractaspis engaddensis*	Peptide	Endothelin receptors	Agonist	Arrhythmias	15 μg/kg	Bdolah et al., 1989
GsMtx-4	Spider – tarantula: *Grammostola spatulata*	Peptide	Stretch activated ion channels (SACs)	Antagonist	Inhibits atrial fibrillation	N/A	Bowman et al., 2007

Table 5. Natural cardiotoxic toxins from animals: source, structure, receptors, mode of action, effects on heart and toxicity. (N/A - not applicable).

results in the treatment of cardiovascular disorders were also obtained with GsMtx-4 toxin isolated from tarantula *Grammostola spatulata* venom. This toxin is able to inhibit the stretch activated ion channels (SACs) and consequently inhibits atrial fibrillation. Due to its described properties, it can be used as a framework for developing a new class of anti-arrhythmic drugs, which would be directed against pathophysiologic mechanisms of atrial fibrillation, instead of just dealing with the symptoms as with many current therapies (Hodgson & Isbister, 2009).

6. Conclusion

Severe acute toxic insult caused by natural toxins can cause functional changes in heart tissue physiology or even cardiac cell death. Most of the natural toxins derived from plants, bacteria, phytoplanktonic dinoflagellates, fungi and animals target ionic channels in excitable membranes of cardiac cells or cardiac cell membranes itself, produce alteration in AP (e.g. depolarization, repolarization, alterations in its duration) or significant changes in intracellular ion activity. These changes may lead to reversible or even irreversible life threatening cardiac arrhythmias and eventually heart failure.

7. References

Albuquerque EX., Daly JW. & Witkop B. Batrachotoxin: chemistry and pharmacology. *Science*, Vol. 172, No. 987, (Jun 1971), pp. 995-1002, 0036-8075

Anderson D. (August 2010). The harmful algae page. Available from http://www.redtide.whoi.edu/hab/

Aune T., Sørby R., Yasumoto T., Ramstad H. & Landsverk T. Comparison of oral and intraperitoneal toxicity of yessotoxin towards mice. *Toxicon*, Vol. 40, No. 1, (Jan 2002), pp. 77-82, 0041-0101

Barros SF., Friedlanskaia I., Petricevich VL. & Kipnis TL.Local inflammation, lethality and cytokine release in mice injected with Bothrops atrox venom. *Mediators of inflammation*, Vol. 7, No. 5, (Sep 1998), pp. 339-346, 0962-9351

Bawaskar HS. & Bawaskar PH. Management of the cardiovascular manifestations of poisoning by the Indian red scorpion (Mesobuthus tamulus). *British Heart Journal*, Vol. 68, No. 5, (Nov 1992), pp. 478-480, 0007-0769

Bdolah A., Wollberg Z., Ambar I., Kloog Y., Sokolovsky M. & Kochva E. Disturbances in the cardiovascular system caused by endothelin and sarafotoxin. *Biochemical pharmacology*. Vol. 38, No. 19, (Oct 1989), pp. 3145-3146, 0006-2952

Becker A., Dowdle EB., Hechler U., Kauser K., Donner P. & Schleuning WD. Bibrotoxin, a novel member of the endothelin/sarafotoxin peptide family, from the venom of the burrowing asp Atractaspis bibroni. *FEBS Letters*, Vol. 315, No. 1, (Jan 1993), pp. 100-103, 0014-5793

Berne S., Krizaj I., Pohleven F., Turk T., Macek P. & Sepcić K. Pleurotus and Agrocybe hemolysins, new proteins hypothetically involved in fungal fruiting. *Biochimica et Biophysica Acta*, Vol. 1570, No. 3, (Apr 2002), pp. 153-159, 0304-4165

Bidard JN., Vijverberg HP., Frelin C., Chungue E., Legrand AM., Bagnis R. & Lazdunski M. Ciguatoxin is a novel type of Na+ channel toxin. *Journal of Biological Chemistry*, Vol. 259, No. 13, (Jul 1984), pp. 8353-8357, 1083-351X

Borison HL., McCarthy LE. & Ellis S. Neurological analysis of respiratory, cardiovascular and neuromuscular effects of brevetoxin in cats. *Toxicon*, Vol. 23, No. 3, (1985), pp. 517-524, 0041-0101

Bowman CL., Gottlieb PA., Suchyna TM., Murphy YK. & Sachs F. Mechanosensitive ion channels and the peptide inhibitor GsMTx-4: history, properties, mechanisms and pharmacology. *Toxicon*, Vol. 49, No. 2, (Feb 2007), pp. 249-270, 0041-0101

Brill DM. & Wasserstrom JA. Intracellular sodium and the positive inotropic effect of veratridine and cardiac glycoside in sheep Purkinje fibers. *Circulation Research*, Vol. 58, No. 1, (Jan 1986), pp. 109-119, 1524-4571

Brown BS., Akera T. & Brody TM. Mechanism of grayanotoxin III-induced afterpotentials in feline cardiac Purkinje fibers. *European Journal of Pharmacology*, Vol. 75, No. 4, (Nov 1981), pp. 271-281, 0014-2999

Brown AM., Yatani A., Lacerda AE., Gurrola GB. & Possani LD. Neurotoxins that act selectively on voltage-dependent cardiac calcium channels. *Circulation Research*, Vol. 61, No. 4, (Oct 1987), pp. 16-19, 0009-7330

Bunc M., Drevenšek G., Budihna M. & Šuput D. Effects of equinatoxin II from Actinia equina (L.) on isolated rat heart: the role of direct cardiotoxic effects in equinatoxin II lethality. *Toxicon*, Vol. 37, No. 1, (Jan 1999), pp. 109-123, 0041-0101

Carmeliet E. Cardiac ionic currents and acute ischemia: from channels to arrhythmias. *Physiological reviews*, Vol. 79, No. 3, (Jul 1999), pp. 917-1017, 0031-9333

Chianca Júnior DA., Cunha-Melo JR. & Freire-Maia L. The Bezold-Jarisch-like effect induced by veratridine and its potentiation by scorpion toxin in the rat. *Brazilian Journal of Medical and Biological Research*, Vol. 18, No. 2, (1985), pp. 237-248, 0100-879X

Debnath A., Saha A., Gomes A., Biswas S., Chakrabarti P., Giri B., Biswas AK., Gupta SD. & Gomes A. A lethal cardiotoxic-cytotoxic protein from the Indian monocellate cobra (*Naja kaouthia*) venom. *Toxicon*, Vol. 56, No. 4, (Sep 2010), pp. 569-579, 0041-0101

Dechraoui MY., Naar J., Pauillac S. & Legrand AM. Ciguatoxins and brevetoxins, neurotoxic polyether compounds active on sodium channels. *Toxicon*, Vol. 37, No. 1, (Jan 1999), pp. 125-143, 0041-0101

Dechraoui MY., Wacksman JJ. & Ramsdell JS. Species selective resistance of cardiac muscle voltage-gated sodium channels: characterization of brevetoxin and ciguatoxin binding sites in rats and fish. *Toxicon*, Vol. 48, No. 6, (Nov 2006), pp. 702-712, 0041-0101

Dell'Ovo V., Bandi E., Coslovich T., Florio C., Sciancalepore M., Decorti G., Sosa S., Lorenzon P., Yasumoto T. & Tubaro A. In vitro effects of yessotoxin on a primary culture of rat cardiomyocytes. *Toxicological sciences*, Vol. 106, No. 2, (Dec 2008), pp. 392-399, 1096-6080

Dominguez HJ., Paz B., Daranas AH., Norte M., Franco JM. & Fernández JJ. Dinoflagellate polyether within the yessotoxin, pectenotoxin and okadaic acid toxin groups: characterization, analysis and human health implications. *Toxicon*, Vol. 56, No. 2, (Aug 2010), pp. 191-217, 0041-0101

Fantini E., Athias P., Tirosh R. & Pinson A. Effect of TaiCatoxin (TCX) on the electrophysiological, mechanical and biochemical characteristics of spontaneously beating ventricular cardiomyocytes. *Molecular and Cellular Biochemistry*, Vol. 160, No. 161, (Jul-Aug 1996), pp. 61-66, 1573-4919

Fozzard HA. & Hanck DA. Structure and function of voltage-dependent sodium channels: comparison of brain II and cardiac isoforms. *Physiological Reviews*, Vol. 76, No. 3, (Jul 1996), pp. 887–926, 0031-9333

Frangež R., Meunier F., Molgo J. & Šuput D. Equinatoxin II increases intracellular Ca^{2+} in NG 108-15 cells. *Pflügers archive: European Journal of Physiology*, Vol. 439, Suppl. 3, (2000), pp. R100-1, 0031-6768

Frangež R., Šuput D. & Molgó J. Effects of equinatoxin II on isolated guinea pig taenia caeci muscle contractility and intracellular Ca^{2+}. *Toxicon*, Vol. 51, No. 8, (Jun 2008), pp. 1416-1423, 0041-0101

Friese J., Gleitz J., Gutser UT., Heubach JF., Matthiesen T., Wilffert B. & Selve N. Aconitum sp. alkaloids: the modulation of voltage-dependent Na+ channels, toxicity and antinociceptive properties. *European Journal of Pharmacology*, Vol. 337, No. 2-3, (Oct 1997), pp. 165-74, 0014-2999

Gill DM. Bacterial toxins: a table of lethal amounts. *Microbiological Reviews*, Vol. 46, No. 1, (Mar 1982), pp. 86–94, 0146-0749

Gutser UT., Friese J., Heubach JF., Matthiesen T., Selve N., Wilffert B. & Gleitz J. Mode of antinociceptive and toxic action of alkaloids of Aconitum spec. *Naunyn-Schmiedeberg's archives of pharmacology*, Vol. 357, No. 1, (Jan 1998),pp. 39-48, 0028-1298

Hamilton SL., Yatani A., Hawkes MJ., Redding K. & Brown AM. Atrotoxin: a specific agonist for calcium currents in heart. *Science*, Vol. 229, No. 4709, (Jul 1985), pp. 182-184, 0036-8075

Harvey AL. (1990). Cytolytic toxins. In: *Handbook of Toxinology*, Shier TW and Mebs D, pp. 1-66. Marcel Dekker Inc., New York.

Hodgson WC. & Isbister GK. The application of toxins and venoms to cardiovascular drug discovery. *Current Opinion in Pharmacology*, Vol. 9, No. 2, (Apr 2009), pp. 173-176, 1471-4973

Honda T., Goshima K., Takeda Y., Sugino Y. & Miwatani T. Demonstration of the cardiotoxicity of the thermostable direct hemolysin (lethal toxin) produced by Vibrio parahaemolyticus. *Infection and Immunity*, Vol. 13, No. 1, (Jan 1976), pp. 163-171, 0019-9567

Huang LY., Moran N. & Ehrenstein G. Gating kinetics of batrachotoxin-modified sodium channels in neuroblastoma cells determined from single-channel measurements. *Biophysical Journal*, Vol. 45, No. 1, (Jan 1984), pp. 313-322, 0006-3495

Igarashi T., Aritake S. & Yasumoto T. Mechanisms underlying the hemolytic and ichthyotoxic activities of maitotoxin. *Natural Toxins*, Vol. 7, No. 2, (1999), pp. 71-79, 1056-9014

Juntes P., Rebolj K., Sepcić K., Macek P., Zuzek MC., Cestnik V. & Frangez R. Ostreolysin induces sustained contraction of porcine coronary arteries and endothelial dysfunction in middle- and large-sized vessels. *Toxicon*, Vol. 54, No. 6, (Nov 2009), pp. 784-792, 0041-0101

Kawada T., Akiyama T., Shimizu S., Kamiya A., Uemura K., Sata Y., Shirai M. & Sugimachi M. Large conductance Ca2+-activated K+ channels inhibit vagal acetylcholine release at the rabbit sinoatrial node. *Autonomic Neuroscience: Basic & Clinical*, Vol. 156, No. 1-2, (Aug 2010), pp. 149-151, 1566-0702

Kloog Y., Ambar I., Sokolovsky M., Kochva E., Wollberg Z. & Bdolah A. Sarafotoxin, a novel vasoconstrictor peptide: phosphoinositide hydrolysis in rat heart and brain. *Science*, Vol. 242, No. 4876, (Oct 1988), pp. 268-270, 0036-8075

Kobayashi M., Kondo S., Yasumoto T. & Ohizumi Y. Cardiotoxic effects of maitotoxin, a principal toxin of seafood poisoning, on guinea pig and rat cardiac muscle. *The Journal of Pharmacology and Experimental Therapeutics*, Vol. 238, No. 3, (Sep 1986), pp. 1077-1083, 0022-3565

Koca I. & Koca AF. Poisoning by mad honey: a brief review. *Food and Chemical Toxicology*, Vol. 45, No. 8, (Aug 2007), pp. 1315-1318, 0278-6915

Lalloo DG., Trevett AJ., Nwokolo N., Laurenson IF., Naraqi S., Kevau I., Kemp MW., James R., Hooper L., David R., Theakston G. & Warrell D. Electrocardiographic abnormalities in patients bitten by taipans (Oxyuranus scutellatus canni) and other elapid snakes in Papua New Guinea. *Transactions of the Royal Society of Tropical Medicine and Hygiene*, Vol. 91, No. 1, (Jan-Feb 1997), pp. 53-56, 0035-9203

Legrand AM., Galonnier M. & Bagnis R. Studies on the mode of action of ciguateric toxins. *Toxicon*, Vol. 20, No.1, (1982), pp. 311-315, 0041-0101

Macek P. & Lebez D. Isolation and characterization of three lethal and hemolytic toxins from the sea anemone *Actinia equina* L. *Toxicon*. Vol. 26, No. 5, (1988), pp. 441-451, 0041-0101

Mebs D. & Hucho F. (1990). Toxins acting on ion channels and synapses. : *Handbook of Toxinology*, Shier TW and Mebs D, pp. 493-597. Marcel Dekker Inc., New York.

Moore RE. & Scheuer PJ. Palytoxin: a new marine toxin from a coelenterate. *Science*, Vol. 172, No. 982, (Apr 1971), pp. 495-498, 0036-8075

Nielsen KJ., Schroeder T. & Lewis R. Structure-activity relationships of omega-conotoxins at N-type voltage-sensitive calcium channels. *Journal of Molecular Recognition*, Vol. 13, No. 2, (Mar-Apr 2000), pp. 55-70, 0952-3499

Okuyan E., Usulu A. & Ozan LM. Cardiac effects of "mad honey": a case series. *Clinical Toxicology (Phila)*, Vol. 48, No. 6, (Jul 2010), pp. 528-532, 1556-3650

Onat F., Yegen BC., Lawrence R., Oktay A. & Oktay S. Site of action of grayanotoxins in mad honey in rats. *Journal of Applied Toxicology*, Vol. 11, No. 3, (Jun 1991), pp. 199-201, 0260-437X

Pignier C., Rougier JS., Vié B., Culié C., Verscheure Y., Vacher B., Abriel H. & Le Grand B. Selective inhibition of persistent sodium current by F 15845 prevents ischaemia-induced arrhythmias. *British Journal of Pharmacology*, Vol. 161, No. 1, (Sep 2010), pp. 79-91, 0007-1188

Purkerson SL., Baden DG. & Fieber LA. Brevetoxin modulates neuronal sodium channels in two cell lines derived from rat brain. *Neurotoxicology*, Vol. 20, No. 6, (Dec 1999), pp. 909-920, 0161-813X

Rangel-Santos A., Dos-Santos EC., Lopes-Ferreira M., Lima C., Cardoso DF. & Mota I. A comparative study of biological activities of crotoxin and CB fraction of venoms from Crotalus durissus terrificus, Crotalus durissus cascavella and Crotalus durissus collilineatus. *Toxicon*, Vol. 43, No. 7, (Jun 2004), pp. 801-810, 0041-0101

Rebolj K., Batista U., Sepčić K., Cestnik V., Macek P. & Frangez R. Ostreolysin affects rat aorta ring tension and endothelial cell viability in vitro. *Toxicon*, Vol. 49, No. 8, (Jun 2007), pp. 1211-1213, 0041-0101

Renaud JF., Kazazoglou T., Lombet A., Chicheportiche R., Jaimovich E., Romey G. & Lazdunski M. The Na^+ channel in mammalian cardiac cells. Two kinds of tetrodotoxin receptors in rat heart membranes. *The Journal of Biological Chemistry*, Vol. 258, No. 14, (Jul 1983), pp. 8799-8805, 0021-9258

Santos PE., Souza SD., Freire-Maia L. & Almeida AP. Effects of crotoxin on the isolated guinea pig heart. *Toxicon*, Vol. 28, No. 2, (1990), pp. 215-224, 0041-0101

Santostasi G., Kutty RK., Bartorelli AL., Yasumoto T. & Krishna G. Maitotoxin-induced myocardial cell injury: calcium accumulation followed by ATP depletion precedes cell death. *Toxicology and Applied Pharmacology*, Vol. 102, No. 1, (Jan 1990), pp. 164-173, 0041-008X

Sauviat MP. Muscarinic modulation of cardiac activity. *Journal de la Société de Biologie*, Vol. 193, No. 6, (1999), pp. 469-480, 1295-0661

Sauviat MP., Marquais M. & Vernoux JP. Muscarinic effects of the Caribbean ciguatoxin C-CTX-1 on frog atrial heart muscle. *Toxicon*, Vol. 40, No. 8, (Aug 2002), pp. 1155-1163, 0041-0101

Selwood AI., Ginkel R., Wilkins AL., Munday R., Ramsdell JS., Jensen DJ., Cooney JM. & Miles CO. Semisynthesis of S-desoxybrevetoxin-B2 and brevetoxin-B2, and assessment of their acute toxicities. *Chemical Research in Toxicology*. Vol. 21, No. 4, (Apr 2008), pp. 944-950, 0893-228X

Sepcić K., Berne S., Potrich C., Turk T., Maček P. & Menestrina G. Interaction of ostreolysin, a cytolytic protein from the edible mushroom Pleurotus ostreatus, with lipid membranes and modulation by lysophospholipids. *European Journal of Biochemistry*, Vol. 270, No. 6, (Mar 2003), pp. 1199-1210, 0014-2956

Scott PM., Coldwell BB. & Wiberg GS. Grayanotoxins. Occurrence and analysis in honey and a comparison of toxicities in mice. *Food and Cosmetics toxicology*, Vol. 9, No. 2, (Apr 1971), pp. 179-184, 0015-6264

Sket D., Drašlar K., Ferlan I. & Lebez D. Equinatoxin, a lethal protein from Actinia equina. II. Pathophysiological action. *Toxicon*, Vol. 12, No. 1, (Jan 1974), pp. 63-68, 0041-0101

Sosa S., Del Favero G., De Bortoli M., Vita F., Soranzo MR., Beltramo D., Ardizzone M. & Tubaro A. Palytoxin toxicity after acute oral administration in mice. *Toxicology Letters*, Vol. 191, No. 2-3, (Dec 2009), pp. 253-259, 0378-4274

Su Z., Sheets M., Ishida H., Li F. & Barry WH. Saxitoxin blocks L-type ICa. *The Journal of Pharmacology and Experimental Therapeutics*, Vol. 308, No. 1, (Jan 2004), pp. 324-329, 0022-3565

Swiss ED. & Bauer RO. Acute toxicity of veratrum derivatives. *Proceedings of the Society for Experimental Biology and Medicine*. Vol. 76, No. 4, (Apr 1951), pp. 847-849, 0037-9727

Templeton CB., Poli MA. & LeClaire RD. Cardiorespiratory effects of brevetoxin (PbTx-2) in conscious, tethered rats. *Toxicon*, Vol. 27, No. 9, (1989), pp. 1043-1049, 0041-0101

Terao K., Ito E., Oarada M., Murata M. & Yasumoto T. Histopathological studies on experimental marine toxin poisoning. The effects in mice of yessotoxin isolated from Patinopecten yessoensis and of a desulfated derivative. *Toxicon*, Vol. 28, No. 9, (1990), pp. 1095-1104, 0041-0101

Tirapelli CR., Ambrosio SR., da Costa FB. & de Oliveira AM. Diterpenes: a therapeutic promise for cardiovascular diseases. *Recent Patents on Cardiovascular Drug Discovery*. Vol. 3, No. 1, (Jan 2008), pp. 1-8, 2212-3962

Tubaro A., Dell'ovo V., Sosa S. & Florio C. Yessotoxins: a toxicological overview. *Toxicon*, Vol. 56, No. 2, (Aug 2010), pp. 163-172, 0041-0101

Tubaro A., Sosa S., Carbonatto M., Altinier G., Vita F., Melato M., Satake M. & Yasumoto T. Oral and intraperitoneal acute toxicity studies of yessotoxin and homoyessotoxins in mice. *Toxicon*. Vol. 41, No. 7, (Jun 2003), pp. 783-792, 0041-0101

Wang SY. & Wang GK. Voltage-gated sodium channels as primary targets of diverse lipid-soluble neurotoxins. *Cellular Signalling*, Vol. 15, No. 2, (Feb 2003), pp. 151-159, 0898-6568

Williams DL. Jr., Jones KL., Colton CD. & Nutt RF. Identification of high affinity endothelin-1 receptor subtypes in human tissues. *Biochemical and Biophysical Research Communications*, Vol. 180, No. 2, (Oct 1991), pp. 475-480, 0006-291X

Xu Q., Huang K., Gao L., Zhang H. & Rong K. Toxicity of tetrodotoxin towards mice and rabbits. *Wei sheng yan jiu*, Vol. 32, No. 4, (Jul 2003), pp. 371-374, 1000-8020

Zhang P., Lader AS., Etcheverry MA. & Cantiello HF. Crotoxin potentiates L-type calcium currents and modulates the action potential of neonatal rat cardiomyocytes. *Toxicon*, Vol. 55, No. 7, (Jun 2010), pp. 1236-1243, 0041-0101

Zorec R., Tester M., Maček P. & Mason WT. Cytotoxicity of equinatoxin II from the sea anemone Actinia equina involves ion channel formation and an increase in intracellular calcium activity. *The Journal of Membrane Biology*, Vol. 118, No. 3, (Dec 1990), pp. 243-249, 0022-2631

Žužek MC., Maček P., Sepčić K., Cestnik V. & Frangež R. Toxic and lethal effects of ostreolysin, a cytolytic protein from edible oyster mushroom (Pleurotus ostreatus), in rodents. *Toxicon*, Vol. 48, No. 3, (Sep 2006), pp. 264-271, 0041-0101

2

Role of Nitric Oxide in Isoproterenol-Induced Myocardial Infarction

Victoria Chagoya de Sánchez et al.*
Departamento de Biología Celular y Desarrollo,
Instituto de Fisiología Celular,
Universidad Nacional Autónoma de México,
Mexico

1. Introduction

Myocardial infarction (MI) is an important cause of mortality around the world, resulting from an ischemic necrosis induced by a vascular occlusion. In general, MI occurs unexpectedly and the clinical syndrome previous to MI is difficult to detect. Animal models of MI are very useful in the study of prevention, diagnosis and therapy design for human MI [Smith & Nuttall., 1985]. MI induced by ligation of the left anterior descending coronary artery is the animal model most frequently used; however, the anesthesia and surgical procedures affect the conditions in which the infarction occurred [Wang et al., 2006]. Therefore, MI in animal models studies should be induced in conscious animals with intact reflexes for greater clinical relevance. Myocardial infarction induced by isoproterenol (ISO) using toxic concentration of this β-adrenergic agonist drug, originally described by Rona [Rona et al., 1959] has been used by several groups to study the cardiotoxic effects of this molecule [Stanton et al,1969]. This model becomes relevant if we consider that increased adrenergic activation plays a role as a trigger of acute myocardial infarction. In addition, the stress associated to MI in patients, increases catecholamine blood levels, which in turn, augment contraction force of the heart and ATP utilization favoring an energetic unbalance [Wallace & Klein, 1969, Ueba et al, 1973].

We have used ISO-induced MI, which is a non-invasive experimental model, to study the mechanisms involved in MI in the steps previous and posterior to infarction [Chagoya de Sánchez et al., 1997]. Myocardial lesions induced by ISO are related to its cardiac stimulating properties [Chappel et al.,1959]. Our group has characterized histological, physiological and biochemical alterations in a long term model (0-96h) of ISO administration to rats [Chagoya de Sánchez et al., 1997]. Animals treated with ISO showed an infarct-like damage of the circumferential type in the subendocardium at the apex region of the left ventricle that

*Lucía Yañez-Maldonado[1], Susana Vidrio-Gómez[1], Lidia Martínez[1], Jorge Suárez[4], Alberto Aranda-Fraustro[2], Juan Carlos Torres[3] and Gabriela Velasco-Loyden[1]
[2]*Departamento de Patología, Instituto Nacional de Cardiología, "Ignacio Chávez", Mexico*
[3]*Departamento de Farmacología, Instituto Nacional de Cardiología, "Ignacio Chávez", Mexico*
[4]*Current address: Department of Medicine, University of California, San Diego, CA, USA*

occurred at 12-24h after ISO administration. MI lesion was defined by: 1) histological criteria looking for coagulative necrosis and fiber fragmentation, 2) physiological and biochemical criteria, 3) functionally by a continuous telemetric ECG recordings and 4) the increase of serum marker enzymes specific for myocardial damage. These results lead us to define three stages of myocardial damage induced by ISO, preinfarction (0-12 h), infarction (12-24 h) and postinfarction (24-96 h).

During the physiological characterization of the ISO model, the first functional events observed after 2 minutes of ISO administration were a 70% increase in heart rate and a 40% and 30% decrease in diastolic and systolic blood pressure respectively, which lasted from 3 minutes to 6 h after ISO administration, inducing a functional hypoxia that resulted in a MI. Ultra structural changes in mitochondria were evident from the first hour of treatment but functional alterations in isolated mitochondria, like oxygen consumption, respiratory quotient, ATP synthesis and membrane potential appeared at 6 h of drug administration. However, an important decrease in mitochondrial protein (50%) was noticed after 3 h of treatment and was maintained during the whole study, but the energy imbalance, reflected by a decrease in energy charge and in the creatine phosphate/creatine ratio, was observed after 30 minutes of the treatment. All these alterations reached a maximum at the onset of infarction. Partial recovery of some of these parameters was observed during post-infarction period (24-96h) but it was not the case for ATP synthesis, oxygen consumption, total adenine nucleotides, and mitochondrial protein [Chagoya de Sánchez et al., 1997]. These results showed the critical role of mitochondrial function in the energy unbalance at the onset of MI induced by ISO.

Early changes in Ca^{2+} overload and their consequences are crucial in ISO cardiotoxicity [Fleckenstein et al.,1974, Bloom & Davis, 1972; Barry & Bridge, 1972]. Prolonged hypoxia and the inotropic action of ISO on the cardiac muscle make it very likely that oxidative stress and Ca^{2+} overload could be involved in the mechanism of ISO-induced MI. Deregulation of intracellular Ca^{2+} homeostasis modifies the cell redox state generating oxidative stress [Choudhary & Dudley, 2002]. Knowing that myocardial Ca^{2+} overload and oxidative stress are well documented effects of ISO-induced MI, we investigated the correlation between oxidative stress and intracellular calcium handling in our model [Díaz-Muñoz et al., 2006]. Analysis of total calcium content in sub cellular fractions, revealed that the mitochondrial fraction presented a significantly elevated Ca^{2+} content (80%) after 30 minutes of ISO treatment reaching a peak at 6h (220%) and returning towards normal values after the MI (24-48h). These results showed a good correlation with the energy unbalance previously commented.

The oxidative stress in the ISO-induced myocardial infarction was evaluated studying lipid peroxidation, the free radical generating systems, antioxidant enzymes and the glutathione system [Díaz-Muñoz et al., 2006]. Oxyradical generation during myocardial ischemia occurs mainly through the xanthine oxidase and the activated neutrophils [Ray & MaCord, 1982; Reimer et al., 1989] In addition, ISO oxidation also generates superoxide anions [Yates et al., 1981]. In our model, a large amount of superoxide anions are formed during the preinfarction phase by inhibition of superoxide dismutase and catalase, just after MI there is an increase in the activity of both enzymes inactivating the superoxide ion. The nitroradicals during MI are related with nitric oxide formation quantified by the stable products nitrite and nitrates ions. Lipid peroxidation was clearly increased after 6-96 h of ISO treatment as a consequence of ion superoxide formation during the pre-infarction period And the nitric oxide (NO) generated throughout the experimental period. The glutathione cycle, studied by the content of GSH and GSSG and the activities of GSH-peroxidase and GSH-reductase, was decreased during the three stages of ISO-induced cardiotoxicity. Thus, confirming the importance of the oxidative stress generated by an increase in ROS and RNS as well as a decrease in antioxidant defenses in this experimental model, reaching a maximum at 24-48 h [Díaz-Muñoz et al., 2006].

Niric oxide is a small biological molecule generated as gaseous free radical that participates in multiple physiological and pathological processes. It is a very reactive molecule with a life span of a few seconds that diffuses freely across membranes. To date, NO is considered as an important messenger molecule. In 1987 Moncada's group [Palmer et al., 1987] showed that the endothelium derived relaxing factor (EDRF) was the nitric oxide that is biosynthesized from L-arginine [Palmer et al., 1988]. Later on, it was shown that NO formation is not limited to vascular tissue but into numerous cells. Apparently, it is a general mechanism of intercellular communication in order to activate the guanylate cyclase [Berrazueta et al., 1990]. NO is also a main regulator of the immune activity and functions as neurotransmitter in the central nervous tissue as physiological messenger [Lowestein & Snyder,1992] but it also has an important cytotoxic activity in vivo [Kröncke et al., 1997]. Physiological NO is synthesized by the constitutive nitric oxide synthase (eNOS, or III) for short periods of time (seconds or minutes). Cytotoxic NO is synthetized by the inducible nitric oxide synthase (iNOS or II) which produces NO for large periods of time, hours or days [Laurent et al., 1996] as occurs in macrophages activation.

NO action can be direct or indirect [Espey et al., 2000; Wink & Mitchell, 1998]. In the direct one, NO interacts rapidly with the biological blank as occurs in the activation of the guanylate cyclase. In this case, NO reacts directly with the iron of the hemo group of the active center of the enzyme generating GMPc, which activates a cGMP dependent protein kinase resulting in the relaxation of the smooth muscle and vasodilatation, diminished heart contraction and stimulation of ionic pumps [Ignarro, 1990; Kröncke, 1997]. On the other hand, indirect effects are related to oxygen and nitrogen reactive species generating peroxynitrites ($ONOO^-$). These compounds are responsible for the cytotoxicity that induces DNA fragmentation or lipid oxidation. Peroxynitrtites induce damage of the I-IV segments of the respiratory chain in the mitochondria as well as damage of Mn dependent superoxide dismutase (SOD-Mn) increasing the generation of H_2O_2 and superoxide anion which results in a dysfunctional mitochondria [Brown, 1999]. NO in the extracellular medium will react with oxygen and water to form nitrites and nitrates.

Nitric oxide is produced by three isoforms of nitric oxide synthases in the heart; endothelial (eNOS), inducible (iNOS) and neuronal (nNOS). Cardiac myocytes express the three isoforms although eNOS is mainly expressed in the endothelial cells. eNOS is constitutively expressed and can be stimulated with the increase of cytosolic calcium and phosphorylation [Cale & Bird, 2006]. In contrast, iNOS is a cytokine–inducible isoenzyme. In healthy heart, physiological amounts of NO may help to sustain cardiac inotropy [Krenek et al., 2009]. It is our hypothesis that in the ISO-induced MI model, the hypotensive effect observed after ISO administration, in the preinfarct stage [Chagoya de Sánchez, 1997], is mediated by NO and might be critical for the MI development. The main goal of this study is to investigate the role of NO in the development of MI using an inhibitor of its synthesis L-NAME (nitro-L-arginine methyl ester). We examined the relative role of eNOS and iNOS on IM-induced pathological changes of histological, physiological, biochemical and molecular parameters as well as energy state of heart. Preinfarction, infarction and postinfarction stages were analysed.

2. Material and methods

Enzymes, coenzymes, isoproterenol, L-NAME and the kits for the assessment of enzyme activities were from Sigma Chemical Co (St. Louis, MO). eNOS and iNOS antibodies were obtained from Santa Cruz Biotechnology (Santa Cruz, CA). All other reagents were obtained from Merck (Mexico).

2.1 Animal treatment

Male Wistar rats (250-300g, body weight) were injected subcutaneously (s.c.) at 9 AM with a single dose of isoproterenol hydrochloride (67mg/kg body weight). Control animals were injected with saline solution. Animals were euthanized at 0.5, 1, 3, 6, 12, 24, 48, 72, and 96 h after treatment, with exception of the animals used for hemodynamic parameters by radiotelemetry. Blood samples were taken to obtain serum. A heart sample was used for histological studies; other sample was taken for perchloric extracts and for analysis of the expression of the nitric oxide synthases. Other set of experiments in similar conditions were performed for Langendorff preparations to evaluate NO formation. L-NAME was administered i.p. at the dose of 110 mg/kg of body weight one hour before the ISO treatments. All procedures were conducted in accordance to the Federal Regulation for Animal Care and Experimentation (Ministry of Agriculture, SAGAR, Mexico).

2.2 Histological studies

The heart was removed immediately after death and slices were cut from the apex, fixed with 10% neutral buffered formaline. After embedding tissue in paraffine 4 μm thickness sections were stained with hematoxilin-eosine and Masson's trichrome. A qualitative evaluation was made with a light microscope considering elongation, ondulation of the fibers, formation of contractile bands as a characteristic of the pre infarction stage, and the presence o macrophages, fibroblasts and collagen fibers as a post infarction stage.

2.3 Hemodynamic studies

These parameters were studied by radiotelemetry in freely moving conscious animals with a Data Sciences International equipment (Brockway and Hassier 1993), using a TL11M2-C50-PXT implant to monitor blood systolic and diastolic pressure, and heart rate. To implant transmitters, rats were anesthetized with an i.p. injection of ketamine plus xylazine at 80 and 10 mg/kg body weight respectively, surgical conditions as previously described [Chagoya de Sánchez et al., 1997]. Animals were allowed to recover at least for one week. Twenty four-hours recordings were taken as control of the parameters to be studied. Afterwards, ISO was s.c. administered. L-NAME was administered one hour before ISO administration in the corresponding groups.

2.4 Biochemical studies

Nitric oxide formation was measured in isolated perfused hearts as described previously [Suárez et al., 1999]. Briefly, animals were anesthetized with sodium pentobarbital (63 mg/ kg of body weight). The heart was removed and retrogradely perfused via a non-recirculating perfusion system at constant flow. Perfusion medium was Krebs-Henseleit solution equilibrated with 95% O_2 -5% CO_2 at 37°C and pH of 7.4, with 2μM oxihemoglobin solution for NO further quantification. Once the heart had been connected, it was maintained 30 minutes (perfusion flow rate of 25 ml/min for 5 minutes, then the following 25 minutes at 10 ml/min) and cardiac frequency was stabilized at 1 Hz. Perfusion flow rate was controlled by a peristaltic pump and 3 samples spaced by 5 minutes were taken from the coronary arteries. NO was measured indirectly in a double bean spectrophotometer (DW2000, SLM Aminco, Urban Illinois USA) quantifying the metahemoglobin produced as a function of NO generated in the coronary arteries [Kelm & Schrader, 1988]. NO serum levels were measured indirectly by the quantification of nitrites and nitrates ions with the Grieiss reagent [Shultz et al., 1991]. NO synthase activity was measured by monitoring the conversion of [^{3}H]-Arginine to [^{3}H]-Citrulline using a NOS Activity Assay Kit (Cayman Chemical Co, Ann Arbor, MI) and [^{3}H]-Arginine (PerkinElmer, Inc, Boston, MA) according to the manufacturer´s instructions. Briefly, 40 μg of heart homogenate were used for the assay, and the reaction was carried out for 30 min at 37 °C. Serum levels of myocardial-damage enzyme markers were measured from blood samples taken from the neck of the rat at the time of euthanasia. Creatine phosphokinase (CK) (EC2.7.3.2) and its heart isoenzyme (CK-MB), as well as alpha-hydroxybutyrate dehydrogenase (alpha-HBDH, EC 1.1.1.30) were determined using conventional diagnostic kits. Aspartate aminotransferase (AST, EC 2.6.1.1) and lactic dehydrogenase (LDH, EC1,1,1,27) were measured by the method of Bergmeyer and Bernt [1965] and [Bergmeyer etal. 1965]. Energy metabolism in the heart was evaluated measuring adenine nucleotides ATP, ADP and AMP and energy parameters as total adenine nucleotides and energy charge. For adenine nucleotide determination, 300mg of the heart were extracted with 8% perchloric acid, after centrifugation the sample was neutralized with 4M K_2 CO_3 Adenine nucleotide were quantified by reversed-phase high performance liquid chromatography [Hoffman& Liao, 1977]. Energy charge was calculated according to Atkinson [1968].

2.5 Protein expression by western blotting

Apical part of the left ventricle were homogenized in 50 mM Tris, pH 7.4, 1mM EDTA, containing a mixture of protease inhibitors. Homogenates were centrifuged at 10,000 g for 15 min, and the supernatant was used as whole cell protein. Protein samples (20 μg of protein/well) were electrophoresed in SDS-polyacrylamide gels and transferred to PDVF membranes. Membranes were blocked for 1 h with 5% nonfat dry milk in TBST (50 mM Tris, 150 mM NaCl at pH 7.4, and 0.05% Tween 20). Proteins were detected by incubating membranes overnight at 4°C with the following primary antibodies: anti-eNOS and anti-iNOS from Santa Cruz Biotechnology (Santa Cruz, CA), anti-phospho-eNOS (Ser-1177) (Cell

Signaling Technology, Danvers, MA). Primary antibody binding was detected with the respective horseradish peroxidase-conjugated secondary antibody (Santa Cruz Biotechnology, Santa Cruz, CA). Densitometric analysis of bands was performed with the Quantity One software (Bio-Rad).

3. Results

3.1 Histological studies

Histological evaluation of the myocardial lesion induced by isoproterenol treatment with and without L-NAME is shown on Table 1. The ISO-induced lesion is localized in the apical region of the left ventricle. In the presence of L-NAME, ISO-induced lesion maintained the same localization but it was extended to the subepicardial zone with less intensity. The pre-infarct lesions; elongation and ondulation of the fibers and necrosis and contraction bands were prolonged for 24h. The infarct lesions persisted for 48 h and the post infarction initiated early at 24 h with a slight decrease. Although the damaged fibers were similar in both groups, no necrosis was observed at the pre infarction stage suggesting that acute phase of necrosis at 6 h observed in the ISO group decreased and was extended for a longer period in presence of L-NAME. A diminished presence of polymorphonuclear cells and macrophages indicates a minor cellular lesion in the group treated with L-NAME demonstrating a different histological profile for each group.

	Time of ISO treatment (hours)							Time of ISO-L-NAME treatment (hours)						
Type of damage	3	6	12	24	48	72	96	3	6	12	24	48	72	96
Elongation and ondulation of fibers	+++	++	+	-	-	+	+	++	++	+++	++	+	-	-
Necrosis and contraction bands	+	+++	++	+	-	-	-	++	+	++	+++	+	+	++
Coagulative necrosis	-	-	+	++	-	-	-	-	+/-	+	++	+	-	-
Fragmentation of myofibrils	-	-	-	+	++	-	-	-	-	+/-	+	++	++	-
Polymorphonuclear cells	-	+	++	+++	+	-	-	-	-	+	++	+	-	-
Macrophages	-	-	-	+	+++	++	+	-	-	-	+	++	++	+
Fibroblasts and collagen fibers	-	-	-	-	+	++	+++	-	-	-	+	++	+++	++
Edema	-	+	++	+++	++	+	-	+	+	+++	++	+	-	+/-

Table 1. Histological evaluation of the myocardial lesion by isoproterenol (ISO) with and without L-NAME. Animals received an s.c. administration of ISO. L-NAME was administrated 1 hour before. They were euthanized after ISO administration. Total damage with ISO was taken as 100%. Score code is: (+)= 25%; (++)= 50%; (+++)= 75%; (-)= not observed.

3.2 Physiological studies

Blood pressure and heart rate were monitored continuously by telemetry, the results are shown in the Figure 1. To study the effect of L-NAME it was administered i.p. 1 h before ISO, its effect was detected in the pre-ISO lecture, the initial ISO effect was observed at time 0. A) Heart rate shows a strong and immediate increase from 279 to 450 b.p.m. during the first minutes of ISO administration. A further small increase (20%) was observed in the group of animals treated with L-NAME until 48h of treatment. B) Changes in systolic blood pressure show the hypotensive effect of ISO previously described (Chagoya de Sánchez et al., 1997). The group treated with L-NAME showed an increase in systolic pressure from 85 to 155 mmHg. ISO administration induced a diminution towards normal values followed by an increase to 140mmHg at 3 h of treatment returning to control values at 24 h. C) Similar profile was observed with diastolic pressure but the hypertensive effect (180 mmHg) was more evident. L-NAME administration did not significantly affect the effect of ISO increasing the heart rate but significantly reduced the hypotensive effect of ISO.

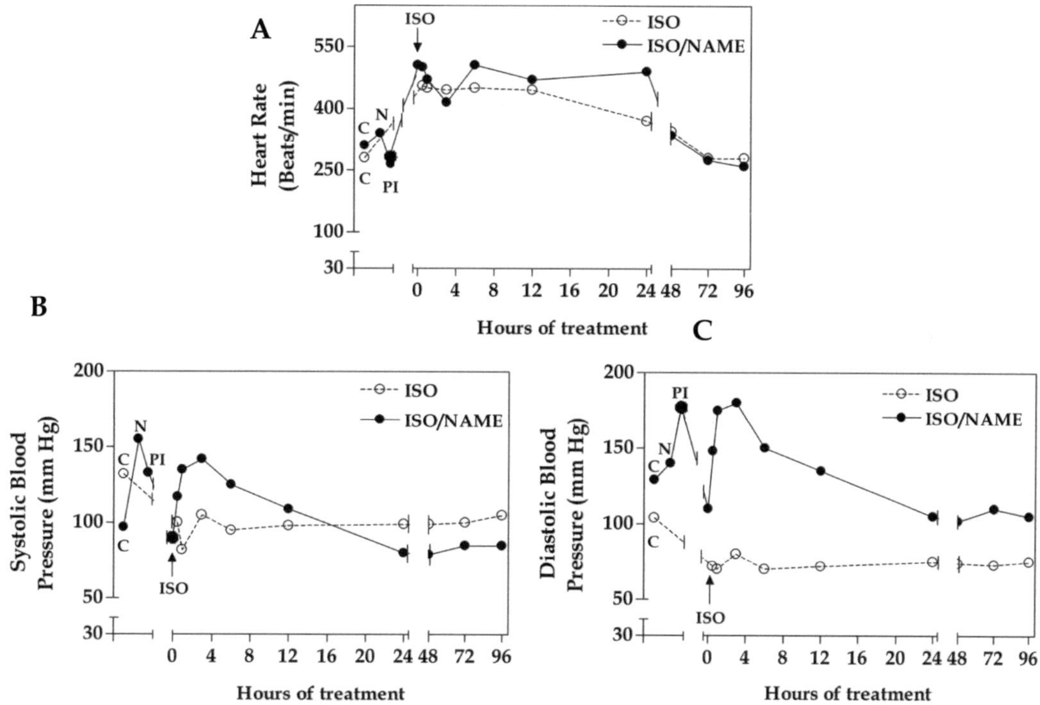

Fig. 1. In vivo effect of L-NAME on changes induced by isoproterenol on heart rate and blood pressure. Rats received (i.p) NAME one hour before isoproterenol injection (s.c) at time 0, as described in Material and methods. The response was monitored continuously by a telemetry system. C= Control, N= NAME and PI= Pre-ISO. A) Time course of the variation in heart rate (b.p.m.; beats per minute) B) Systolic pressure (mmHg) and C) Diastolic pressure (mmHg). Values are from a representative experiment of five.

3.3 Biochemical studies

3.3.1 Marker enzymes of myocardial damage (CK, CK-MB, α-HBDH, AST, LDH)

Were measured in serum of the experimental animals at the time of infarction that is at 12 h after ISO treatment in the presence or absence of L-NAME. Results are presented in the Table 2. ISO-induced cardiac lesions caused a 2 to 10-fold increase in marker enzymes including specific enzymes of cardiac origin like CK-MB which increased almost 4-fold with respect to its control values. Enzymes representative of cell necrosis, as LDH, showed a tenfold augmentation. Animals treated with L-NAME and ISO showed a significant reduction in the level of marker enzymes mainly CK-MB and LDH indicating diminished myocardial damage at that time in the group of animals treated with L-NAME.

Enzymes	Without treatment	ISO	ISO/NAME
CK	110 ± 9.2	220 ± 23 $P < 0.005$	80 ± 2.4 $P < 0.001$
CK MB	104 ± 6.5	389 ± 50.0 $P < 0.001$	160 ± 3.5 $P < 0.005$
α-HBDH	22 ± 1.9	50 ± 8.0 $P < 0.01$	44 ± 3.9 $P < 0.5$
AST	110 ± 7.0	260 ± 16.8 $P < 0.001$	220 ± 10.0 $P < 0.1$
LDH	120 ± 5.6	1 180 ± 13.0 $P < 0.001$	102 ± 2.0 $P < 0.001$

Table 2. Effect of isoproterenol and L-NAME on serum levels of marker enzymes of myocardial damage at the time of infarction (12h). Values are average activity of the different enzymes in serum samples of the rats (n=5) ± standard error. P value of the isoproterenol column represents a comparison with the control group without treatment and the P value of the ISO-NAME group is the significance of the L-NAME/ISO group vs. ISO group.

3.3.2 Energy metabolism

The influence of L-NAME on the changes in energy metabolism produced by isoproterenol (Chagoya de Sánchez et al., 1997) is shown in Table 3. Values at time 0 were obtained in animals without treatment. Values of the Pre-ISO group correspond to the group that received L-NAME treatment one hour before ISO administration. The energy unbalance generated by ISO treatment is clearly observed by the statistically significant decrease in ATP levels along the three stages of cardiotoxicity; pre infarction, infarction and post infarction, being more decreased at 24 h during the infarction period. These changes are also accompanied by a diminution of ADP and an increase in AMP levels resulting in low levels of total adenine nucleotides in the heart with decreased energy charge (E.C.= [ATP]+ 1/2 [ADP]/ [ATP]+[ADP]+[AMP] (AN = total adenine nucleotides), being 0.86 a normal value). Animals treated with L-NAME also presented an energy unbalance ATP and ADP levels were higher than those observed in the ISO group. AMP levels increased only at 3 and 6 h and an interesting observation is that during the pos infarction stage energy parameters (ATP, total adenine nucleotides and energy charge) recovered towards normal values.

3.3.3 NO formation

We evaluated NO release in isolated perfused hearts from experimental animals at different times of ISO treatment (Fig 2). An increase in NO release was observed since 0.5 h reaching a maximum at 6 and 12 h of ISO treatment. NO release levels returned to control values from 24 to 96 h. L-NAME inhibitory effect on ISO-induced NO release was evident since

Time of Treatment	ATP		ADP		AMP		AN		EC	
Hours	ISO	ISO/NAME	ISO	ISO/NAME	ISO	ISO/NAME	ISO	ISO/NAME	ISO	ISO/NAME
Pre-ISO	-	4.9 ± .40	-	2.5 ± .22	-	1.3 ± .20	-	7.99 ± .33	-	0.71 ± .01
0	6.2 ± .50	-	2.7 ± .10	-	0.4 ± .08	-	9.1 ± .59	-	0.8 ± .01	-
3	3.0 ± .20*	3.9 ± .60	3.1 ± .40	2.8 ± .66	1.4 ± .20*	2.1 ± .16*#	7.3 ± .73*	8.0 ± .99	0.6 ± .01*	0.6 ± .008*
6	2.7 ± .20*	2.6 ± .10*	2.0 ± .05*	2.2 ± .11	1.5 ± .12*	1.5 ± .08	5.6 ± .17*	5.7 ± .16*	0.61 ± .02*	0.61 ± .01*
12	2.6 ± .18*	2.6 ± .20*	1.8 ± .27*	1.9 ± .05*#	1.4 ± .37*	1.2 ± .29	5.6 ± .49*	6.0 ± .66*	0.61 ± .05*	0.57 ± .02*#
24	1.5 ± .10*	2.7 ± .05*#	1.0 ± .08*	1.5 ± .03*#	0.9 ± .15*	1.1 ± .08	3.3 ± .09*	4.8 ± .03*#	0.6 ± .02*	0.67 ± .01*#
48	3.4 ± .10*	3.9 ± .60	1.3 ± .05*	2.0 ± .16*#	0.4 ± .04*	1.1 ± .04#	5.0 ± .09*	6.5± .66#	0.77 ± .005*	0.71 ± .02*#
72	3.2 ± .05*	6.4 ± .40*#	1.9 ± .10*	3.0 ± .16*#	1.1 ± .07*	1.2 ± .01	4.3 ± .16*	9.6± .49*#	0.67 ± .005*	0.81 ± .01*#
96	2.3 ± .10*	4.0 ± .20*#	1.5 ± .16*	2.3 ± .27#	0.4 ± .04	1.5 ± .33#	4.2 ± .33*	7.3 ± .33#	0.72 ± .03*	0.70 ± .04*

Table 3. Effect of L-NAME on changes of rat heart adenine nucleotides in the ISO-induced infarction. AN (adenine nucleotides) is de sum of adenine nucleotides; EC, energy charge (ATP+1/2 ADP/AN) values are the means ± SEM, n=4, *p<0.05 ISO vs. 0 or ISO/NAME vs. Pre-ISO, #p<0.05 ISO-NAME vs. ISO.

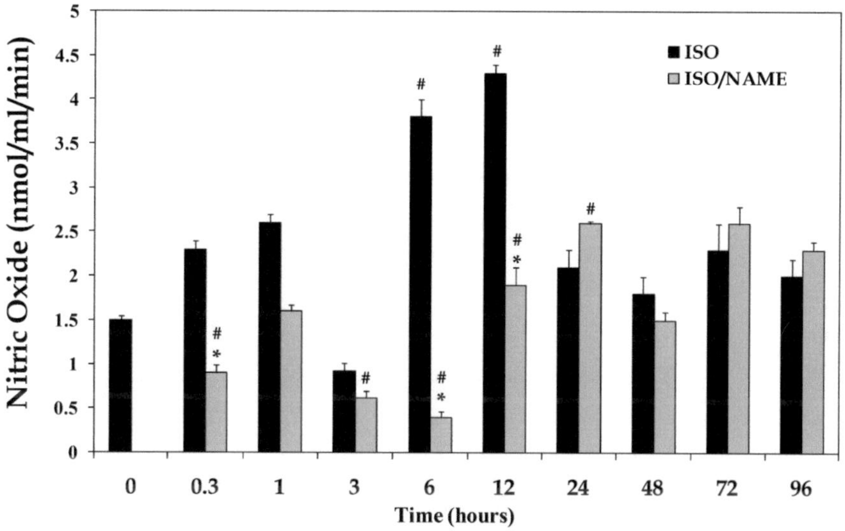

Fig. 2. Effects of isoproterenol and L-NAME on NO release. NO release in perfused hearts from treated rats at different times. Values are mean ± S.E n=5. Dark bars are isoproterenol treatment and gray bars L-NAME + isoproterenol.# p ≤ 0.05 ISO or ISO/NAME group vs Control (Time 0). * p ≤ 0.05 ISO/NAME group vs ISO.

0.5h with a maximal effect at 6-12 h of ISO treatment. After this time, the amount of NO released was similar in both groups suggesting the end of the inhibitory effect of L-NAME. Fig 3, shows nitric oxide synthases activity of the constitutive form (eNOS) and the inducible form (iNOS). ISO treatment gradually increased the activity of both isoforms during the pre infarction and infarction period. The maximal increase was at 24 h for eNOS and 12 h for iNOS. After this time, during the postinfarction, there was an important decrease on both isoforms. Animals treated with L-.NAME showed a gradual diminution of eNOS activity (3, 24 h). After this time the activities of the isoforms reach normal values. The increase in nitric oxide release during the pre infarction periods are the result of an increase in the activity of eNOS and iNOS and L-NAME decreased NO release by decreasing eNOS activity during the preinfarction-infarction stages since no significant change was observed in iNOS activity.

Protein expression of constitutive and inducible NO synthases in the presence of ISO and ISO+ L-NAME are shown in Fig 4. Small changes in the eNOS protein expression were observed during the preinfarction stage and more important ones during the post infarction Decreased eNOS protein levels were evident at 3, 12, and 24 h in the presence of L-NAME and no appreciable changes during the post infarction. eNOS is activated by phosphorylation in serine 1177. An increase in p-eNOS was observed after ISO treatment (1,3,6 h) with a diminution at (12,24,h). Treatment with L-NAME markedly decreased p-

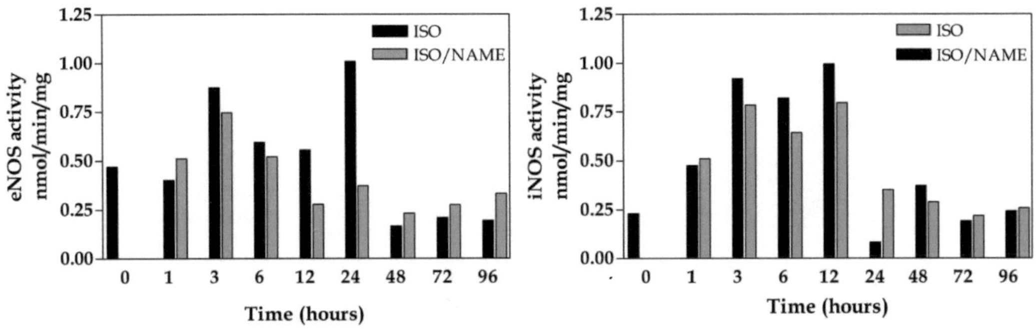

Fig. 3. The activity of constitutive and inducible (eNOS, iNOS) nitric oxide synthases. Values shown represent typical results of one experiment. Four experiments were performed.

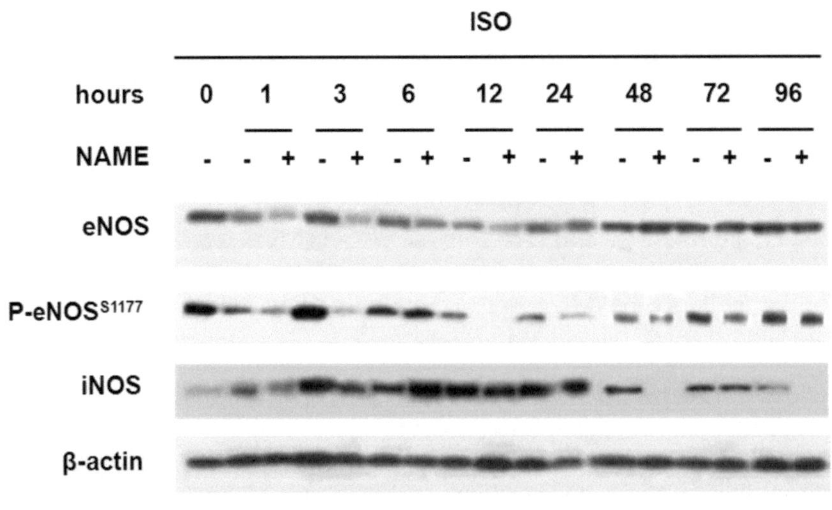

Fig. 4. Western blot analysis of a representative experiment (from three) of eNOS, P-eNOS ^{s1177}, iNOS protein expression.

eNOs (S1177) at 3, 12, and 24 h. At 6h eNOS is phosphorylated and must be active, however, there is an important reduction in NO release in the presence of L-NAME. iNOS expression was not detected in the control group. However, after ISO treatment, there was a gradual increase until 12 h with an important decrease after infarction which reached almost the control value at 96 h. A similar profile was observed in the group treated with L-NAME with differences at 6, 12, 48, and 96 h. NO serum levels were measured indirectly quantifying nitrites and nitrates (Fig 5). Although the same tendency as in isolated perfused hearts was observed, increased NO release during infarction (12, 24 h) was more clearly observed in the ISO-NAME group.

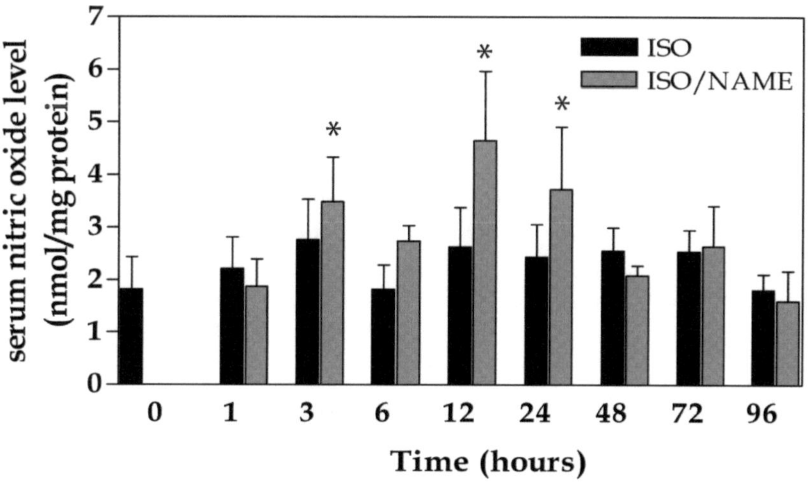

Fig. 5. $NO_2 + NO_3$ in serum from both groups. Values are the mean ± SE, n=3.
* p values > 0.05 ISO/NAME group vs control (Time 0)

4. Discussion

The role of nitric oxide in cardiovascular diseases is complex and controversial, mainly due to its multiple physiological and pathological effects which depend on the amount of NO synthetized by the nitric oxide synthases, their allosteric modulators, the metabolic conditions of the cells, redox and energy state, and the different experimental models used. A major physiological role of nitric oxide is the regulation of vascular tone. In this case the activity of endothelial eNOS is crucial since endothelial dysfunction is characterized by impairment of nitric oxide bioavailability which induces hypertension and cardiovascular diseases [Török, 2008]. In pathological conditions there is an increase in oxidative stress. Nitric oxide reacts with superoxide (O^{2-}) to produce peroxynitrites, highly cytotoxic nitrogen species, that induce DNA fragmentation, and damage of segments of the respiratory chain inducing dysfunctional mitochondria [Brown, 1999]. In the experimental model of myocardial infarction induced by isoproterenol studied here, we observed this dual actions of nitric oxide: 1) the marked diminution of systolic and diastolic pressure after 2 minutes of ISO treatment [Chagoya de Sanchez et al. 1997], suggesting the participation of the nitric oxide and 2) the cytotoxic action reflected in energy unbalance, dysfunctional mitochondria, oxidative stress, with increased levels of nitrites and nitrates as indicative of NO formation [Díaz-Muñoz et al, 2006).

In order to determine the role of nitric oxide in the ISO-induced MI, we used an inhibitor of endothelial nitric oxide synthase; L-NAME (N^G-nitro-L-arginine methyl ester) [Sander et al. 1999; Frandsen et al. 2001] and systolic and diastolic blood pressure and heart rate were evaluated (Fig 1). The drastic decrease in systolic and diastolic blood pressure caused by isoproterenol could be related to an increase in nitric oxide release due to an overexpression of eNOS induced by isoproterenol as previously described [Krenek et al. 2006]. This idea was confirmed by our results that clearly showed a marked increase in NO release after ISO administration during the pre infarction stage (0.5- 12 h). These results correlated with the increase in eNOS activity and protein expression of total eNOS. In addition, the activated form phosphorylated eNOS at Ser-1177 was increased during the pre infarction and infarction stages. During post-infarction phase, the expression of total and activated phosphorylated enzyme corresponds to a moderate increase in nitric oxide. This effect of isoproterenol is partially prevented by the presence of L-NAME and a decrease of 30 to 90% in NO release was observed (Fig2A). This reduction in NO release was also related to a decrease in eNOS activity and protein expression of total and phosphorylated (eNOS, P-eNOS^{s1177}. The eNOS-mediated NO generation is a highly regulated cellular event with multiple regulatory factors such as gene expression, translational modifications, intracellular localization, cofactors and phosphorylation [Govers & Rabelink, 2001). This could be the case for the result obtained at 3h of ISO administration in which NO release was low with elevated activity and expression of total and active form of eNOS. Isoproterenol also induced an increase of iNOS activity from 1-12 h of treatment reaching control values at the post infarction stage. Treatment with L-NAME induced a non-significant decrease in its activity and expression. The decrease in NO release and inhibition of eNOS in the presence of L-NAME lead us to the conclusion that the increase in systolic and diastolic pressure (Fig 1) contributes to improve heart function. The maintenance of the diastolic pressure is very important for a good perfusion of the heart through the coronary arteries. These effects were maintained throughout pre-infarction, infarction and post-infarction suggesting a decrease of cardiotoxicity induced by isoproterenol. This possibility was also tested measuring marker enzymes of myocardial damage in serum at the time of infarction (Table 1). The dramatic drop in CK-MB and LDH serum levels suggests that in the presence of L-NAME, the magnitude of myocardial damage was reduced. Previously it was shown that isoproterenol-induced MI is accompanied by a marked energetic unbalance through the 3 cardiotoxicity periods with no recovery in the post infarction stage. An interesting finding was that in the presence of L-NAME, at 48 h of ISO treatment in the post infarction stage, induced a recovery of energy balance which occurred increasing ATP, total adenine nucleotides and energy charge (Table 2). The indirect assessment of nitric oxide in serum also reflects the increase in NO at the infarction stage and it is mainly generated by iNOS when inflammatory cytokine levels are elevated as previously suggested [Gaballa et al., 1999]. Inhibition of eNOS by L-NAME blocks vessel dilation inducing a more extended lesion increasing the number of damaged cells. At same time, inflammatory cell migration diminishes by the vessel constriction induced by L-NAME resulting in less inflammation.

5. Conclusion

In summary, the present study shows that NO plays an important role in the installation and progression of the myocardial infarction induced by isoproterenol. The increased generation of nitric oxide was evidenced from 0.5 h until 12h of isoproterenol administration these likely resulted from an increase in the activity of both eNOS and iNOS. The first action seem to be a consequence of isoproterenol triggered signaling cascade action on the enzyme and the second one from subsequent inflammatory processes. The increase in eNOS is responsible for the hypotensive effect of ISO decreasing the systolic and diastolic pressure since the first 2 minutes of its administration. The consequent hypoperfusion induced an energy unbalance possibly due to the chronotropic and inotropic effects of isoproterenol which generates an increase in energy consumption. These effects demand an increase in mitochondrial function generating oxidative stress with ion superoxide formation, which in the presence of NO, will generate peroxynitrites resulting in mitochondrial damage and cellular death. All above contribute to myocardial infarction and the dysfunctional mitochondria prevents recovery of energy balance at the post infarction stage. Experiments in the presence of L-NAME (NO inhibitor) clearly showed a diminution of the acute phase of infarct, the inflammatory process and the reduction of the hypotensive action of ISO. As a result, there was an important increase in diastolic pressure and perfusion of the heart through the coronary arteries, diminishing the oxidative stress and a recuperation of energy balance which contributed to ameliorate myocardial function. The infarction observed in the presence of L-NAME is likely involved by the inflammation process that is not affected significantly by L-NAME treatment. These results clearly show the action of NO in isoproterenol-induced myocardial infarction and suggest the importance to assess the role of NO in pre infarction and early post infarction stages in patients. It is possible that the therapeutic modulation of NO release might prevent the cytotoxic actions of the excessive NO release which facilitate the recovery of the patient at the post infarction stage.

6. Clinical perspective

Myocardial ischemia/reperfusion is the major threat to cardiac myocytes in acute myocardial infarction. In spite of early interventions like reperfusion therapy, myocardial damage can not be avoided. Consequently, additional options to enhance myocardial resistance to ischemia/reperfusion are needed. Increasing nitric oxide action has been considered a possibility to enhance myocardial perfusion during myocardial infarction. However, nitric oxide action may lead to adverse effects. We now add data on the beneficial effect of inhibiting nitric oxide action by using L-NAME during development of myocardial infarction. Inhibition of nitric oxide release diminished the inflammatory process and reduced the hypotensive action of isoproterenol. As a result, there was an important increase in diastolic pressure and perfusion of the heart. These effects diminished the oxidative stress and helped to improve energy balance which contributed to better recovery of the myocardial function. Hence, increasing nitric oxide action as a therapeutic regimen in acute myocardial infarction is likely to be less successful if the distinct phases of myocardial infarction development are not considered. Undoubtedly, nitric oxide-modulation of coronary vessel tone is a therapeutic target in myocardial infarction. In the present work, we demonstrated that inhibition of nitric oxide action can be beneficial depending of the infarction stage. Development of new therapeutic strategies focused to manipulate nitric oxide action in pre-infarction, infarction and post-infarction is necessary to alleviate this important cardiac disease.

7. Acknowledgment

This study was partially supported by grants from Dirección de Asuntos del Personal Académico (DGAPA IN-296589) and Consejo Nacional de Ciencia y Tecnología (M9109-0710). The authors acknowledge critical comments from Dr. Adolfo García-Sáinz as well as the assistance of M.C. Rebeca Pérez Cabeza de Vaca, and secretarial assistance of Miss Rosario Villaseñor.

8. References

Atkinson D.E. (1968) The energy charge of the adenylate pool as a regulatory parameter. Interaction with feedback modifiers. Biochemistry 7: 4030-4034, 1968.

Bergmeyer H.U. & Bernt E. (1965) Glutamate-oxaloacetate transaminase. Colorimetric determination with with 2,4 -dinitrophenyl-hydrazine. In Methods of enzymatic analysis, p 837 Edited by H.U: Bergmeyer. Academic Press, New York.

Bergmeyer, HU., Bernt, E. & Hess, B. (1965) Lactic dehydrogenase. In Methods of enzymatic analysis, p 736. Edited by H.U. Bergmeyer. Academic Press, New York.

Berrazueta J.R., López Jaramillo P., Moncada S. (1990) EL óxido nítrico: de vasodilatador endógeno a mediador endógeno. Revista Española de Cardiología 43: 421-431.

Brown G.C. (1999) Nitric oxide and mitochondrial respiration. Biochim. Biophys. Acta 1411: 351-369.

Cale J.M. & Bird I.M. (2006) Dissociation of endothelial nitric oxide synthase phosphorylation and activity in uterine artery endothelial cell. Am J Physiol Heart Circ Physiol 290: H1433-H1445.

Chagoya de Sánchez V., Hernández-Muñoz R., López-Barrera F., Yañez L., Vidrio S., Suárez J., Cota-Garza M.D., Aranda-Frausro A., Cruz D. (1997) Sequential changes of energy metabolism and mitochondrial function in myocardial infarction induced by isoproterenol in rats: a long-term and integrative study. Can. J. Physiol. Pharmacol 75: 1300-1311.

Diaz-Muñoz M., Älvarez-Perez M.A., Yañez L., Vidrio S., Martínez L., Rosas G., Yañez M., Ramírez S., Chagoya de Sánchez V. (2006) Correlation between oxidative stress and alteration of intracellular calcium handling in isoproterenol-induced myocardial infarction. Mol Cell Biochem 289: 125-136.

Chappel C.I., Rona G., Balzs T. (1959) Comparison of cardiotoxic action.of certain sympathomimetic amines. Can J BIochem Physiol 37:35-42.

Espey M.G., Miranda K.M., Feelisch M., Fukuto J., Grisham M.B., Vitek M.P. and Wink D.A. (2000) Mechanism of cell death governed by the balance between nitrosative and oxidation stress. Ann. NY Acad. Sci. 899: 209-221.

Frandesen U, Bangsbo J, Sander M, Hoffner L, Betak A, Saltin B & Hellsten Y (2001) Excercise-induced hyperaemia and leg oxygen uptake are not altered during effective inhibition of nitric oxide synthase with N^G-nitro-L-arginine methyl ester in humans. J. Physiol 531:257-264.

Govers, R. & T.J: Rabelink (2001) Cellular regulation of endothelial nitric oxide synthase. Am J Physiol, Renal Physiol 280: F193-F206.

Hoffman N.E., & Liao J.C. (1977) Reversed phase high performance liquid chromatography separations of nucleotides in the presence of solvophobic ions. Anal. Chem 49:22313-2234.

Ignarro L.J. (1990) Biosynthesis and metabolism of endothelium-derived nitric oxide. Annu, Rev Pharmacol. Toxicol 30: 535-560.

Kelm M., Schrader J. (1988) Nitric oxide release from the isolated guinea heart. Eur. J. Pharmacol. 155: 317-321.

Krenek P, Kimas J. Krolakova M, Gasova A, Plandorova J, Kucerova D, Fecenkova A. Svec P, Kyselovic J. (2006) Increased expression of endothelial nitric oxide synthase and caveolin-1 in the aorta of rats with isoproterenol-induced cardiac hypertrophy .Can J Physiol Pharmacol 84: 1245-1250.

Krenek P., Kmecova J., Kucerova D., Bajuszova Z., Musil P., Gazova A., Ochodnicky P., Klimas J. & Kyselovic J. (2009) Isoproterenol-induced heart failure in the rat is associated with nitric oxide-dependent functional alterations of cardiac function. European J Heart Failure 11: 140-146

Kröncke Klaus-D., Fehsel K. and Kolb Bachofen V. (1997) Nitric Oxide: Cytotoxicity versus Cytoprotection. How, Why, and Where? Nitric Oxide: Biology and Chemistry 1: 107-120. (Ignarro L.J. Annu. Rev Pharmacol. Toxicol 30: 535-560, 1990

Laurent M., Lepoivre M., and Tenu J.P. (1996) Kinetic modeling of the nitric oxide gradient generate in vitro by adherent cells expressing inducible nitric oxide synthase. Biochem J. 314: 109-113.

Palmer R.M.J., Ferrige A.G., Moncada S. (1987) Nitric oxide release accounts for the biological activity of endothelium-derived relaxing factor. Nature 327: 524-526.

Palmer R.M., Ashton D.S., Moncada S. (1988) Vascular endothelial cell synthesize nitric oxide from L-arginine. Nature 333: 664-666.

Rona G., Chapel C.I., Balazs T., Gaudry R. (1959) An infarct-like myocardial lesion and other toxic manifestations produced by isoproterenol on the rat. Arch Pathol 67:443-455.

Sander M, Chavoshan B. & Victor R.G. (1999) A large blood pressure raising effect of nitric oxide synthase inhibition in humans, Hipertensiόn 33: 937-942.

Shultz PJ, Taych MA, Marletta MA, Raij L. (1991) Synthesis and action of nitric oxide in rats glomerular mesangial cells. Am J PHysiol 261: F600-F606.

Stanton H.C., Brenner G., Mayfield E.D. (1969) Studies on isoproterenol-induced cardiomegaly I rats. Am Heart J 77:72-80.

Suárez J., Torres C., Sánchez L., del Valle L. & Pastelin G. (1999) Flow stimulates nitric oxide release in guinea pig heart. Role of stretch-activated ion channels. Biochem Biophys Res Comm, 261: 6-9.

Ueba Y., Ito Y., Mori K., Tomomatsu T. (1973) Studies of catecholamine metabolism in myocardial infarction. Singapore Medical J. 14: 351-352.

Wallace A.C. and Klein R.F. (1969) Role of catecholamines in acute myocardial infarction. The Am J of Med Scs 258:139-143.

Wink D.A. & Mitchell, J.B. (1998) Chemical biology of nitric oxide :Insights into regulatory, cytotoxic and citoprotective mechanisms of nitric oxide. Free Rad. Biol. Med 25:434-456.

3

Cardiac Complications of Cancer Treatment

Beata Mlot and Piotr Rzepecki
Military Institute of Medicine,
Poland

1. Introduction

Nowadays improvement in overall survival in patients suffered from cancer is observed. It is caused by using more effective treatments. The often observed side effect of anti-cancer therapy is cardiotoxicity. The decision about further treatment in cancer patients can be affected by the risk of development of this complication.

This chapter presents examples of proven cardiac toxicity associated with oncology treatment. It describes cytotoxic drugs used in chemotherapy, new anticancer agents from the group of molecular targeted therapy, radiotherapy and supportive treatment in oncology.

Drug-induced cardiomyopathy, which is a consequence of oncological treatment may be asymptomatic or present with acute or chronic heart failure, myocardial infarction, arrhythmia or sudden cardiac death. [1]

Drug-induced toxicity can be divided depending on the time of onset:

- acute: namely, that appeared in the course of cancer therapy,
- chronic: that is to say, that occurred within 12 months of completion of oncological treatment and
- chronic delayed: that is appearing 5 years after the end of treatment. [1]

2. Cytostatics with confirmed myocardial toxicity: Anthracycline antibiotics, nitrogen mustard-derivatives (cyclophosphamide and ifosfamide), 5-fluorouracil and mitomycin C. [1,2]

2.1 Anthracycline antibiotics

Anthracycline antibiotics are compounds isolated from fungi Streptomyces percetus and Streptomyces caesius.

2.1.1 The mechanism of anticancer action of anthracyclines

- incorporation to the structure of DNA, leading directly to inhibit transcription, protein production and replication problems,
- formation of additional abnormal bonds between nitrogen bases of DNA strands, which causes disruption of DNA and RNA synthesis and impaired DNA repair mechanisms,

- interference in the process of separating the strands of DNA and helicase activity, inhibition of key enzymes in the synthesis of DNA topoisomerase I and II,
- formation of free radicals that damage DNA, causing lipid peroxidation and accumulation of proapoptotic ceramide,
- induction of apoptosis via activation of p53. [3,4,5]

2.1.2 Clinical application of anthracyclines

Due to antitumor activity of anthracycline antibiotics they are incorporated into many therapeutic regimens in both solid tumors and hematological cancers. For example, doxorubicin is used to treat breast cancer, lymphoma, Ewing sarcoma, small cell lung cancer and soft tissue sarcomas. Daunorubicin is used primarily to treat acute myeloid and lymphoblastic leukemias. [6]

The cardiotoxicity of anthracycline antibiotics has been already documented in the seventies and affects all currently used anthracyclines [2]:

- doxorubicin,
- daunorubicin,
- epirubicin,
- esorubicin,
- aklarubicin,
- idarubicin
- and mitoxantrone, derivative-anthracycline.

The newer generation of antibiotics are derivatives of liposomal anthracycline doxorubicin, which are characterized by lower cardiotoxicity compared to their predecessors. [1,2]

2.1.3 Risk factors for cardiotoxicity after treatment with anthracyclines

Toxicity of anthracycline antibiotics depends on the dose. Most published reports showed that, the possibility of permanent myocardial damage is significantly increased beyond the cumulative dose of anthracyclines.

The cumulative doses significantly increasing the risk of permanent damage of heart muscule are as follow:

- doksorubicin-550mg/m2 (450 mg/m2 when radiotherapy was used or when

other risk factors of cardiotoxicity are present),

- daunorubicin-600mg/m2,
- epirubicin-1000 mg/m2,
- esorubicin-1900 mg/m2,
- aklarubicin-2000-3000 mg/m2,
- mitoxantrone-160 mg/m2. [2]

Other risk factors of cardiotoxicity associated with anthracycline antibiotics treatment include:

- individual susceptibility of the patient,

- genetic polymorphism associated with drug transport and metabolism of free radicals,
- age (over 65 years and under 4 years),
- black race,
- Down syndrome,
- prior mediastinal irradiation of ionizing radiation dose > 20Gy,
- previous cytotoxic therapy with potentially cardiotoxic drugs,
- pre-existing heart disease (valvular, ischemic origin, etc.),
- hypertension,
- diabetes,
- liver disease, [1,2]
- higher risk for chronic heart failure is observed in women,
- late coronary events are more common in men. [7]

2.1.4 Mechanism of cardiotoxicity action of anthracyclines

Mechanisms of anthracyclines cardiotoxicity with the pathogenesis of cardiomyopathy and heart failure are not fully explained.

One hypothesis assumes that the cardiotoxic effect of anthracyclines is a consequence of damage of mitochondria by these drugs. They bind to cardiolipin forming part of the inner mitochondrial membrane. This results in unbalanced electron transport in the respiratory chain, leading to depletion of ATP and phosphocreatine stores resulting in a decrease in myocardial contractility. Doxorubicin-cardiolipin complex also causes the formation of free hydroxyl radicals and hydrogen peroxide, which contributes to further damage to cell membranes and DNA. [2] The biopsy of the myocardium after therapy with anthracylines revealed myocyte vacualization, reduce amount of myofibrils, an increased number of lysosomes and mitochondria swelling. [8] Billigham scale is used in order to evaluate the histological severity. [9]

At present the most intensive examination of factors involved in the pathogenesis of anthracycline cardiomyopathy is cardiomyocyte apoptosis. Anthracyclines induce myocyte death through changes in protein expression of Bax (a protein with Bcl-2 family, cytochrome c release through mitochondrial pore opening) and Bcl-Xl (a protein with Bcl-2 family block cytochrome c release). [10,11]

The role of iron ions is significant as well. Iron is necessary for the conversion of O2-and H2O2 into the highly reactive hydroxyl radical (OH), and other toxic compounds. They can cause death of cardiomyocytes. It is also believed that the anthracycline antibiotics disturb cellular iron homeostasis in cardiomyocytes. It is plausible that change in the dynamics of release and storage of iron ions in the intracellular resources contribute to the death of heart muscle cells. In addition, it is believed that anthracyclines reduce iron release from ferritin, thus affect important metabolic processes dependent on iron. Iron is essential for DNA synthesis and cytochromes. However, accumulation of iron in ferritin is a protective mechanism against apoptosis by slowing the reaction of free radicals. [12,13]

Another possible mechanism of anthracyclines cardiotoxicity is the influence of anthracyclines on the calcium homeostasis. Before leading to apoptosis, oxidative stress can induce mitochondrial permeability transition with alterations in mitochondrial calcium transport. Changes in calcium transport can lead to tissue injury, cell killing and impaired cardiac contraction. In vitro doxorubicin treatment caused an irreversible decrease in mitochondrial calcium loading capacity. Moreover, anthracyclines can stimulate the release of calcium from isolated cardiac and skeletal muscle sarcoplasmic reticulum vesicles. This is strengthened by the observation of Rossi *et al.* who found a protective effect of the calcium blocking agent verapamil on doxorubicin induced cardiotoxicity in rats. This effect would be due to the calcium blocking capacities of verapamil inhibiting the intracellular calcium overload and antagonizing the effect of doxorubicin on mitochondria. However, others have demonstrated an increase in cardiotoxicity when doxorubicin was given in combination with verapamil. Different mechanisms for this effect are postulated. One is based on the capacity of verapamil to inhibit the function of P-glycoprotein and increase intracellular cytotoxic drug concentrations. This may be useful in overcoming resistance to chemotherapeutic drugs in cancer cells, but it could also lead to toxic effects in normal structures such as cardiac cells. Some studies showed in vitro increased doxorubicin accumulation in rat cardiomyocytes when incubated with a combination of verapamil and doxorubicin. Akimoto *et al* did not show an increased cellular anthracycline uptake but they found additive cardiotoxicity by verapamil due to its selective inhibition of cardiac actin gene expression, a similar effect which was demonstrated before with doxorubicin alone. The exact role of the changing capacities of doxorubicin on calcium regulation and its implications for cardiotoxicity remains to be elucidated. [2]

Recently, clinical trials evaluated the effect of anthracyclines on dysfunction of cardiac stem cells. These are undifferentiated cells, who renews themselves and differentiates into cardiac muscle cells and coronary vessels both in vitro and in vivo. Cardiac stem cells resulting in the surface receptor c-kit have been identified in the adult mammalian heart muscle. There is the evidence that the loss of cardiac stem cells with impaired production of daughter cells may be responsible for the development of anthracycline cardiomyopathy. Moreover it has been found that stem cells show efficacy in the treatment of experimentally induced heart failure. [14,15,16]

Other potential etiologies of development of anthracycline cardiomyopathy, reported in the literature are:

- effect of anthracyclines on the enzymatic antioxidant system cells, via reducition of the activity of glutathione peroxidase (GS-PX1) and the amount of copper-zinc superoxide dismutase (CuZnSOD) in cardiomyocytes,
- membrane lipid peroxidation,
- disruption of titin* (protein associated with myosin, and which is incorporated into the structure of sarcomeric),

* Titin, also known as connectin, is a protein that in humans is encoded by the TTN gene. Titin is a giant protein that functions as a molecular spring which is responsible for the passive elasticity of muscle. It is composed of 244 individually folded protein domains connected by unstructured peptide sequences. These domains unfold when the protein is stretched and refold when the tension is removed. Titin is important in the contraction of striated muscle tissues. It connects the Z line to the M line in the sarcomere. The protein contributes to force transmission at the Z line and resting tension in the I band region. It limits the range of motion of the sarcomere in tension, thus contributing to the passive stiffness of muscle.

- abnormal calcium homeostasis and cardiac contractility, reduction in expression of contractile proteins and proteins regulating intracellular calcium movement,
- inactivation of mitochondrial creatine kinase and abnormal structure of dystrophin. [17,18,19]

Acute cardiotoxicity associated with anthracyclines may occur after either first or initial few infusions of drug. It is not dose depend and presents as sinus tachycardia. It may result in myocarditis, with or without pericarditis.

The ECG changes include:

- voltage decrease.
- widening of QRS complexes.
- small R wave progression [anterior wall of heart].
- nonspecific T wave changes.

Acute cardiotoxicity associated with anthracyclines despite its the transient nature can cause life-threatening complications such as myocardial infarction, pulmonary edema, hypotension and serious arrhythmias. [20]

Chronic anthracycline cardiotoxicity occurs during the first year after treatment [10% of patients treated with anthracyclines]. It is dose-dependent. Most commonly it is manifested as exacerbation of heart failure, decrease in ejection fraction, cardiac arrhythmias, and development of dilated cardiomyopathy. A history of treatment with anthracyclines may be associated with long-term risk of cardiac complications in both children and adults. [20]

Mitoxantrone is a derivative of anthracycline-like structure similar to doxorubicin and contributes to the occurrence of left ventricular dysfunction. It has been used in the induction of remission in acute myeloid leukemia, in breast cancer and ovarian cancer resistant to chemotherapy as well as prostate cancer resistant to hormonotherapy. In the assessment of 80 patients treated with mitoxantrone, clinical congestive heart failure (CHF) was diagnosed in 1.5% of them. The risk of cardiac complications increases after the total dose of 160 mg/m2. Reduction of left ventricular EF [LVEF] was observed in patients with prior history of diseases of the cardiovascular system and with previous exposure to anthracyclines. [21]

Mechanism of cardiotoxicity action of anthracyclines is shown in Table nr 1.

2.2 Cardiotoxicity of taxanes

Cardiac complications may be caused by another group of cytostatic drugs used in oncology- the taxanes.

2.2.1 Mechanism of antitumor action of taxanes

The mechanism of antitumor action of this relatively new group of cytostatics are:

- Stabilization of microtubules, causing cell cycle blockage at the stage of mitosis.
- In addition, docetaxel can induce apoptosis by blocking the antiapoptopic action of BCL-2 gene, and by influencing the activation of the p53 gene.

At the level of myocytes	• apoptosis of cardiomyocytes as a result of changes in protein expression of Bcl-2, • mitochondrial damage, • decreasing the activity of glutathione peroxidase (GSH-PX1) and the amount of copper-zinc superoxide dismutase (CuZnSOD), • abnormal cellular iron homeostasis in cardiomyocytes, • direct DNA damage of cardiomyocytes, membrane lipid peroxidation, disruption of titin, disturbances of calcium homeostasis and cardiac contractility, reduced expression of contractile proteins and proteins regulating intracellular calcium movement, inactivation of mitochondrial creatine kinase and abnormal structure of dystrophin.
At the level of cardiac stem cells (SKM)	• induction of apoptosis and inhibition of proliferation of SKM through increased oxidative DNA damage and telomere shortening.

Table 1. Mechanisms of cardiotoxicity action of anthracyclines

2.2.2 Clinical application of taxanes

Taxanes are used primarily in chemotherapy of solid tumors, including lung cancer, hormone-refractory prostate cancer, bladder cancer, stomach cancer, breast cancer or ovarian cancer. [22]

2.2.3 Risk factors for cardiotoxicity after treatment with taxanes

Cardiac risk factors included were age, hypertension, diabetes and prior radiotherapy to the chest wall. [2,22,23]

Docetaxel shows no increase in cardiac toxicity when combined with doxorubicin. This is in line with the observation that a pharmacokinetic interaction with doxorubicin as described for paclitaxel has not been observed. [2,22]

2.2.4 Mechanism of cardiotoxicity of taxanes

During administration of paclitaxel, whether or not combined with cisplatin, various cardiac disturbances are reported like brady- and tachyarrhythmias, atrioventricular and bundle branch blocks and cardiac ischemia. Hypotension is also reported, probably as a result of a hypersensitivity reaction. When evaluating three phase I and one phase II studies performed at the John Hopkins Institute it appeared that 5% (n = 7) of the patients showed overt cardiac disturbances as ventricular tachycardia and atrioventricular conduction abnormalities. Asymptomatic bradycardia occurred in 29% of patients receiving maximal tolerable doses (110-250 mg/m^2) of paclitaxel in the phase II study. These disturbances did not lead to clinical symptoms. The abnormalities usually started several hours following the initiation of paclitaxel therapy and resolved after discontinuation. This evident time relationship and the fact that most patients had no cardiac risk factors supports the assumption of causality between paclitaxel and the observed cardiac rhythm disturbances. [2,22,23]

Another concern with the use of taxoids has been the development of congestive heart failure in patients treated with a combination of doxorubicin and taxoids. The cardiotoxicity associated with taxoids seems to be mild in most cases. However, in clinical trials patients with prior history of cardiac disturbances were often excluded. Therefore, the rate of cardiotoxicity in this group of patients is difficult to estimate. Study in patients with major cardiac risk factors revealed that paclitaxel could be safely administered as single therapy or in combination with a platinum agent such as cisplatin or carboplatin. Cardiac risk factors included unstable angina, severe coronary artery disease, congestive heart failure and atrial fibrillation. [2,22,23]

Paclitaxel is formulated in a cremophor EL vehicle to enhance the drug solubility and it is suggested that the vehicle and not the cytotoxic drug itself is responsible for the cardiac disturbances. However, the cardiac rhythm disturbances are not reported with use of other drugs containing cremophor EL such as cyclosporin. The possible mechanism by which cremophor EL would cause cardiotoxicity is massive histamine release. Indeed, stimulation of histamine receptors in cardiac tissue in animal studies has resulted in conduction disturbances and arrhythmias. An alternative explanation for paclitaxel induced cardiotoxicity could be the induction of cardiac muscle damage by affecting subcellular organelles. [2]

Enhanced cardiac toxicity has been found in combined therapy of paclitaxel and doxorubicin. At doses of doxorubicin exceeding 380 mg/m^2, the toxicity increased in combination therapy compared to doxorubicin single therapy. A pharmacokinetic interaction appears to be responsible for this effect as paclitaxel has been found to decrease doxorubicin hepatic elimination and lead to increased plasma concentrations of doxorubicin. This effect depends on the interval and sequence of drug administration as well as the duration of the paclitaxel infusion. [2,22]

A similar effect has been shown for epirubicin. Baldini et al. [23] evaluate cardiac safety of two different schedules of epirubicin and paclitaxel in advanced breast cancer. Patients were enrolled into a multicenter randomized phase III trial. They received epirubicin 90 mg/m2 plus paclitaxel 200 mg/m2 (3-h infusion) on day 1 every 3 weeks for eight courses (arm A), or epirubicin 120 mg/m2 on day 1 every 3 weeks for four courses followed by four courses of paclitaxel 250 mg/m2 on day 1 every 3 weeks (arm B). Baseline median left ventricular ejection fraction was 60% in arm A and 65% in arm B; after four courses, figures were 57 and 60%, respectively. After eight courses, the median left ventricular ejection fraction in arm A declined to 50% while no further reduction was detected in arm B by adding four courses of high-dose paclitaxel. Seven episodes of congestive heart failure were observed during treatment in arm A. The risk of congestive heart failure or impairment in the cardiac function correlated only with the cumulative dose of epirubicin. No impact on cardiotoxicity can be attributed to high-dose paclitaxel. [23]

2.3 Cardiotoxicity of nitrogen mustard derivatives of cyclophosphamide [CTX] and ifosfamide [IFO]

2.3.1 Cyclophosphamide

2.3.1.1 Mechanism of antitumor action of cyclophosphamide

These drugs are alkylating agents. Their biological active metabolities are responsible for their action. Cyclophosphamide and ifosfamide are alkylating oxazaphosphorine agents that need to be metabolized in vivo in the liver to form the active cytotoxic agent phosphoramide mustard. They contain many chloroethyl groups and therefore may create cross-binding of the DNA chain, causing damage that is difficult to repair. [22]

2.3.1.2 Clinical application of cyclophosphamide

Cyclophosphamide has a very wide range of indications:

- acute myeloid leukemia,
- acute lymphoblastic leukemia,
- chronic lymphocytic leukemia,
- Hodgkin, non-Hodgkin lymphomas,
- lung, breast, ovarian and bladder cancers,
- sarcomas,
- retinoblastoma.

2.3.1.3 Risk factors for cardiotoxicity after treatment with cyclophosphamide

Cardiotoxicity of this drug depends on its dose. Described complications of the cardiovascular system occur after administration of 120 to 200 mg/kg of cyclophosphamide. [24] Some sources indicate that cardiotoxicity of cyclophosphamide may be present in 3% of patients who received a dose of less than 1.55 g/m2/daily and in 25% who received cyclophosphamide at a daily dose greater than 1.55 g/m2/daily. [25]

2.3.1.4 Mechanism of cardiotoxicity of cyclophosphamide

Cardiac complications observed in patients treated with CTX were as follows:

- ECG abnormalities in the form of low-voltage QRS wave,
- progressive heart failure,
- myocarditis or pericarditis which sometimes lead to cardiac tamponade requiring urgent pericardiocentesis.

In 90% of patients with confirmed adverse effect of cyclophosphamide on the heart muscle, there were no clinical signs of cardiac toxicity of this drug. In these cases, ones observed mild pericarditis, and slight changes in the ECG that did not require treatment and resolved spontaneously without leaving any complications. They were ST-segment abnormalities and supraventricular arrhythmias. [25-27] The Harvard Medical School studied the cardiotoxicity of cyclophosphamide, depending on the dose in the preparatory regimen before bone marrow transplantation. Cyclophosphamide (CTX) cardiotoxicity may be a lethal complication of bone marrow transplantation. Previous echocardiographic studies have reported that left ventricular dysfunction due to CTX occurs in over 50% of patients undergoing transplantation. To evaluate the cardiotoxicity of new dosing protocols that included twice-daily rather than once-daily CTX, 44 bone marrow transplantation patients were prospectively evaluated with serial ECGs and echocardiograms. Twenty-six patients received a once-daily lower-dose protocol (mean total 87 +/- 11 mg/kg), and 18 patients received a twice-daily higher-dose (mean total 174 +/- 34 mg/kg) CTX regimen. In the higher-dose CTX group, significant reductions in summed ECG voltage (-20%) (P less than 0.01) and increases in left ventricular mass index (LVMI) (+10%) (P less than 0.05) were detected in the first week following therapy. These changes resolved by the third week following CTX and were significantly greater than the changes noted in the lower-dose group. However, LVEF did not change significantly in either group. Five patients developed clinical cardiotoxicity (four- pericarditis; one- congestive heart failure); four of the five patients were in the higher-dose group (P = 0.14). Only a prior history of congestive heart failure or a baseline EF less than 50% was an independent correlate of clinical cardiotoxicity (P less than 0.05). Thus, dose-dependent cardiotoxicity following the use of CTX for bone marrow transplantation presents as reversible decreases in ECG voltage and increases in left ventricular mass. This likely reflects myocardial edema or hemorrhage. However, systolic dysfunction is much less common with these new twice-daily dosing regimens when compared with earlier studies of high-dose once-daily CTX.

It has been proven that the cardiotoxicity of cyclophosphamide is a result of its biologically active metabolites such as 4-hydroxy cyclophosphamide (HCY), o-carboxyetyl-nitrogen mustard (CEPM), deschloroetyl-cyclophosphamide (DCCY), 4-keto-cyclophosphamide (KetoCY) and hydroxypropyl nitrogen-mustard (HPPM). [21,29] Endothelial damage by toxic metabolites of cyclophosphamide results in extravasation of blood and damage to the vessel wall myocytes resulting in intravascular hematoma with subsequent swelling. Symptoms of congestive heart failure usually appear within two weeks after drug administration. In patients in whom it is rapid, it can lead to death within a few weeks. There is evidence that the severity of the toxicity of cyclophosphamide depends on the personal attributes associated with the intensity of metabolism of this drug. [21]

2.3.2 Ifosfamide

Ifosfamide (IFO) is a structural isomer of cyclophosphamide.

2.3.2.1 Mechanism of antitumor action of ifosfamide

Mechanism of action this drug is the same like cyklophosphamide.

2.3.2.2 Clinical application of ifosfamide

This cytostatic is used to treat lung cancer, germ cell tumors, sarcomas and lymphomas, may also lead to cardiac complications.

2.3.2.3 Risk factors for cardiotoxicity after treatment with ifosfamide

The risk of congestive heart failure depends on the dose ifosfamide and increases from 8% to 67% at doses ranging from 10 g/m2 to 18 g/m2. An additional risk factor in these cases is the development of renal failure with subsequent overload the body's fluids.

2.3.2.4 Mechanism of cardiotoxicity of ifosfamide

In 15% of patients receiving a dose of this cytostatic up to 10g /m2 may experience the following variations in the ECG:

- supraventricular tachycardia,
- changes in ST-T.

The development of congestive heart failure (from mild stagnation in the circulation to a cardiogenic shock of lesser severity) occurs 6 to 23 days after starting therapy, with improvement within 4 to 7 days after discontinuation of cytostatic and appropriate treatment. Usually, it is fully reversible. Cardiac tamponade or pericardial effusion is extremely rare. There were reports of various types of arrhythmias after various doses of ifosfamide:

- extrasystoles supraventricular or ventricular,
- supraventricular tachycardia,
- atrial fibrillation,
- atrial flutter,
- acute ventricular arrhythmias.

In addition, there were changes in the passage from the ST-T ECG and QRS voltage reduction. In a study of patients treated with fractionated doses of ifosfamide (doses ranging from 6.5 to 10 g/m2) 15% of them developed symptoms of acute cardiac toxicity in the form of supraventricular arrhythmias and changes in ST-T. The symptoms were reversible after discontinuation of treatment. In one patient re-use of ifosfamide led to the development of arrhythmias resistant to treatment. [30-34]

The possible causes of cardiac complications associated with cyclophosphamide and ifosfamide are electrolyte imbalance. The development of severe hypokalemia was described in four patients treated with ifosfamide with mesna supply. Three patients received ifosfamide at a dose of 5g /m2, and one at a dose of 4g /m2. One patient was treated with ifosfamide + mesna only, others also received mitoxantrone plus etoposide or doxorubicin and vindesine, or methotrexate and etoposide. In none of these patients other causes of hypokaliemia were found. Hypokaliemia appeared between 2 and 12 days after application of ifosfamide with mesna. One death was observed due to cardiac arrest in a patient with a potassium level of 2.2 mEq/l. In the remaining patients, the lowest potassium levels ranged from 1.7 to 2.6 mEq/l. [35-37]

Mechanism of cardiotoxicity action of nitrogen mustard derivatives is showen in Table nr 2.

• endothelial damage by toxic metabolites for example: 4-hydroxy cyclophosphamide (HCY), o-carboxyetyl-nitrogen mustard (CEPM), deschloroetyl-cyclophosphamide (DCCY), 4-keto-cyclophosphamide (KetoCY) and hydroxypropyl-nitrogen mustard (HPPM), • electrolyte disturbances including hypokalemia

Table 2. Mechanisms of cardiotoxicity action of cyclophosphamide and ifosfamide

2.4 Cardiotoxicity of 5-fluorouracil [5-Fu]

Another chemotherapeutic agents with potentially cardiotoxic action are 5-fluorouracil (5-Fu) and its prodrug capecitabine-(4-pentoksykarbonylo-5-deoxy-5-fluorocytydyna).

2.4.1 Mechanism of antitumor action of 5-fluorouracil and capecitabine

The mechanism of antitumor action of 5-Fu is the inhibition of DNA synthesis by the active metabolite - phosphodeoksyrybonucleotide (FdUMP). In addition, 5-Fu forms additional metabolite- (5-FUTP), which can be incorporated into RNA. Thus it blocks the processing of RNA and its function.

2.4.2 Clinical application of 5-Fu and capecitabine

They are the main cytostatics used in the treatment of epithelial cancers, especially: breast, head, neck and gastrointestinal tract. [38]

2.4.3 Risk factors for cardiotoxicity after treatment with 5-Fu and capecitabine

The incidence of 5-Fu cardiotoxicity is 7.6% with mortality ranging between 2.2% and 13%. [38] Cardiac toxicity of 5-fluorouracil is dose-dependent. A cumulative dose threshold for severe heart effects has been calculated between 1.5 and 7g. [39] The risk of cardiac ischemia appears to vary ranging from 1-68% in the patients treated with high-dose infusions of 5-fluorouracil. [40] Cardiac complications after administration of a bolus occur with a frequency of 1.6-3%, while after 4-5 days of continuous infusions at a frequency of 7.6-15%.

2.4.4 Mechanism of 5-fluorouracil cardiotoxicity

The most often cardiac symptoms are:

- chest pain,
- ST-T wale changes,
- arrhytmias (for example atria fibrylattion),
- asymptomatic bradycardia,
- hypotension,
- cardiogenic shocks,
- cardiac failure,
- acute coronary syndrome.

But most common finding is reversible ST-T wave changes. [41] Fidan et al. [42] described a 46-year-old patient with stomach cancer, in whom the administration of 5-Fu in the bolus as the adjuvant chemoradiotherapy attack of ventricular fibrillation occurred. It was accompanied by a decrease in EF to 40%. This complication is extremely rare after administration of 5-Fu in the bolus. It has been proved that the administration of the drug in the form of short-term injection is safer than continuous infusions. [42]

The literature describes several potential mechanisms of toxicity of 5-Fu on the cardiovascular system. Many authors claim that the basic mechanism is due to coronary artery spasm. Ischemia could be because of direct tonic effect on the vascular endothelium involving NO synthase, which leads to coronary vasospasm. The other mechanism of vasospasm endothelial vasoconstriction is via protein kinase C. The hypothesis that endothelin-1 (ET1) release could be involved in 5-Fu cardiotoxicity has never been substantiated. 5-Fu can also damage endothelium, causing thrombus formation and vascular endothelial release of vasoactive substances. A reduction of antioxidant defense capacities in myocardial tissues and modulation of the immune response are other potential causes of 5-Fu cardiotoxicity. The administration of 400 mg/kg/day of 5-Fu to guinea-pigs reduced the activity of the cardiac enzymes: superoxide dismutase and glutathione peroxidase. Concomitantly there was an increase in the activity of catalases and malondialdehyde concentrations. Interestingly, an increase in malondialdehyde concentrations is consistently observed in myocardial ischemia and this increase is prevented or reversed by calcium inhibitors. A proliferation of the sarcoplasmic reticulum with vacuolizations similar to that occurring with anthracyclines was also reproted with 5-Fu. [38,43] According to Labianca et al.,[44] the global incidence of heart lesions associated with 5-Fu is higher in patients with a cardiac history in comparison to patients with no cardiac history (4.5 versus 1.1%). [44] The risk of 5-Fu cardiotoxicity was increased in 5-Fu-treated patients receiving mediastinal radiotherapy. [45] However Tsibiribi et al. [43] described cardiac complications in 16 out of 1350 patients treated with 5-Fu with a negative history of diseases of the cardiovascular system. Ten patients complained of angina pectoris. Two were asymptomatic, but had electrocardiographic changes indicative of myocardial ischemia. Three patients had clinical symptoms without EKG changes. Heart failure was observed in one patient. [43]

2.4.5 Mechanism of cardiotoxicity of capecitabine

While cardiac events associated with the use of 5-Fu are a well known side effect, capecitabine-induced cardiotoxicity has been only rarely reported. Capecitabine is an orally active prodrug of 5-Fu and breast cancer and colon cancer exhibits antitumor efficacy comparable to 5-Fu. Capecitabine is converted to the active 5-Fu by the action of a series of enzymes. One of these enzymes, thymidine phosphorylase (TP), has higher concentrations in tumor tissue than in normal tissue. This suggests that the activation occurs preferentially in tumor tissue, providing a favorable ratio for toxicity and radiosensitization. [46] In a retrospective analysis performed on studies of patients unergoing chemotherapy for metastatic breast and colon cancer, the incidence of cardiotoxicity with capecitabine was found to be comparable to that of 5-Fu. [47] Wijesinghe et al [48] reported an acute coronary syndrome in a patient with no history of cardiovascular disease who had been on capecitabine for only 2 days. [48] Kosmas et al documented myocardial infarction, electrocardiographic abnormalities, and ventricular extrasystoles in patients on capecitabine. [49] Furthermore, Goldsmith et al recently reported exercise-induced global myocardial ischemia with an ejection fraction of 36% in a patient with normal coronary arteries and resting left ventricular function who was on capecitabine for recurrent breast cancer. [50] For the first time cardiac arrhythmia in the form of symptomatic bradycardia described Ang C et al. [51] Capecitabine should be considered a drug with cardiotoxic potential even in the absence of prior cardiac history. It is believed that 5-Fu or its metabolites were responsible for cardiotoxicity after capecitabine administration. Coronary artery vasospasm, direct toxicity to the myocardium, thrombogenic effects and autoimmune phenomena have been proposed as plausible mechanisms. [52]

The mechanisms of cardiotoxicity of 5-Fu and capecitabine is shown in Table nr 3.

5-fluorouracil	coronary artery vasospasm, modulation of immune response, direct myocardial injury,
capecitabine	coronary artery vasospasm, direct toxicity to the myocardium, thrombogenic effects, autoimmune phenomena,

Table 3. The mechanisms of cardiotoxicity of 5-Fluorouracil and capecitabine

2.5 Cardiotoxicity of mitomycin C

There are reports of potentially cardiotoxic activity of mitomycin C. It is a antibiotic with antitumor cytotoxic activity. It is used in multi-drug regimens chemotherapy in the therapy of: stomach, colon, pancreatic, small cell lung, breast, cervical, advanced endometrial and squamous cell cancers of head and neck. [2]

2.6 Cardiotoxicity of cisplatin

2.6.1 Mechanism of antitumor action of cisplatin

Its effect is to create cross-linkages between adjacent strands of DNA and within the same thread. The formation of these cross-linkages prevents DNA replication and cell division. Also exerts influence on the metabolic functions of starting the process of cell apoptosis.

2.6.2 Clinical application of cisplatin

Cisplatin is a platinum substance and used in the treatment of many tumors (i.e. testicular cancer).

2.6.3 Mechanism of cardiotoxicity of cisplatin

Several cases of acute myocardial infarction after cisplatin therapy are reported. In a retrospective study 87 long term survivors of metastatic testicular cancer treated with cisplatin were evaluated for the occurrence of cardiovascular events. A significantly increase in cardiac events as well as an unfavorable cardiovascular risk profile were observed. [2]

Several factors have been suggested to be involved like vascular damage, alterations in platelet aggregation and hypomagnesemia. In experiments on human platelets cisplatin was able to trigger platelet aggregation and/or enhance thromboxane formation by platelets. Activation of an arachidonic pathway in platelets by cisplatin seemed to be involved. Raynaud phenomenon has been described in patients receiving cisplatin-based therapy. [2]

3. Cardiotoxicity of antineoplastic agents belonging to the so-called molecular targeted therapy

Molecular targeted therapy plays an increasingly important role in cancer therapy. This kind of treatment is also at risk of complications development including cardiac events. The most common symptoms associated with cardiac toxicity of molecular targeted therapy include hypertension, thromboembolic complications and dilated cardiomyopathy. Despite these symptoms treatment is better tolerated compared to other cytostatics. Most of the complications are reversible and respond to symptomatic treatment. Due to the fact that some of these drugs are used in combination with chemotherapy, reported side effects are the result of overlapping toxicities. Due to the relatively short experience with this type of therapy we cannot answer the question about the consequences of targeted therapy. [53]

This group of drugs of proven cardiac toxicity can be divided into:

- small molecule tyrosine kinase inhibitors (sunitinib, sorafenib, imatinib, lapatinib, dasatinib),

- proteasome inhibitors (bortezomib),
- monoclonal antibodies directed against the receptor or tyrosine kinase ligands (trastuzumab, bevacizumab). [54]

3.1 Small molecule tyrosine kinase inhibitors

This group of drugs bind to the part of the receptor complex, which is a tyrosine kinase. They are transmembrane proteins whose extracellular part acts as a both receptor and associated ligands at the same time [for example vascular endothelial growth factor (VEGF), platelet-derived (PDGF) etc.]. Intracellular domain of this protein has a catalytic activity. Key tyrosine kinases responsible for the pathogenesis of malignancy are associated with: vascular endothelial factor, FLT-1 and FLT-3-like tyrosine kinase fms, KDR kinase insert domain-containing receptor and for platelet-derived growth factor, stem cell factor receptor and RET-protonkogen. The emergence of the cancer cells will result from mutation and constant activation of these receptors.

Tyrosine kinase inhibitors block the activity of individual cells pathway-receptor signal transmission from membrane through cytoplasm to nucleus. They inhibit the activity of transcription factors and the expression of proteins responsible for fundamental processes of cancer cell development.

3.1.1 Sunitinib (SU 011248)

3.1.1.1 Mechanism of antitumor action of sunitinib

Sunitinib is an oral antiangiogenic small molekule tyrosine kinase inhibitor. It inhibits VEGFR-1 to VEGFR-3, stem cell factor receptor, platelet-derived growth factor receptor PDGFR-2-alfa and PDGFR-beta, RET, colony-stimulating factor-1 receptor, and fetal liver tyrosine kinase receptor 3 FLT-3. [55]

3.1.1.2 Clinical application of sunitinib

Sunitinib was approved by the European Medicines Agency (EMEA) for the treatment of advanced kidney cancer and / or metastatic kidney cancer and for the treatment of unresectable and / or metastatic GIST after failure of imatinib treatment due to resistance to imatinib or intolerant. [56]

3.1.1.3 Mechanism of cardiotoxicity of sunitinb

Sunitinib causes hypertension. In phase I clinical trials the incidence of CTC grade >=3 hypertension was 7.3%. [57] In single-agent phase II clinical trials with sunitinib the rates of grade 1-2 and grade 3 hypertension were 8.4% and 7.5% respectively. [58] In phase III clinical trials which established the efficacy of sunitinib in gastrointestinal stroma tumors (GISTs) and renal cell carcinoma grade 3 hypertension was more frequent in the sunitinib group than in the placebo group (3% versus 0%) or the interferon group (8% versus 1%). [59,60]

In phase I clinical trials of sunitinib two of 55 patients developed left ventricular dysfunction and heart failure. [57] In the phase II clinical trials of sunitinib in renal cell carcinoma 8.9% of patients developed a reduction in LVEF. [58] Grade 3 reductions in

LVEF were seen in a phase III trial of renal cell carcinoma. [60] In another retrospective analysis 11% of the patients with GISTs had heart failure and left ventricular dysfunction, 18% of patients had a myocardial infarction and/or asymptomatic elevations in troponin. [61] At the University of Stanford among 48 patients treated with sunitinib within 22-435 days after initiation of therapy in 7 (15%) patients experienced left ventricular III / IV grade according to the CTCAE (Common Terminology Criteria For Adverse Events). Despite the discontinuation of sunitinib heart failure maintained in 3 patients. Not without significance in this group of patients had a history of the burden from cardiovascular diseases as the 3 subjects had a history of heart failure, while another 2 patients were burdened with coronary artery disease. [62] In the University of Texas at 2.7% (6 / 224) of patients treated with sunitinib develop symptoms of heart failure during therapy in a one year. It is important that none of the reported patients prior to study entry had any heart disease. Five of the reported patients, who developed heart failure in the III and stage IV NYHA, required discontinuation of study drug. In one patient after the study drug dose reduction and after symptomatic treatment of heart failure symptoms subsided. [63]

Only a few cases of thromboembolic complications were reported. In phase I trials 2 of 55 patients developed myocardial infarction and pulmonary embolism. Two patients experienced pulmonary embolism and one experienced cerebrovascular accident in phase II studies. [57] These events were rare in phase III studies. [59,60]

The mechanism of cardiotoxicity associated with sunitinib therapy is not entirely clear. There are various hypotheses on this subject. It is shown that sunitinib induces the development of hypertension. It is not confirmed, that this is the way of the development of cardiac systolic dysfunction. Sunitinib inhibits cardiac PDGFR receptor. It is known that the number of active receptors and their signals transmitted to the interior have the great impact on survival of cardiomyocytes. Another hypothesis assumes that the mechanism of sunitinib cardiotoxicity may be related to inhibition of activating protein kinase (AMPK) and the kinase from the group of ribosomal S6 kinase (RSK 1). It is known that heart muscle cells require to function properly a large amount of energy. Thus they can be sensitive to inhibition of AMPK kinase, which acts as a regulating factor of the energy levels of ATP. Metformin used in diabetes, which activates AMPK kinase, does not protect against cardiac toxicity of treatment with sunitinib. [64] In addition, sunitinib treatment does not affect the level of cellular ATP. It is proven that the use of the dexrazoksan protection does not protect cardiomyocytes against the negative action of sunitinib. There are suggestions that the mechanism of toxicity of sunitinib is not associated with oxidative processes. Perhaps the non-selective inhibition of the kinase and blocking other pathways contribute to the development of drug-induced cardiotoxicity. [64]

3.1.2 Sorafenib (BAY 439006)

3.1.2.1 Mechanism of antitumor action of sorafenib

Sorafenib is an oral small molecule tyrosine kinase inhibitor designed to inhibit C-type Raf kinase (c-RAF), FLT-3, KIT, and B-type Raf kinase (b-RAF), VEGFR-2, VEGFR-3 and PDGFR. [55]

3.1.2.2 Clinical application of sorafenib

On the basis of multicenter clinical trials have shown that the use of sorafenib causes a statistically significant prolongation of progression-free survival of of patients with kidney cancer with prior ineffective immunotherapy.

3.1.2.3 Mechanism of cardiotoxicity of sorafenib

It has been proven that sorafenib may increase the risk of acute coronary syndrome, including myocardial infarction. An independent review of two studies by the FDA indicated that the incidence of ischemia/infarction was higher in the sorafenib group (2.9%) than in the placebo group (0.4%). [65] In another study the incidences of cardiac ischemia and infarction was significantly higher in the sorafenib arm (3% versus <1%). [66] In addition, sorafenib therapy may contribute to the occurrence of hypertension as with other targeted therapies that inhibit angiogenesis. In single-agent and combination phase I clinical trials of sorafenib the incidence of grade 3-4 hypertension was 3%. [67] In phase II studies with sorafenib 12% of patients developed grade 1-2 and 13.8% developed grade 3 hypertension. [68] In a phase III trial of sorafenib versus placebo in renal cell carcinoma hypertension was the most frequent serious adverse event but led to drug discontinuation in <1% of patients. The incidence of hypertension was significantly higher than in the placebo group: grade 2 10% versus 2% and grade 3-4 4% versus <1% , respectively. [66]

Similarly in a phase III trial in hepatocellular carcinoma patients grade 3 hypertension was more frequent in the sorafenib arm, but the difference did not reach the level of statistical significance. [69] Sorafenib-associated thrombotic events were infrequent (phase I trials, grade 3 thrombotic events 0.8%). No grade 3-4 thromboembolic events were noted in single-agent phase II studies or in phase III studies. [55] Perhaps the mechanism of cardiotoxicity of this drug results from inhibition of serine-threonine kinases RAF1 and BRAF. RAF1 inhibition blocks the activity of apoptosis signal regulating kinase 1 (ASK1) and mammalian stearin kinase 2 (MST2), which are involved in the mechanisms of formation of oxidative stress associated with tissue damage. It is still unclear the blockade by the sorafenib RAF1 or its effect on the signal transmission pathway of RAF1 to ASK1 and MST2 is at fault. [64]

3.1.3 Imatinib

3.1.3.1 Mechanism of antitumor action of imatinib

Imatinib strongly inhibits the tyrosine kinase Bcr-Abl, by blocking the transfer of a phosphate group from ATP molecules to the substrate protein tyrosine. Preventing this interaction blocks the ability to activate protein kinase transmitting proliferative signals to the nucleus and induces apoptosis of leukemia cells in patients with chronic myelogenous leukemia (CML) and acute lymphoblastic leukemia (ALL) with the Philadelphia chromosome. Imatinib also inhibits receptor tyrosine kinases platelet activation factor (PDGF), stem cell factor (SCF), Steel factor (c-KIT) and inhibits the cellular processes activated by PDGF and SCF. [70]

3.1.3.2 Clinical application of imatinib

This drug is used in the treatment of patient with chronic myelogenous leukemia and acute lymphoblastic leukemia.

3.1.3.3 Mechanism of cardiotoxicity of imatinib

O`Brief et al [71] reported ten individuals who developed severe congestive heart failure while on imatinib. They showed that imatinib-treated mice develop left ventricular contractile dysfunction. Transmission electron micrographs from humans and mice treated with imatinib showed mitochondrial abnormalities and accumulation of membrane whorls in both vacuoles and the sarco- (endo-) plasmic reticulum, findings suggestive of a toxic myopathy. With imatinib treatment, cardiomyocytes in culture show activation of the endoplasmic reticulum (ER) stress response, collapse of the mitochondrial membrane potential, release of cytochrome *c* into the cytosol, reduction in cellular ATP content and cell death. Retroviral gene transfer of an imatinib-resistant mutant of c-Abl, alleviation of ER stress or inhibition of Jun amino-terminal kinases, which are activated as a consequence of ER stress, largely rescues cardiomyocytes from imatinib-induced death. Thus, cardiotoxicity is an unanticipated side effect of inhibition of c-Abl by imatinib. [71]

In turn, international and randomized phase III study involving 1106 patients with newly diagnosed chronic myeloid leukemia with Philadelphia chromosome, who are in chronic phase, severe cardiac failure and left ventricular dysfunction was reported in 0.7% of patients receiving imatinib, compared to 0,9% of patients treated with interferon alpha (IFN) with cytosine arabinoside (Ara-C). However, in the IRIS study, after imatinib treatment of heart failure incidence was 1% of patients. [72]

Cardiac toxicity of imatinib may be due to inhibition by this drug tyrosine kinase c-Abl. It was confirmed that by the action of imatinib in response to oxidative stress occur:

- activation of the endoplasmic reticulum (ER),
- decreased mitochondrial membrane potential,
- release of cytochrome c into the cytosol,
- decrease in cell ATP and ultimately cell death. [71]

3.1.4 Dasatinib

3.1.4.1 Mechanism of antitumor action of dasatinib

Dasatinib is a potent inhibitor of the tyrosine kinase Bcr-Abl. Also it blocks a number of other tyrosine kinases, including compounds belonging to the families: scr, c-kit and PDGFR eEPHA 2.

3.1.4.2 Clinical application of dasatinib

This drug is used in the treatment of CML and Ph + ALL patients who had developed resistance to imatinib.

3.1.4.3 Mechanism of cardiotoxicity of dasatinib

There have been reports of congestive heart failure and cardiac arrhythmias in patients during dasatinib therapy. This medicine may also cause QT prolongation. Treatment with dasatinib may increase the risk of pulmonary arterial hypertension. Patients who reported the occurrence of pulmonary hypertension during treatment with dasatinib usually received other cardiotoxic drugs or suffered from other chronic diseases. In these patients improved hemodynamic and clinical parameters after discontinuation of treatment dasatinib was reported. [73]

3.1.5 Lapatinib (GW572016)

3.1.5.1 Mechanism of antitumor action of lapatinib

Lapatinib is an oral dual tyrosine kinase inhibitor selective for inhibition of EGFR/ErbB1 and HER2/ErbB2.

3.1.5.2 Clinical application of lapatinib.

This small molecule represents one of the most promising target therapies in breast cancer that overexpressed HER2. It is used in trastuzumab-refractory breast cancer.

3.1.5.3 Mechanism of cardiotoxicity of lapatinib

Perez et al. reviewed the cardiotoxicity data of lapatinib in 3558 patients, including 1674 breast cancer patients, already treated with the drug alone or in combination with other agents. A total of 1090 patients had >6 months exposure to lapatinib. Evaluation of cardiac left ventricular ejection fraction (LVEF) was done every 8 weeks while patients were receiving therapy, in addition to follow-up for any cardiac clinical events. A preliminary analysis of patients treated with lapatinib to date revealed that incidence of symptomatic

• Tyrosine kinase inhibitors (TKIs) have revolutionized the treatment of several malignancies, converting lethal diseases into manageable, if not curable, chronic diseases. This is essential to limit toxicities of these agents. • The goal of tumor-cell killing by TKIs must be balanced against cardiotoxicity, because in some instances tumor cell death and preservation of cardiomyocyte health may be mutually exclusive. • Cardiomyocytes are contractile and have an extremely high demand for ATP. As a result, they might be particularly susceptible to agents that perturb mitochondrial function, either as a primary or secondary effect. Therefore, alterations in mitochondrial function could have a role in the cardiotoxicities of some currently approved agents. • Very few clinical trials have examined cardiotoxicities of TKIs in a prospective fashion with predefined cardiac endpoints, including left ventricular function. Therefore, there is a wide gap in our knowledge regarding the types, and risk of, cardiotoxicity for most of these agents. • Some current kinase targets in cancer are not expressed in cardiomyocytes. Therefore have little or no direct role in cardiomyocyte survival. The current generation of TKIs is inherently non-selective, and the purposeful design of multitargeted TKIs might allow a single agent to be more effective, and to be used in more types of cancer, but with this comes an increased risk of cardiotoxicity. In some cases this will probably be due to inhibition of 'bystander' targets that are not essential for the killing of tumour cells but that are involved in cardiomyocyte survival. • Identification of the kinase responsible for cardiotoxicity of an agent is important for future drug design. Future kinases should avoid this kinase. Thus, greater selectivity of individual agents may require the use of more agents to treat a particular cancer, but cardiotoxicity as an 'off-target' effect should be minimized.

Table 4. Tyrosine kinase inhibitors- SUMMARY

and asymptomatic decreased LVEF among 1674 breast cancer patients was 1.3% and was also 1.3% among 1453 patients with non- breast malignancies. Lapatinib- associated LVEF decrease was symptomatic in 0.1%, generally reversible/nonprogressive. Average duration of LVEF decrease was 40 days. The other studies conducted so far showed that the cardiotoxicity associated with lapatinib is not severe, is reversible, and usually patients can continue lapatinib therapy, when symptomatic treatment has been started. [54]

3.2 Bortezomib

Recent case reports provide alarming signals that treatment with bortezomib might be associated with cardiac events.

3.2.1 Mechanism of antitumor action of bortezomib

Bortezomib is a reversible proteasome inhibitor.

3.2.2 Clinical application of bortezomib

It is used in treatment of patients suffering from multiple myeloma or mantle cell lymphoma.

3.2.3 Mechanism of cardiotoxicity of bortezomib

Nowis et al. [74] reported that bortezomib treatment leads to left ventricular contractile dysfunction in rats manifested by a significant drop in left ventricle ejection fraction. It is important that in this study rats were not treated with other drugs. Dramatic ultrastructular abnormalities of cardiomyocytes, especially within mitochondria, were accompanied by decreased ATP synthesis and decreased cardiomyocyte contractility. [74] Bortezomib induced cardiac effects seem to be reversible. The risk of cardiotoxicity after bortezomib is higher in patients which have previously cardiac problems or being concomitantly treated with other chemotherapeutics including cardiotoxic anthracyclines. In a recent phase III clinical study of bortezomib was used in combination with pegylated liposomal doxorubicin, LVEF ejection fraction was reported to decrease in 7% of patients treated with bortezomib. [75] In another clinical study, grade 3 to 4 cardiac heart failure was reported in 2 cases (one fatal) receiving bortezomib in combination with doxorubicin. [76]

3.3 Monoclonal antibodies directed against the receptor or tyrosine kinase ligands

3.3.1 Trastuzumab

3.3.1.1 Mechanism of antitumor action of trastuzumab

Trastuzumab is a monoclonal antibody selectively connecting to the extracellular domain of HER-2 receptor, which belongs to the family of epidermal growth factor receptors. Overexpression of this receptor is found in approximately 20-25% of breast cancers. It is presence is associated with poor prognosis and shorter overall survival time. [22]

3.3.1.2 Clinical application of trastuzumab

Trastuzumab improves response rate and survival in women with metastatic breast cancer with known overexpression of the HER-2 receptor. Also the use of trastuzumab concurrently with adjuvant chemotherapy significantly improves the relapse-free survival and overall survival in women with overexpressing HER-2 receptor in localized form of breast cancer. [22]

3.3.1.3 Risk factors for cardiotoxicity after treatment with trastuzumab

The risk factors associated with trastuzumab cardiotoxicity include:

- history of hypertension,
- diabetes,
- obesity,
- older age,
- past radiotherapy prior therapy with anthracyclines.

It was proven that the risk of cardiomyopathy after trastuzumab (as opposed to anthracycline antibiotics) does not depend on the total dose of drug. Contrast, cardiac dysfunction associated with trastuzumab therapy is completely reversible after discontinuation of the drug and after symptomatic treatment and leaves without residual effects in the structure of cardiac muscle. [77]

3.3.1.4 Mechanism of cardiotoxicity of trastuzumab

Cardiotoxicity associated with trastuzumab was analyzed only in the phase III trials, sporadic cases relate to assessment of phase II trials, because nobody knows whether this drug may cause clinically significant cardiac complications. No patients were monitored in terms of efficiency of the cardiovascular system during trastuzumab therapy.

Cardiac complications, grade IV NYHA (New York Heart Association) was observed in 2% of patients treated with trastuzumab in the first line, in 4% of patients treated with trastuzumab because of resistance to previous treatment, in 2% of patients treated with concomitant paclitaxel and trastuzumab (compared to 1% of patients the group receiving paclitaxel alone) and in 16% of patients receiving chemotherapy: adriamycin with cyclophosphamide (AC) plus trastuzumab (compared to 4% in the group receiving chemotherapy alone AC). Symptoms of heart failure occurred in 75.5% of patients (83 in the group of 110 patients). In 79% of cases symptomatic treatment of heart failure has proved effective. [77]

Based on 7 studies: phase II and III, Cardiac Review and Evaluation Committee (CREC) conducted a retrospective analysis of cardiac events associated with trastuzumab therapy. One analysis was based on international study 222 women who received trastuzumab in the second or third line treatment of metastatic breast cancer. Patients were previously treated with anthracyclines (94% women), taxanes (67% women), radiotherapy (71% women), hormonal therapy (57% women). Cardiac complications were seen in 10 patients (4.7%), including 3 patients after treatment with trastuzumab. 9 patient out of all who develop complication (n=10) had been treated with anthracylines previously. Most of the cardiac complications in this study were clinically significant. There was one death following a ventricular arrhythmia, in a patient after previous treatment with anthracyclines with reduced baseline left ventricular ejection fraction. [78]

Another study conducted by CREC concerned randomized, international phase III study comparing trastuzumab in combination with chemotherapy to chemotherapy alone in 469 patients with metastatic breast cancer. The symptoms of cardiotoxicity were observed in

27% of patients who received trastuzumab with anthracyclines and cyclophosphamide compared to 8% of patients after treatment with chemotherapy alone (anthracycline and cyclophosphamide without trastuzumab). In 13% of patients treated with paclitaxel with trastuzumab cardiac complications occurred. Continuation of trastuzumab did not affect the severity of dysfunction of the cardiovascular system in most patients. The symptomatic treatment was effective. [78]

Further analysis concerned three trials [338 patients] where trastuzumab monotherapy was used. It was estimated that the risk of cardiotoxicity associated with trastuzumab was 4%. 3% of patients had grade 3 and 4 toxicity according to Common Toxicity Criteria (CTC). [78]

Mechanism of cardiotoxicity induced by trastuzumab is still not fully clear. But role of inhibition of normal cardiac repair pathways by this drug seem to be probable. Her-2 heterodimerizes to Her-4, leading to autophosphorylation of the Her-2 tyrosine kinase domain. [79] This complex, which is the antitumor target of trastuzumab, is also active in cardiac repair. The complex is activated by neuregulin 1, which is secreted in paracrine fashion by cardiac endothelial cells that are under stress. [79] Activation of the complex leads to multiple downstream effects. In turn they lead to hypertrophy of cardiac myocytes in vivo. In mice, deletion of Her-2 results in a dilated cardiomyopathy. [80] Chien proposed a model in which various types of cardiac stress such as mechanical strain, anthracyclines, or hypoxia trigger two competing pathways of cardiac myocyte survival (mediated by neuregulin-1 or gp 130 cytokines) or apoptosis. The clinical outcome depends on which process prevails. In this model, treatment with trastuzumab blocks the survival pathway by preventing Her-2/Her-4 heterodimerization, thus shifting the balance to apoptosis. The result is decreased cardiac contractility and CHF. [81]

Mechanism for inducing cardiotoxicity by trastuzumab is presented in Table nr 5.

• by the presence of HER-2 receptor on cardiomyocytes, • blocks the cardiac survival pathway by preventing Her-2/Her-4 heterodimerization, • induced apoptosis of cardiomyocytes, • cased hypertrophy of cardiac myocytes,

Table 5. Mechanism of cardiotoxicity of trastuzumab

3.3.2 Bevacizumab

3.3.2.1 Mechanism of antitumor action of bevacizumab

Bevacizumab is a recombinant humanised IgG monoclonal antibody specifically binds to vascular endothelial growth factor (VEGF) and blocking its connection to the membrane receptor and thereby inhibits the process of neoangiogenesis.

3.3.2.2 Clinical application of bevacizumab

Bevacizumab is adjunct to cytotoxic drug combination. It is approved for use in colon, lung, renal and breast cancer.

3.3.2.3 Mechanism of cardiotoxicity of bevacizumab

Based on the research phase I and II found that the possible side effects of bevacizumab are:

- bleeding,
- thromboembolism,
- proteinuria,
- hypertension.

The presence of hypertension was reported in 5-7% of patients participating in clinical trials. It was also observed [in rare cases] development of encephalopathy associated with hypertension and subarachnoid haemorrhage. Patients after treatment with anthracyclines and radiotherapy are at increased risk for cardiac complications during or after treatment with bevacizumab. In patients previously treated with anthracyclines followed by mediastinal radiotherapy, the incidence of left heart failure was about 4%. When anthracyclines and radiotherapy were used at the same time heart failure was observed in 14% of patients. [54]

In a randomized study breast cancer patients receiving paclitaxel with bevacizumab compared to patients receiving paclitaxel alone the risk of hypertension 3 and 4 level rose to about 15%, thromboembolic events up to about 2.5%, proteinuria to about 3.1% and cardiac function the left ventricle to 1.4%. One patient receiving bevacizumab with paclitaxel died of a myocardial infarction. [54]

4. Cardiotoxicity of anagrelide

1. Mechanism of antitumor action of anagrelide.

Anagrelide works by inhibiting the maturation of platelets from megakaryocytes. The exact mechanism of action is unclear, although it is known to be a phosphodiesterase inhibitor. It is a potent inhibitor of phosphodiesterase-II. It inhibits PDE-3 and phospholipase A2.

2. Clinical application of anagrelide.

This medicine is a standard treatment of thrombocythemia in chronic myeloproliferative disorders: essential thrombocythaemia (ET), polycythemia vera (PV) and bone marrow fibrosis.

3. The mechanism of cardiotoxicity of anagrelide.

The mechanism of cardiotoxicity of this drug is not fully known. It may be due to medicine`s positive inotropic effect or consequence of vasodilatation and tachyarrhythmia induced by anagrelide. During the treatment following can occur: palpitations and tachycardia, less common- congestive heart failure, hypertension, arrhythmia, atrial fibrillation and the occasional- angina, myocardial infarction, cardiomegaly, cardiomyopathy, pericardial effusion, and orthostatic hypotension. [82]

Anagrelide was found as a cause of cardiomyopathy in 2000 at the Mayo Clinic [Rochester, USA]. The data were collected from 434 patients suffered from essential thrombocythaemia and polycythemia vera. Investigators confirmed by echocardiography the development of idiopathic cardiomyopathy during treatment of these chronic myeloproliferative disorders with anagrelide in 11 patients. The decrease in LVEF was significant from 35% (two persons) to 10% (one person). Discontinuation of treatment with anagrelide resulted in an increased LVEF. [82]

Cardiotoxicity of anagrelide also confirmed case of 50-year-old man diagnosed with essential thrombocythaemia. Due to the increasing resistance to first-line treatment the patient was treated with anagrelide in a dose gradually increasing up to 2.5 mg twice a day. The patient developed clinical features of congestive heart failure, NYHA IV. LVEF was 18%. ECG findings were typical for myocardial ischemia but troponin T level was normal. Coronary angiography was performed revealing normal in which the coronary arteries. Treatment of anagrelide was stopped, hydroxyurea therapy was started again. Patients received symptomatic therapy of heart failure: diuretics and ACE-inhibitors with good response. Hydroxyurea therapy once again proved to be ineffective. Doctors were decided to join hydroxyurea of anagrelide at a reduced dose 0.5 mg twice a day. Modification of treatment was effective, the level of platelets decreased to the normal limits, the symptoms of heart failure was absent. ECHO, made by 2 and 8 months after starting treatment with anagrelide [low doses] and hydroxyurea, showed increasing LVEF from 40 to 50%. [83]

These observations confirm that the use of anagrelide is not absolutely safe to the cardiovascular system. Cardiomyopathy, during anagrelide treatment is rare but clinically significant. Therefore, patients with a history of heart disease should be treated with anagrelide with caution, when potential benefits exceed risk of this kind therapy. [82,83]

Mechanism of cardiotoxicity associated with the action of anagrelide is showen in Table nr 6.

• by positive inotropic effects, • by vasodilatation, • by tachyarrythmias,

Table 6. The mechanism of cardiotoxicity of anagrelide

5. Cardiotoxicity of High Dose Chemotherapy (HDC) followed by Hematopoietic Stem Cell Transplantation (HSCT)

Hematopoietic stem cell transplantation (HSCT) has now become the treatment of choice for large number of malignant and non-malignant diseases. Cardiac complications may result from high-dose chemotherapy or irradiation administered during the conditioning phase of bone marrow and blood stem cell transplantation (BMT). Cardiac complications of high-dose cyclophosphamide and total body irradiation (TBI) or other intensive conditioning regimens administered prior to bone marrow and stem cell transplantation (BMT) have been well documented. Clinically, patients present with congestive heart failure and pancarditis. Hemorrhagic perimyocarditis with endothelial damage and microthrombi in capillaries as well as acute fibrinous pericarditis. Several other cytotoxic drugs such as busulfan, carmustine or cytarabine used in pre-BMT regimens may cause significant cardiotoxicity. Acute myocardial infarction and various cardiac arrhythmias including cardiac arrest as a consequence of infusion of cryopreserved marrow have been reported during the acute phase of BMT. Pretreatment with anti-tumor antibiotics including anthracyclines and prior mediastinal irradiation may increase the risks of adverse cardiac sequelae after BMT, but identification of the risk factors and effective strategies for cardiologic prescreening have not been well established. Although cardiac complications associated with BMT have been documented in several series, the incidence of reported cardiotoxicity has varied among investigators, probably reflecting patient selection, differences in BMT preparative regimens and lack of universal grading system for cardiotoxic events. [84-87]

Cardiac complications associated with exposure to the conditioning factors can be acute, with a relatively short or long period of latency after HSCT. [84-87]

To assess the frequency of clinically serious cardiac toxicity related to the acute phase of bone marrow transplantation (BMT), investigators from University of Minnesota retrospectively examined life-threatening or fatal cardiotoxicity identified using the complications records of their transplant center clinical database. All serious cardiac toxicity events within 100 days of BMT except those attributable to septic shock, pneumonitis or multi-organ failure were reviewed. During the first 100 days after transplantation 628 cardiac complications experienced and divided by four-level scale cardiac toxicity [86]:

- Stage I- asymptomatic cardiomegaly, mild ECG changes, not requiring treatment, asymptomatic stroke in the pericardium,
- Stage II- moderate changes in the ECG, which require and well respond to routine treatment, congestive heart failure responsive to afterload reduction in the treatment of diuretics and digitalis, pericarditis,
- Stage III: severe abnormalities in the ECG with no or partial response to medical intervention, congestive heart failure, requiring drugs with isotropic, cardiogenic shock, reducing the voltage wave QRS&> 50%, pericardial tamponade.
- Stage IV- death following cardiac toxicity.

Of 2821 BMT patients at the University of Minnesota between 1977 and 1997, 26 were identified as having suffered major or fatal (n = 13) cardiotoxicity (0.9%, 19 adults and seven children). Rapidly progressive heart failure resulted in death of 11 patients, one patient had fatal pericardial tamponade, and one had an acute ventricular fibrillation arrest. The remaining 13 patients (50%) had life-threatening cardiotoxicity including four patients with pericardial tamponade and nine patients with cardiac arrhythmias. Overall, we observed that acute, major cardiotoxic events attributable to BMT are uncommon, occurring with a frequency of 1%. These data suggest that with appropriate pre-transplant clinical evaluation, high-dose cyclophosphamide and irradiation in the BMT preparative phase does not result in frequent, clinically relevant short-term cardiac toxicity. [86]

The most common late complications of HSCT include valvular dysfunction, conduction disturbances, pericarditis and cardiomyopathies. Are also observed vascular complications, which include: coronary heart disease, cerebral vascular dysfunction and disease. [84-87]

Investigators from City of Hope National Medical Center [87] examined the independent roles of pre-hematopoietic cell transplantation (HCT) therapeutic exposures, transplantation-related conditioning, and comorbidities (pre- and post-HCT) in the development of late congestive heart failure (CHF) after HCT. This was a nested case-control design. Individuals with late CHF (diagnosed 1 year after HCT) were identified from a cohort of 2,938 1 year survivors who underwent transplantation at City of Hope National Medical Center, Duarte, CA. This cohort formed the sampling frame for selecting controls (without CHF) matched for age and year of HCT, donor source (allogeneic v autologous), and length of follow-up. Sixty patients with late CHF were identified; median age at HCT was 45.3

years (range, 16.6 to 68.6 years); median time to CHF was 3.0 years (range, 1.03 to 18.9 years); 68% received autologous HCT. Median ejection fraction was 36.9% (range, 15% to 53%). Compared with matched controls (n = 166), patients with late CHF received more cycles of pre-HCT chemotherapy (8.6 v 4.9 cycles; P= 0.01), had greater body mass index at HCT (28.4 v 26.2 kg/m^2; P= 0.01), greater lifetime anthracycline exposure (285.3 v 175.6 mg/m^2; P= 0.01), and were more likely to have multiple chronic comorbidities (30.0% v 13.9%; P= 0.01). Multivariable analysis revealed number of pre-HCT chemotherapy cycles (odds ratio [OR] 1.2; P= 0.01), anthracycline dose 250 mg/m^2 (OR 3.2; P= 0.05), and two or more chronic comorbidities (OR 4.3; P= 0.01) to be independently associated with late CHF. Pre-HCT exposure to anthracyclines and presence of comorbidities are primarily risk associated with late CHF after HCT. Conditioning-related therapeutic exposure does not contribute significantly to the risk. These results form the basis for identifying high-risk individuals for targeted surveillance, as well as developing preventive strategies in the form of aggressive management of comorbidities. [87]

Considering all of the above the important factors affecting the occurrence of cardiotoxic high dose chemotherapy complications include exposure to high doses of cyclophosphamide, total body irradiation, prior anthracycline therapy, the presence of dimethyl sulfoxide (DMSO) in intravenous products, infectious complications associated with neutropenia. The risk of cardiac complications after HSCT is also influenced by patient age, type of therapy applied and previous medical history. [84]

Dimethyl sulphoxide (DMSO) is cells protective factor, preventing the crystallization of water and damage to cell membranes collected stem cells, which are subjected to freezing in liquid nitrogen at temperatures below -120 degrees C. Cardiotoxicity associated with DMSO may result in hypotension, requiring fluid infusion or even inotropic drugs. Ones also reported cardiac arrhythmias such as atrial fibrillation, or bradycardia, and incidents of acute coronary syndromes. Cardiotoxicity associated with DMSO is rare. Wether DMSO is responsible for these has been questioned. [84,85] Recent reports of similar acute cardiac events despite DMSO depletion have led to the suggestion that perhaps the complications seen following infusion may be more a product of the amount of infused granulocytes, rather than DMSO. [84]

Infectious complications during early post-transplant neutropenia or prolonged immunosuppression for GVHD prophylaxis are common problems following HSCT. Overwhelming sepsis can lead to cardiopulmonary failure, necessitating prolonged intubation and cardiac inotropic support, potentially causing subclinical cardiotoxicity or other end-organ compromise that may not be evident until years following HSCT. [84]

The Tichellis study [84] provided preliminary evidence for an association between GVHD and the development of arterial disease. There are emerging data to suggest that chronic GVHD could play a role in the development of cardiovascular disease. Cardiac side effects of chronic GVHD, while rare, likely occur as a result of direct organ lymphocytic infiltration. Increased levels of circulating tumor necrosis factor alfa [TNF alfa] may impair muscle electrical activity and compromise myocardial contractility. Furthermore, increased amounts of inflammatory markers, such as TNF alfa and interleukin-6, could perpetuate endothelial injury, contributing to premature arterial events in long-term survivors after allogeneic HSCT. Treatment of GVHD is not without cardiovascular consequences.

Prolonged treatment with calcineurin inhibitors and steroids can lead to myocardial hypertrophy, as well as increase the likehood of cardiovascular disease risk factors such as hypertension, diabetes, and renal insufficiency. [84]

6. Carditoxicity of radiotherapy

In anticancer treatment, radiotherapy plays an important role. It can also damage the heart muscle. Due to the location of the heart in human body, mediastinal radiotherapy poses the highest risk of cardiac complications. This form of treatment is commonly used in lymphoma, breast, esophageal and lung cancers. In connection with the expected long period of survival of patients with Hodgkin lymphoma and breast cancer the risk of complications from cardiovascular diseases is the highest. The maximum potential safe dose of ionizing radiation on the heart area are as follows [88]:

- approximately 60 Gy when 25% or less heart volume is irradiated,
- about 45 Gy, while 65% of the volume of the heart is irradiated with a standard fractionation at 2 Gy per day.

Early cardiac complication after radiation therapy is acute pericarditis, which usually occurs within a few weeks after treatment. The most common late effect of radiotherapy on cardiovascular system is coronary artery disease. It usually appears within 10-15 years after radiation. Ones have been shown that ionizing radiation can initiate or accelerate the atherosclerotic process, this phenomenon refers mainly to people with other risk factors for cardiovascular disease. On others cardiac structures radiotherapy also has a negative effect, but to a lesser extent. It may lead to development of restrictive cardiomyopathy, cardiac diastolic dysfunction, impaired contractile function [that occurs after mated treatment with anthracyclines], aortic stenosis, QT prolongation, persistent tachycardia [damage of autonomic nervous system]. [88]

Risk factors for acute or chronic cardiac complications after radiation therapy include [88]:

- irradiated volume of the heart (cardiac risk is proportional to the irradiated volume of the heart),
- patient age (younger age at the time of exposure to ionizing radiation is a risk factor for vascular disease),
- time of exposure (the majority of published reports that the need for a minimum of 10 years to the risk of death from heart attack increased above 10%),
- dose and technique of application of ionizing radiation (it is considered that the total radiation dose in the case of mediastinal radiotherapy, increasing the risk of cardiovascular disease is> 35-40 Gy, whereas a fractional dose> 2 Gy per day) and
- prior chemotherapy (especially anthracycline-based regimens).

7. Cardiotoxicity of antagonists of 5-HT3 receptor

Potentially cardiotoxic drugs, inevitably associated with oncology therapy, are also antagonists of 5-HT3 receptor. Chemotherapy, especially given in high doses causes of nausea and vomiting, which are very burdensome for the patient with neoplastic disease. The mechanism of vomiting is the release of large amount of serotonin, stimulating 5-HT3 receptors located on nerve endings centripetal parasympathetic system. Parasympathetic system also innervates the heart muscle, which explains the cause of the cardiac complications associated with this class of drugs. [89]

Results of the review of clinical trials with MEDLINE database from the period 1963-2002 for cardiotoxicity antagonists 5-HT3 receptor were as follows [89-91]:

- ECG changes (PR, QRS, QT, QTc, JT) were small, reversible, clinically insignificant and dependent on the selected group of patients,
- ECG changes occurred most frequently between 1 and 2 hours after administration of dolasetron, ondansetron and granisetron and returned to normal within 24 hours, no evidence of acute, clinically significant cardiac complications.

Based on these data it was concluded that the benefits of this class of drugs greatly outweigh their adverse effects on the cardiovascular system. [91]

Considering the high risk of cardiac complications due to oncological treatment, it is important to establish standards of conduct with patients undergoing cancer therapy proven to cardiac toxicity.

8. References

[1] Ewer MS, Von Hoff DD, Benjamin RS. A historical perspective of anthracycline cardiotoxicity. Heart Fail Clin 2011; 17: 363-372.

[2] Schimmel K, Richel D, van den Brink R, Guchelaar HJ. Cardiotoxicity of cytotoxic drugs. Cancer Treat Rev 2004; 30: 181-191.

[3] Pommier Y, Leo E, Zhang H, Marchand C. DNA topoisomerases and their poisoning by anticancer and antibacterial drugs. Chem Biol. 2010; 17: 421-433.

[4] Binaschi M, Bigioni M, Cipollone A, Rossi C, Goso C, Maggi CA, Capranico G. Anthracyclines: selected New developments. Curr Med Chem Anticancer Agents. 2001; 1: 113-130.

[5] Minott G, Cairo G, Monti E. Role of iron in anthracycline cardiotoxicity: new tunes for an old song? FASEB J 1999; 13: 199-212.

[6] Sieswerda E, van Dalen EC, Postma A. Medical interventions for treating anthracycline-induced symptomatic and asymptomatic cardiotoxicity duriong and after treatment for childhood cancer. Cohrane Database Syst Rev 2011.

[7] Armenian Saro H., Bhatia S. Cardiovascular disease after hematopoietic cell transplantation- lessons learned. Haematologica 2003; 93: 1132-1136.

[8] Singal PK, Li T, Kumar D, et al. Adriamycin-induced heart failure: mechanizm and modulation. Mol Cell Biochem. 2000; 207: 77-86.

[9] Bristol MR, Mason JW, Billingham ME, Daniels JR. Dose-effect and structure-function relationchips In doxorubicin cardiomyopathy.Am. Heart J. 1981; 102: 709-18.

[10] Wang L, Ma W, Markovich R, et al. Regulation of cardiomyocyte apoptotic signaling by insuline- like growth factor I. Circ Res 1998; 83: 516-522.

[11] Kim Y, Ma AG, Kitta K, Fitch SN et al. Anthracycline-induced suppression of GATA-4 transcription factor: implication in the regulation of cardiac myocyte apoptosis. Mol Pharmacol. 2003; 63: 368-377.

[12] Minotti G. Sources and role of iron in lipid peroxidation. Chem Res Toxicol. 1993; 6: 134-146.

[13] Cairo G, Recalcati S, Pietrangelo A, Minotti G. The iron regulatory proteins: targets and modulators of free radical reactions and oxidative damage. Free Radic Biol Med. 2002; 32: 1237-1243.

[14] Beltrami AP., Barlucchi L, Torella D, et al. Adult cardiac stem cells are multipotent and support myocardial regeneration. Cell.2003; 114: 763-776.

[15] Linke A, Muller P, Nurzynska D, et al. Stem cell in the dog heart are self-renewing, clonogenic, and multipotent and regenerate infarcted myocardium, improving cardiac function. Proc. Natl. Acad. Sci. USA. 2005; 102: 8966-8971.

[16] Bearzi C, Rota M, Hosoda T, et al. Human cardiac stem cells. Proc. Natl. Acad. Sci. USA. 2007; 104: 14068-14073.

[17] Gille L, Nohl H. Analyses of the molecular mechanism of adriamycin induced cardiotoxicity. Free Radiac Biol Med. 1997; 23: 775-782.

[18] Doroshow JH, Locker GY, Myers CE. Enzymatic defences of the mouse heart against reactive oxygen metabolites. J Clin Invest. 1980; 65: 128-135.

[19] Li T, Danelisen I, Signal PK. Early changes in myocardial antioxidant enzymes in rats treated with adriamycin. Mol Cell Biochem. 2002; 232: 19-26.

[20] Stiefelhagen P. Cardiotoxicity of chemotherapy. An increasing problem in oncology and cardiology. Med Monatsschr Pharm 2011; 34: 96-99.

[21] Feenstra J., Grobbee D.E., Remme W.J, et al. Drug- Induced Heart Failure. J Am Coll Cardiol. 1999; 33: 1152-1162.

[22] Eisenhauer EA, Vermorken JB. The taxoids. Comparative clinical pharmacology and therapeutic potential. Drugs 1998;55:5-30.

[23] Baldini E, Prochilol T, Salvadoril B, et al. Multicancer randomized phase III trial of epiribicin plus paclitaxel vs epirubicin followed by paclitaxel in metastatic breast cancer patients: focus on cardiac safety. Br J Cancer 2004; 91: 45-49.

[24] Burt R.K., Wilson W.H. Conditioning (preparative) regimens. In: Bone Marrow Transplantation. Burt R.K., Deeg H.J., Lothian S.T. (eds.). R.G. Landes Company 1998; 95-97.

[25] Simon TL, Snyder EL, Solheim BG, Stowell CP, Strauss RG and Petrides M (eds.). Rossi`s principles of transfusion medicine, 4th edn.. Blackwell Publishing, Singapore, 2009.

[26] Blume KG, Forman SJ, Appelbaum FR (eds.).Thomas' Hematopoietic Cell Transplantation Third Edition. Blackwell Publishing; Massachusetts 2004.

[27] Apperley J, Carreras E, Gluckman E, Gratwohl A, Masszi T. (eds.): Haematopoietic stem cell transplantation. Forum Service Editore, Genoa 2008.

[28] Braverman A.C., Antin J.H., Plappert M.T., et al. Cyclophosphamide cardiotoxicity in bone marrow transplantation a prospective evaluation of new dosing regimens. J Clin Oncol. 1991; 9: 1215-1223.

[29] McDonald G.B., Slaterry J.T., Bouvier M.E, et al. Cyclophosphamide metabolism, liver toxicity, and mortality following hematopoietic stem cell transplantation. Blood. 2003; 101: 2043-2048.

[30] Kandylis K, Vassilomanokalis M, Tsoussis S, et al. Ifosfamide cardiotoxicity in humans. Cancer Chemother Pharmacol 1989; 24: 395- 396.

[31] Wandt H, Birkmann J, Seifert M, et al. Localized cerebral edema after high-dose chemotherapy and ABMT for germ cell tumor. Bone Marrow Transplant 1993; 11: 419- 420.
[32] Quezado Z, Wilson WH, Cunnion RE, et al. High-dose ifosfamide is associated with severe, reversble cardiac dysfunction. Ann Intern Med 1993; 118; 31-36.
[33] Cunnion RE, Cottler-Fox M. Cardiac complications of marrow transplantation. Semin Respir Crit Care Med 1996; 17: 409- 415.
[34] Morandi P, Ruffini PA, Benvenuto GM, et al. Cardiac toxicity of high-dose chemotherapy. Bone Marrow Transplant 2005; 35: 323-334.
[35] Culine S, Ghosn M, Droz JP. Inappropriate antidiuretic hormone secretion induced by ifosfamide. Eur J Cancer 1990; 26: 922.
[36] Kirch C, Gachot B, Germann N, et al. Reccurent ifosfamide- induced hyponatremia. Eur J Cancer 1997; 33: 2438- 2439.
[37] Husband DJ, Watkin SW. Fatal hipokalemia associated with ifosfamide/ mesna chemotherapy. Lancet 1998; 1: 1116.
[38] Bagai RK, Spiro TP, Daw HA. 5-fluorouracil- induced cardiotoxicity during chemotherapy for adenocarcinoma of the small bowel. GI Cancer Research 2009; 3: 167-170.
[39] Weidmann B., Jansen W., Heider A., Niederle N. 5-fluorouracil cardiotoxicity with left ventricular dysfunction under different dosing regimens . Am J Cardiol 1995; 75: 194-195.
[40] Hong R.A, Lemura T., Sumida K.N, et al. Review. Cardio-Oncology. Clin Cardiol 2010; 33: 733-737.
[41] Talapatra K, Rajesh I, Rajesh B, et al. Transient asymptomatic bradycardia in patients on infusional 5-fluorouracil. J Can Res Ther 2007;3:169-171.
[42] Fidan E, Fidan S, Yildiz B, et al. Bolus fluorouracil induced syncope and pulseless ventricular tachycardia: a case report. Hippokratia 2011, 15, 1: 93-95.
[43] Tsibiribi P., Descotes J., Lombard-Bohas C. et al. Cardiotoxicity of 5-fluorouracil in 1350 patients with no prior history of heart disease. Bull Cancer 2006; 93: E27-E30.
[44] Labianca R., Beretta G., Glenici M, et al. Cardiac toxicity of 5-fluorouracil . Study of 1083 patients. Tumori 1982; 68: 505-510.
[45] Anand AJ. Fluorouracil cardiotoxicity. Ann Pharmacother 1994; 28: 374-378.
[46] Miwa M.,Ura M., Nishiada M., et al. Design of a novel oral fluoropyrimidine carbamate, capecitabine, which generates 5-fluorouracil selectively in tumours by enzymes concentrated in human liver and cancer tissue. Eur J Cancer 1998; 34: 1274-1281.
[47] Van Cutsem E, Hoff PM, Blum Jl et al. Incidence of cardiotoxicity with the oral fluoropyrimidine capecitabine is typical of that reported with 5-fluorouracil. Ann Oncol 2002; 13: 484-485.
[48] Wijesinghe N, Thompson PI, McAlister H. Acute coronary syndrome induced by capecitabine therapy. Heart Lung Circ 2006; 15: 337-339.
[49] Kosmas C, Kallistratos MS, Kopterides P., et al. Cardiotoxicity of fluoropyrimidines in different schedules of administration: a prospective study. J Cancer Res Clin Oncol 2008; 134: 75-82.
[50] Goldsmith YB, Roitacher N, Baum MS. Capecitabine-induced coronary vasospasm.J Clin Oncol 2008; 17: 3802-3804.

[51] Ang C., Kornbluth M., Thirlwell M.P, Rajan RD. Capecitabine- induced cardiotoxicity: case report and review of the literature. Curr Oncol 2010; 17: 59-63.
[52] Senturk T, Kanat O, Evrensel T, Aydinlar A. Capecitabine-induced cardiotoxicity mimicking myocardial infarction. Neth Heart J 2009; 17: 277-280.
[53] Theodoulou M., Seidman A.D. Cardiac effects of adjuvant therapy for early breast cancer. Semin Oncol 2003; 30: 730-739.
[54] Bilancia D, Rosati G, Dinota A, et al. Lapatinib in breast cancer. Ann Oncol 2007; 18 (suppl 6): vi26-vi30.
[55] Vaklavas C., Lenihan D., Kurzrock R., Tsimberidou A.M. Anti-vascular endothelial growth factor therapies and cardiovascular toxicity: What are the important clinical markers to target? The Oncologist 2010; 15: 130-141.
[56] Menna P, Salvatorelli E, Minotti G. Cardiotoxicity of antitumor drugs. Chem Res Toxicol 2008; 21: 978-989.
[57] Britten CD, Kabbinavar F, Hecht JR et al. A phase I and pharmacokinetic study of sunitinib administered daily for 2 weeks, followed by a 1-week off period. Cancer Chemother Pharmacol 2008;61:515–524.
[58] Motzer RJ, Michaelson MD, Redman BG et al. Activity of SU11248, a multitargeted inhibitor of vascular endothelial growth factor receptor and platelet-derived growth factor receptor, in patients with metastatic renal cell carcinoma. J Clin Oncol 2006;24:16 –24.
[59] Demetri GD, van Oosteron AT, Garrett CR et al. Efficacy and safety of sunitinib in patients with advanced gastrointestinal stromal tumour after failure of imatinib: Arandomised controlled trial. Lancet 2006; 368: 1329-1338.
[60] Motzer RJ, Hutson TE, Tomczak P et al. Sunitinib versus interferon alfa in metastatic renal-cell carcinoma. N Engl J Med 2007;356:115–124.
[61] Chu TF, Rupnick MA, Kerkela R et al. Cardiotoxicity associated with tyrosine kinase inhibitor sunitinib. Lancet 2007;370:2011–2019.
[62] Khakoo A.Y., Kassiatis C.M., Plana J.C., et al. Heart failure associated with sunitinib malate. A multitargeted receptor tyrosine kinase inhibitor. Cancer 2008; 112: 2500-2508.
[63] Force T., Krause D.S.,Van Etten RA. Molecular mechanisms of cardiotoxicity of tyrosine kinase inhibition. Cancer 2007; 7: 332-344.
[64] Deininger M, Buchdunger E, Druker BJ. The development of imatinib as a therapeutic agent for chronic myeloid leukemia. Blood 2005; 105: 2640-2653.
[65] Kane RC, Farrell AT, Saber H et al. Sorafenib for the treatment of advanced renal cell carcinoma. Clin Cancer Res 2006;12:7271–7278.
[66] Escudier B, Eisen T, Stadler WM et al. Sorafenib in advanced clear-cell renal-cell carcinoma. N Engl J Med 2007;356:125–134.
[67] Siu LL, Awada A, Takimoto CH et al. Phase I trial of sorafenib and gemcitabine in advanced solid tumors with an expanded cohort in advanced pancreatic cancer. Clin Cancer Res 2006;12:144 –151.
[68] Akaza H, Tsukamoto T, Murai M et al. Phase II study to investigate the efficacy, safety, and pharmacokinetics of sorafenib in Japanese patients with advanced renal cell carcinoma. Jpn J Clin Oncol 2007;37:755–762.

[69] Llovet JM, Ricci S, Mazzaferro V et al. Sorafenib in advanced hepatocellular carcinoma. N Engl J Med 2008;359:378 -390.
[70] Kerkela R., Grazette L., Yacobi R., et al. Cardiotoxicity of the cancer therapeutic agent imatinib mesylate. Nat Med 2006; 12: 908-916.
[71] O`Brief S.G., Guilhot F., Larson R.A., et al. Imatinib compared with interferon alfa and low dose cytarabine for newly diagnosed chronic phase chronic myelogenous leukemia. N Engl J Med 2003; 348: 994-1004.
[72] Sacha T. Molekularne mechanizmy opornosci na imatinib. Acta Haematol Pol. 2003; 34: 263-275.
[73] Product Characteristics Sprycel; December 2010.
[74] Nowis D., Maczewski M., Mackiewicz U., et al. Cardiotoxicity of the anticancer therapeutic agent bortezomid. Am J Pathol 2010; 176: 2658-2668.
[75] Orlowski R.Z., Nagler A., Sonneveld P., et al. Rhandomized phase III study of pegylated liposomal doxorubicin plus bortezomid compared with bortezomid alone in relapsed or refractory multiple myeloma: combination therapy improves time to progression. J Clin Oncol 2007; 25: 3892-3901.
[76] Palumbo A, Gay F, Bringhen S et al. Bortezomid, doxorubicin and dexamethasone in advanced multiple myeloma. Ann Oncol 2008; 19: 1160-1165.
[77] Perez E., Rodeheffer R. Clinical cardiac tolerability of trastuzumab. J Clin Oncol 2004; 22: 322-329.
[78] Keefe D.L. Trastuzumab- associated cardiotoxicity. Cancer 2002; 95: 1592-1600.
[79] Lemmens K, Segers VF, Demolder M, et al: Role of neuregulin-1/ErbB2 signaling in endothelium-cardiomyocyte cross-talk. J Biol Chem 2006; 281:19469-19477.
[80] Crone SA, Zhao YY, Fan L, et al: ErbB2 is essential in the prevention of dilated cardiomyopathy. Nat Med 2002; 8:459-465.
[81] Chien KR:Herceptin and the heart: a molecular modifier of cardiac failure.N Engl J Med 2006; 354:789-790.
[82] Jurgens D., Moreno-Aspitia A.,Tefferi A. Anagrelide-associated cardiomyopathy in polycythemia vera and essential thrombocythemia. Haematologica 2004; 89: 1394-1395.
[83] Wong R.S.M., Lam L.W.K., Cheng G. Successful rechallenge with anagrelide in a patient with anagrelide-associated cardiomyopathy. Ann Hematol 2008; 87: 683-684.
[84] Armenian S.H., Bhatia S. Cardiovascular disease after hematopoietic cell transplantation- lessons learned. Haematologica 2008; 93: 1132-1136.
[85] Antin J. H., Yolin Raley D. Manual of stem cell and bone marrow transplantation. Cambridge University Press ; New York, 2009.
[86] Murdych T., Weisdorf D.J. Serious cardiac complications during bone morrow transplantation at the University of Minnesota, 1977-1997. Bone Marrow Transplant 2001; 28: 283-287.
[87] Armenian SH, Sun CL, Francisco L, et al. Late congestive heart failure after hematopoietic cell transplantation. J Clin Oncol 2008; 26: 5537-5543.
[88] Senkus E, Jassem J. Cardiovascular effects of systemic cancer treatment. Cancer Treat Rev. 2011; 37:300-11.
[89] Ettinger D.S. Preventing chemotherapy-induced nusea and vomiting. Semin Oncol 1995; 22: 6-18.

[90] Goodin S.,Cunningham R. 5-HT3 receptor antagonists for the treatment of nausea and vomiting. A reappraisal of their side-effect profile. Oncologist 2002; 7: 424-436.
[91] Navari R.M., Koeller J.M. Electrocardiographic and cardiovascular effects of the 5-HT3 receptor antagonists. Ann Pharmacother 2003; 37: 1276-1286.

4

Neuregulin1-ErbB Signaling in Doxorubicin-Induced Cardiotoxicity

David Goukassian, James P. Morgan and Xinhua Yan*
Cardiovascular Medicine, St. Elizabeth's Medical Center and Tufts University School of Medicine, Boston, USA

1. Introduction

This chapter will review basic and clinical findings regarding the cardioprotective role of Neuregulin1-ErbB signaling against the cardiotoxicity of doxorubicin, a widely used chemotherapeutic agent. In 2001, *The New England Journal of Medicine* published the results from clinical trials in breast cancer patients using Trastuzumab, a monoclonal antibody that blocks the ErbB2 receptor. These studies showed that the incidence of New York Heart Association (NYHA) class III/IV heart failure was 16% in patients who were concurrently treated with doxorubicin and Trastuzumab compared to 3% and 2% respectively in patients who were treated with doxorubicin or Trastuzumab alone (Slamon et al., 2001). These results for the first time suggest that the ErbB signaling has cardioprotective effects against doxorubicin-induced cardiotoxicity. Since then, a significant amount of basic and clinical research has been conducted to investigate the mechanisms of the ErbB signaling pathway in protecting the heart from doxorubicin-induced toxicity. At the same time, studies have been performed searching for factors that stimulate ErbB signaling to protect the heart from doxorubicin. Although ErbB receptors have at least 13 ligands, Neuregulin1 proteins have become the focus of this search (Yarden and Sliwkowski, 2001a). Studies from cardiomyocyte culture, animal models and clinical trials have demonstrated that Neuregulin1 may be effective for preventing or treating doxorubicin-induced cardiotoxicity.

2. Doxorubicin-induced cardiotoxicity

2.1 Background

The anthracycline drug doxorubicin was discovered about 40 years ago and continues to be used as a first line antineoplastic drug (Outomuro et al., 2007a; Moretti et al., 2009). Doxorubicin is effective for the treatment of a wide variety of cancers in children and adults, such as leukemia, lymphoma, breast, lung and colon cancers (Outomuro et al., 2007a; Anderson and Sawyer, 2008). Doxorubicin has significantly improved survival of childhood cancer patients, in which the survival rate is now approaching 75% (Curry et al., 2006). There are an estimated 300,000 childhood cancer survivors in the United States (Jemal et al.,

* Corresponding Author

2006; Oeffinger et al., 2006). Nearly 60% of them have been treated with doxorubicin or its analogs (van Dalen et al., 2006; Bryant et al., 2007; LoPiccolo et al., 2008). In adult patients, such as breast cancer patients, it is estimated that 30% of them have been treated with doxorubicin (Paik et al., 2000; Pritchard et al., 2006). However, dose-related cardiotoxicity has limited the use of doxorubicin at all in a subset of cancer patients with pre-existing cardiovascular conditions and in cancer patients in general, due to significant risk of developing irreversible heart failure months and years after doxorubicin treatment (Barry et al., 2007a; Outomuro et al., 2007a; Anderson and Sawyer, 2008).

The incidence of doxorubicin-induced cardiotoxicity has been reported to be in a variable range of 0.4 - 41% (Outomuro et al., 2007a). The risk of doxorubicin-induced cardiotoxicity mainly depends on the cumulative dose of the drug administered. The incidence of doxorubicin-induced heart failure is about 3% at a cumulative dose of 400 mg/m^2 , 7.5% at a cumulative dose of 550 mg/m^2 and 18% at 700 mg/m^2 (Von Hoff et al., 1979; Swain et al., 2003; Outomuro et al., 2007a). Other factors, such as age (very young or elderly patients), pre-existing cardiovascular disease, and previous or concurrent use of other anti-cancer cytotoxic or targeted therapies, can increase the risk of doxorubicin-induced heart failure (Von Hoff et al., 1979; Safra, 2003; Outomuro et al., 2007b). Trastuzumab, a monoclonal antibody that blocks the HER2 receptor, is the first drug approved by the US Food and Drug Administration (FDA) for targeted cancer therapy. When Trastuzumab and doxorubicin were concurrently used in breast cancer patients, the incidence of New York Heart Association type III and IV heart failure rose from 2-3% to 16% over a period of 50 months of observation (Slamon et al., 2001).

Doxorubicin can cause acute, subacute and late cardiotoxicity. The acute doxorubicin cardiotoxicity starts within 24 hours of drug infusion, and may present as cardiac arrhythmia, myocarditis and pericarditis (Appelbaum et al., 1976). The long-term prognosis of acute doxorubicin cardiotoxicity is relatively good. Subacute doxorubicin cardiotoxicity occurs weeks and months after the treatment, while late cardiotoxicity can occur 4-20 years after the cessation of the treatment. The onset of chronic doxorubicin cardiotoxicity is insidious; the disease, however, progressively develops to severe and irreversible heart failure (Simsir et al., 2005). Therefore, doxorubicin cardiotoxicity is a Type I chemotherapy-related cardiac dysfunction (CRCD) (Ewer and Lippman, 2005). It is irreversible and presents a life-long threat for cancer survivors (Ewer and Lippman, 2005).

The pathological changes in chronic doxorubicin cardiotoxicity include cardiac hypertrophy, which may be followed with thinning of the ventricular wall (dilated cardiomyopathy), interstitial fibrosis, vascular and mitochondrial degeneration. Morphological changes within the cardiomyocyte include distention of the sarcotubular system (vacuolization), loss of myofibrils, as well as mitochondrial swelling and loss of cristae (Billingham et al., 1978; Mortensen et al., 1986; Rowan et al., 1988; Lipshultz et al., 1991; Mackay et al., 1994; Lipshultz et al., 2005; Barry et al., 2007b).

2.2 Potential mechanisms of doxorubicin-induced cardiotoxicity

There have been several proposed mechanisms for doxorubicin-induced cardiotoxicity:

(1) free radical generation and oxidative stress (Kang et al., 1996; Yen et al., 1996; Kang et al., 1997), (2) increased cardiomyocyte death by necrosis and apoptosis (Childs et al., 2002b; Green and Leeuwenburgh, 2002; Aries et al., 2004; Kalivendi et al., 2005a; Poizat et al., 2005),

(3) inhibition of cardiac specific muscle gene transcription and translation, in combination with an increase in myofibril protein degradation, leading to loss of myofibrils (Lewis and Gonzalez, 1987; Ito et al., 1990; Kurabayashi et al., 1994; Toyoda et al., 1998; d'Anglemont de Tassigny et al., 2004; Lim et al., 2004b), and (4) disturbance of intracellular calcium homeostasis (De Beer et al., 2001; Wallace, 2003). The mechanism of doxorubicin-induced free radical generation and oxidative stress has been reviewed in other chapters of this book as well as comprehensive reviews in the field (Singal et al., 2000; Berthiaume and Wallace, 2007; Simunek et al., 2009). In this chapter, we will focus on the mechanisms that connect the Neuregulin1-ErbB signaling to doxorubicin cardiotoxicity.

2.2.1 Doxorubicin-induced apoptosis in the cardiomyocyte

Studies have been conducted to investigate doxorubicin-induced cardiomyocyte apoptosis in H9c2 rat embryonic cardiomyocytes, neonatal and adult rat cardiomyocytes, as well as in hearts from rats and mice treated with doxorubicin (Childs et al., 2002a; Fukazawa et al., 2003; Liu et al., 2005; Youn et al., 2005; Fu and Arcasoy, 2007; Bian et al., 2009).

Doxorubicin induces apoptosis via both intrinsic and extrinsic pathways. Doxorubicin alters the ratio of pro-apoptotic and anti-apoptotic Bcl-2 family proteins, including Bcl-2, Bad, Bim, Bax, Bak and Bik (Aries et al., 2004; Rohrbach et al., 2005b; Kobayashi et al., 2006); it also causes DNA damage and p53 activation (Liu et al., 2004; L'Ecuyer et al., 2006). All these changes can cause loss of mitochondrial integrity, the leakage of cytochrome c and the activation of caspase 9 (Hengartner, 2000; Green and Leeuwenburgh, 2002). Mitochondrial dysfunction is an early indicator of doxorubicin-induced apoptosis in cardiomyocytes (Green and Leeuwenburgh, 2002). Within the extrinsic pathway, doxorubicin increases Fas and FasL, followed by the activation of caspase 8 (Nakamura et al., 2000; Kalivendi et al., 2005b). The activation of caspase 9 and/or caspase 8 eventually leads to the activation of caspase 3, cleavage of genomic DNA and apoptosis (Hengartner, 2000).

2.2.2 Doxorubicin-induced myofibril loss in cardiomyocytes

Doxorubicin selectively down-regulates cardiac specific muscle gene expressions. These may involve decreases in cardiac muscle gene transcription and translation, as well as increases in selective proteasome degradation of these proteins (Poizat et al., 2000).

Studies have shown that doxorubicin decreases the expression of α-sarcomeric actin, cardiac troponin I (cTnI), and myosin light chain 2 (MLC 2) (Ito et al., 1990). Doxorubicin treatment decreases cardiac troponins in left ventricular tissues of mice and in cultured rat neonatal cardiomyocytes (Bian et al., 2009). Down-regulations of cardiac troponins by doxorubicin are caused by decreased transcription and translation as well as increased caspase and proteasome degradation of these proteins (Bian et al., 2009). Caspase 3, 5, 6 or 10 directly cleaves cardiac troponins, while caspase 9 or 13 may indirectly cause degradation of these proteins (Bian et al., 2009).

Other reports also have shown that doxorubicin inhibits the expression of transcription factors or cofactors that are important for regulation of cardiac-specific gene transcription. These include GATA4, MEF2C, dHAND, Nkx2.5 and p300 (Poizat et al., 2000; Aries et al., 2004). In addition to cardiac genes, GATA4 may also regulate genes that are involved in the process of apoptosis. Overexpression of GATA4 in cardiomyocytes or mouse hearts attenuates doxorubicin-induced apoptosis. On the other hand, GATA4 null mice are more susceptible to doxorubicin cardiotoxicity (Aries et al., 2004).

In addition to myofibril loss, doxorubicin also induces myofibril disarray in cardiomyocytes (Sawyer et al., 2002). Degradation of titin, a myofilament protein, may contribute to this effect of doxorubicin. Titin is a scaffold protein that assembles myofilament proteins into sarcomeres. It regulates cardiomyocyte contractile function via length-dependent activation in stretched sarcomeres during the transition from diastole to systole (Helmes et al., 2003). Doxorubicin activates calcium-dependent proteases calpains which in turn cause titin degradation (Lim et al., 2004a).

2.2.3 Doxorubicin disturbs calcium homeostasis in cardiomyocytes

The sarcoplasmic reticulum Ca^{2+} pump (SERCA2a) plays a pivotal role in intracellular calcium mobilization and thus myocardial contractility. The sarcoplasmic reticulum (SR) orchestrates the movement of calcium during both contraction and relaxation of the heart. Excitation leads to the opening of voltage gated L-type calcium channels, allowing the entry of calcium, which then stimulates the release of a much larger amount of calcium from SR and subsequent contraction. During relaxation, calcium is re-sequestered into SR by SERCA2a and extruded to the extracellular fluid by the sarcolemmal sodium-calcium exchanger (NCX) (del Monte et al., 1999; Wehrens and Marks, 2004). A decrease in SR Ca^{2+} ATPase activity and Ca^{2+} uptake is responsible for the abnormal Ca^{2+} homeostasis in human cardiomyocytes from failing hearts (Schmidt et al., 1998; Schmidt et al., 1999).

Studies have shown that doxorubicin can either increase or decrease cardiomyocyte contractility. The discrepancy of these findings may be caused by different animal and cell culture models, the dosage of doxorubicin, the duration of the treatment and especially the developmental stage of the disease. In the early stage of the disease, doxorubicin tends to induce Ca^{2+} release from SR and increase cardiomyocyte contractility (Brown et al., 1989b; Kim et al., 1989; Ondrias et al., 1990; Kapelko et al., 1996). In the late stage of the disease, doxorubicin inhibits Ca^{2+} regulatory proteins and reduces cardiomyocyte contractility (Ondrias et al., 1990; Dodd et al., 1993; Maeda et al., 1998; Boucek et al., 1999; Chugun et al., 2000; Gambliel et al., 2002; Timolati et al., 2006). In a subacute doxorubicin mouse model, doxorubicin induces an increase in cardiac contractile function as measured by dP/dtmax and dP/dtmin during the first few days after the doxorubicin injection; however, cardiac function declines later on (our unpublished data). These results are consistent with the findings in doxorubicin-treated patients (Brown et al., 1989b; Barry et al., 2007a).

Doxorubicin-induced reduction of cardiomyocyte contractility is often associated with decreased expression of SERCA2a (Dodd et al., 1993; Boucek et al., 1999; Gambliel et al., 2002), suggesting that impaired SERCA2a function may contribute to doxorubicin-induced cardiomyocyte contractile dysfunction.

Studies in mice with cardiomyocyte-specific overexpression of SERCA2a, however, showed that SERCA2a overexpression exacerbated doxorubicin-induced mortality and morphological damage to cardiac tissue (Burke et al., 2003). These results may be caused by constitutive activation of SERCA2a, especially during the early stage of doxorubicin cardiac injury. Increase of SERCA2a activities at the early stage of the disease may further aggravate the adverse effects of doxorubicin on Ca^{2+} homeostasis, thereby exacerbating the disease. On the other hand, activation of SERCA2a at a later stage of the disease may be beneficial.

3. The Neuregulin1-ErbB signaling and its physiological functions in the heart

The Neuregulin1-ErbB signaling pathway is an evolutionally conserved signaling pathway. It is pivotal for the development of various organ systems including the heart. It is also important for maintaining normal physiological functions of these organs. During the past two decades, studies using genetically modified mouse models, and most recently systems biology approaches, have revealed that ErbB receptors and their ligands form a complex signaling network, which includes an input layer, signal-processing layers and an output layer. This signaling system regulates a wide range of functions of the cell. In the heart, a significant number of studies have been performed in this area.

3.1 The ErbB receptor tyrosine kinases

3.1.1 Members of the ErbB receptor family

The ErbB receptors, also known as HER receptors, are epidermal growth factor (EGF) receptor tyrosine kinases (RTKs). Worm *C. elegans* contains one ErbB receptor and one ligand (Aroian et al., 1990). In Drosophila, there are one ErbB receptor and four ligands (Freeman, 1998). In humans, there are four members of this RTK family, which include ErbB1 (also known as EGFR, HER1), ErbB2 (HER2), ErbB3 (HER3) and ErbB4 (HER4) (Citri and Yarden, 2006). There are 13 polypeptide extracellular ErbB ligands, which include Neuregulin proteins, epidermal growth factor (EGF), epiregulin, betacellulin and others (Yarden and Sliwkowski, 2001b). All ErbB ligands contain a conserved epidermal growth factor (EGF)-like domain (Yarden and Sliwkowski, 2001b; Citri and Yarden, 2006). This multilayered and various combinations of ErbB receptors and ligands suggest an apparently more sophisticated and fine-tuned NRG1-ErbB axis-dependent regulation of signal transduction and biological responses in humans.

A unique feature of the ErbB family is that there is no known ligand for the ErbB2 receptor (Klapper et al., 1999), while ErbB3 lacks intrinsic kinase activity (Guy et al., 1994). However, ErbB2 and ErbB3 can form heterodimers to generate potent cellular signals (Citri et al., 2003). The ErbB2 receptor is a preferred heterodimeric partner of the other three ErbB receptors (Graus-Porta et al., 1997). Heterodimers which contain ErbB2 have higher affinity and broader specificity for ligands.

The ErbB receptors are expressed in various types of cells, including epithelial, mesenchymal, neuronal and cardiomyocytes. The ErbB receptors play important roles in organ development and maintaining the normal physiological function of adult tissues. In cancer cells, ErbB receptors are aberrantly expressed and constitutively activated. Therefore, they are major drug targets for cancer therapy (Alimandi et al., 1995; Moasser, 2007). In the developing heart, the ErbB2 and ErbB4 receptors are detected in the cardiac myocardium and endocardium (Erickson et al., 1997; Meyer et al., 1997; Zhao et al., 1998; Fuller et al., 2008; Pentassuglia and Sawyer, 2009; De Keulenaer et al., 2010), while the ErbB3 receptor is expressed in the cardiac endocardium and mesenchyme (Erickson et al., 1997; Camenisch et al., 2002). ErbB2 and ErbB4 are expressed in adult cardiomyocytes (Zhao et al., 1998). Further more, recent studies have shown that adult cardiomyocytes also express the ErbB3 receptor (Camprecios et al., 2011).

3.1.2 The signaling network activated by the ErbB receptors

The ErbB receptors contain an extracellular ligand binding domain, a single transmembrane domain and intracellular kinase domain. Upon ligand binding, ErbB receptors form homo- or heterodimers, which trigger auto- or trans-phosphorylation on tyrosine residues of the receptors. These residues then serve as docking sites for recruiting signaling molecules from the cytosol to the cell membrane, which then activate various signaling pathways.

The dimerization of ErbB receptors induces activation of a wide range of signaling molecules. The PI3K and MAPK pathways are among the most studied. In addition, the ErbB receptors activate other pathways, such as STATs, PLCs and JNK. These molecules further regulate the activities of key transcriptional factors, such as Jun, fos and Myc, leading to the modulation of various aspects of cell function including survival, proliferation, and migration.

Systems biology studies have revealed that this signaling network is highly organized and precisely regulated by multiple layers of regulatory and control mechanisms, which include activation of specific pathways, positive and negative feedback loops and horizontal control by parallel signaling networks.

Phosphoproteomics studies have shown that each ErbB receptor has a specific and preferred binding pattern with signaling molecules (Schulze et al., 2005). The ErbB2 receptor has few binding partners, among which, Shc is the most common partner. The ErbB3 receptor has multiple binding sites for the PI3K subunit p85. ErbB1 and ErbB4 receptors show a diversity of interaction partners including STAT5 and Grb2.

Feedback loops in and outside of this network help maintain homeostasis. For example, ErbB-mediated activation of the MAPK pathway induces the transcription of TGFα and HB-EGF (Schulze et al., 2001), which in turn further activate the ErbB receptors. ErbB activation can also lead to transcription of proteins that inhibit further activation of a particular pathway. For example, ErbB1 receptor activation by EGF causes expression of the suppressor of cytokine signaling (SOCS), which in turn promotes ErbB1 degradation (Kario et al., 2005). In addition, the ErbB signaling can be regulated by G-protein coupled receptors (GPCRs). Studies have shown that thrombin and endothelin have positive effects on the ErbB signaling via activation of matrix metalloproteinases (MMPs), subsequent activation of ErbB ligands, or activation of Src or Pyk2 which phosphorylate ErbB receptors (Dikic et al., 1996; Yarden and Sliwkowski, 2001b; Negro et al., 2006).

3.2 Neuregulin1 proteins

Neuregulin1 proteins were discovered during 1992-1993 by four independent research groups. At the time, two of the groups were searching for a ligand for the oncogene ErbB2 (Holmes et al., 1992; Peles et al., 1992; Wen et al., 1992). One group was searching for a factor that stimulated the proliferation of Schwann cells (Marchionni et al., 1993), and the third was searching for a factor that stimulated the synthesis of muscle receptors for acetylcholine (Falls et al., 1993). Subsequently, it was found that all these factors were encoded by the same gene, which is the Neuregulin1 gene (Burden and Yarden, 1997). Therefore, Neuregulin1 proteins were also called Neu differentiation factor (NDF), heregulins, glial growth factor (GGF), acetylcholine receptor inducing activity (ARIA). Subsequently, three other Neuregulin genes were discovered, which are Neuregulin2, Neuregulin3 and Neuregulin4 (Carraway et al., 1997; Zhang et al., 1997; Harari et al., 1999). However, limited information is available regarding the biological functions of Neuregulin2, 3 and 4 gene encoded proteins. Neureuglin1 proteins bind directly to the ErbB3 and the ErbB4 receptors. The ErbB2 receptor does not bind directly to Neureuglin1; rather it serves as a co-receptor and forms heterodimers with the ErbB3 or the ErbB4 receptor (Falls et al., 1993; Burden and Yarden, 1997).

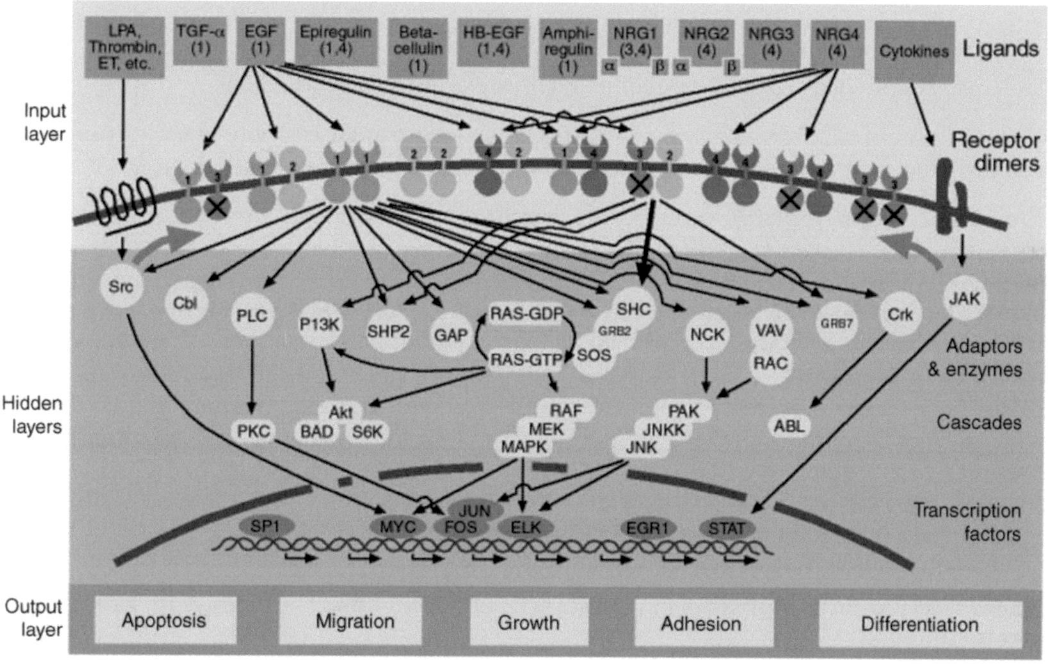

Fig. 1. The ErbB Signaling Network. ErbB receptors and their ligands form a complex signaling network which regulates a wide variety of cell functions. There are four ErbB receptors (ErbB1-ErbB4). The ErbB2 receptor does not bind to any ligand, but is a preferred partner of other ErbB receptors. The ErbB3 receptor is devoid of kinase activity. ErbB2 and ErbB3 can form functional and potent heterodimers. There are at least 13 known ligands for the ErbB receptors, including Neuregulin1 proteins. Ligand binding with the ErbB receptors activates various signaling molecules in the cell. The PI3K and MAPK pathways are among the most studied pathways. Multiple feedback loops exist within and outside of this signaling network. The activation and integration of these pathways lead to the regulation of cell survival, growth, proliferation, migration and differentiation. NRG, Neuregulin; EGF, epidermal growth factor; LPA, lysophosphatidic acid; ET, endothelin; GAP, GTPase activating protein; HB-EGF, heparin-binding EGF; Jak, Janus kinase; PKC, protein kinase C; PLC, phospholipase C; Shp2, Src homology domain-2-containing protein tyrosine phosphatase 2; Stat, signal transducer and activator of transcription. Reprinted by permission from *Nat Rev Mol Cell Biol; 2, 127-137, 2001.*

The Neuregulin1 gene is located on the short arm of the human chromosome 8 (Stefansson et al., 2002). At least 15 Neuregulin1 isoforms are produced by the Neuregulin1 gene as a result of alternative splicing and multiple promoters (Falls, 2003; Hayes and Gullick, 2008). All Neuregulin1 proteins contain the epidermal growth factor (EGF)-like domain, which binds to ligands and also is sufficient for activation of the ErbB receptors. According to the N-terminal structural differences, Neuregulin1 proteins are divided into three types (type I, II and III). Type I Neuregulin1 proteins contain an immunoglobulin (Ig)-like domain, an EGF-like domain, a proteolysis site, a hydrophobic transmembrane domain and a cytoplasmic tail. Like type I Neuregulin1, Type II Neuregulin1 isoforms contain an Ig-like domain and EGF-like domain. In addition, type II isoforms contain a signal peptide, a kringle-like sequence in their N-terminal. Type III isoforms do not have an Ig-like domain; instead, they contain a cysteine-rich domain in the N-terminal part of the protein. Therefore, Type I and II Neuregulin1 proteins are known as Ig-Neuregulin1s. The Type III Neuregulin1 proteins are known as CRD-Neuregulin1s. Other factors that differentiate

Neuregulin1 proteins are the type of EGF-like domain (α, β) and whether the isoform is initially synthesized as a transmembrane or non-membrane protein (Falls et al., 1993).

Type I and II Neuregulin1 proteins are synthesized as secreted proteins or single-pass transmembrane proteins. Proteolytic cleavage of the Ig-Neuregulin1s releases the N-terminal fragment that contains the EGF-like domain to the extracellular space, which may, in turn, bind to the ErbB receptors in a paracrine or autocrine manner. Studies have shown that metalloproteases, such as ADAM17 and ADAM19, are capable of mediating the shedding of Neuregulin1 proteins from cells (Kuramochi et al., 2004; Kalinowski et al., 2010). Type III Neuregulin1 proteins are synthesized as two-pass transmembrane proteins, with a transmembrane domain located at the C-terminal of the EGF domain and a transmembrane domain within the CRD-domain. Cleavage of the type III Neuregulin1 proteins exposes the EGF-like domain of the protein, which may interact with ErbB receptors in a juxtacrine mechanism (Falls et al., 1993).

3.3 Neuregulin-ErbB signaling in developing and adult hearts: Findings in transgenic mouse models

The physiological function of Neuregulin1 proteins and their ErbB receptors have been intensively studied during the past two decades, mainly in transgenic mouse models, as well as in mice treated with recombinant Neuregulin1s and in cell culture. Neuregulin1 proteins are localized in the cardiac endocardium and the endothelium of the cardiac microvasculature (Meyer and Birchmeier, 1995; Lemmens et al., 2006). The ErbB2 and ErbB4 receptors are expressed in cardiac myocardium (Gassmann et al., 1995; Lee et al., 1995) and ErbB3 proteins are expressed in endocardial cushion mesenchyme (Erickson et al., 1997). Neuregulin1s activate ErbB receptors in a paracrine manner (Marchionni, 1995). Studies have demonstrated that Neureuglin-ErbB signaling is essential for cardiac development in embryos and pivotal for protecting adult hearts from stress.

3.3.1 Transgenic mouse models with mutations of the Neuregulin1 gene

Several transgenic mouse models are generated with deletion/disruption of the EGF-like domain, Ig-like domain or the cytoplasmic tail of the Neureuglin1 proteins (Meyer and Birchmeier, 1995; Kramer et al., 1996b; Liu et al., 1998a).

A common phenotype of these transgenic mice is that all homozygous mice die around E10.5 during embryogenesis with the absence or underdevelopment of ventricular trabeculae. EGF-like domain disruption also causes cardiac endocardial cushion defects (Meyer and Birchmeier, 1995). Hearts around E10.5 display depressed contractility, dilatation of the common ventricle, decreased emptying of the ventricle and slow irregular heart rate (Kramer et al., 1996a; Liu et al., 1998b).

In mice with EGF-like domain disruption, the activity of all Neureuglin1s is abolished; while in mice with Ig-like domain deletion, Type III Neuregulin1s are still functional; in mice with cytoplasmic tail disruption, secretive Neuregulin1 proteins are not affected. The Ig-like domain interacts with the extracellular matrix (Kramer et al., 1996a), while the cytoplasmic tail regulates the proteolytic release of the Neuregulin1 extracellular domains (Liu et al., 1998b). Therefore, these studies suggest that Ig-like Neuregulin1s and the release of membrane anchored Neuregulin1s are necessary for cardiac trabeculae formation. They also suggest that Type III Neuregulin1s may not be pivotal for cardiac development. In mice with CRD-Neureuglin1 knockout, no cardiac defects were reported (Wolpowitz et al., 2000).

Recently, Hedhli and colleagues tested whether endothelial-derived Neuregulin1s are important for protecting the heart from ischemia-reperfusion injury (Hedhli et al., 2011). They generated mice with tamoxifen-inducible and endothelium-selective Neuregulin1 gene knockout by cross-breeding mice with VE-cadherin promoter driven Cre-ER (Monvoisin et al., 2006) and mice carrying homozygously floxed alleles of the Neuregulin1 gene (Yang et al., 2001). At the baseline, hearts from these knockout mice showed normal wall thickness, left ventricular chamber size, and systolic function. Cardiac morphology, including capillary density was not different from non-transgenic mice. However, after ischemia-reperfusion, the infarct area, the number of TUNEL positive cells, and the number of infiltrating leukocytes were significantly increased in knockout mice compared with controls. The activation of ErbB4 receptors was decreased in ischemia-reperfusion treated knockout mouse hearts. In addition, injection of a recombinant Neuregulin1 (EGF-like domain) reversed the adverse effects observed in the knockout mice. These results suggested that loss of endothelium-derived Neuregulin1 was the cause of worsening ischemia-reperfusion cardiac injury. This study has identified that Neuregulin1 is one of the protective factors derived from the cardiac endothelium.

3.3.2 Transgenic mouse models with mutations of the ErbB receptors

To understand the physiological roles of the ErbB receptors, transgenic mice with deletion of the ErbB2, ErbB3 or ErbB4 gene were generated (Gassmann et al., 1995; Lee et al., 1995; Erickson et al., 1997; Crone et al., 2002; Ozcelik et al., 2002). Deletion of the ErbB2 or the ErbB4 gene caused a similar cardiac phenotype as that observed in pan-Neuregulin1 knockout mice, which was the underdevelopment of cardiac ventricular trabeculae (Gassmann et al., 1995; Lee et al., 1995; Meyer and Birchmeier, 1995). ErbB2 or ErbB4 knockout mice died around E10.5 due to cardiac defects. Cardiac specific overexpression of the ErbB2 receptor in ErbB2 knockout mice restored normal ventricular trabeculation (Morris et al., 1999). These data suggest that the effects of Neuregulin1 proteins on cardiac development depend on both ErbB2 and ErbB4 receptors. They also suggest that ErbB2 and ErbB4 heterodimers are needed for propagating Neuregulin1 signals in the developing hearts. In mice with the ErbB3 gene knockout, however, the defect of ventricular trabeculation was not observed. Instead, cardiac cushions lacked mesenchyme and cardiac valves were underdeveloped (Erickson et al., 1997). These findings are consistent with the expression pattern of the ErbB3 receptor in the heart.

The studies in mice with ErbB2 cardiac-specific conditional knockout provided further information on the ErbB2 receptor in the adult heart (Crone et al., 2002; Ozcelik et al., 2002). Two independent groups generated these mice by crossbreeding animals carrying the Cre-coding sequence (driven by myosin light chain 2v MLC2v or muscle creatine kinase promoter) and those with the loxP-flanked ErbB2 gene. Loss of the ErbB2 expression was observed perinatally in 50-60% of cardiomyocytes. Cardiac function was initially normal but progressively worsened. At the age of 3 months, these mice developed dilated cardiomyopathy with enlarged ventricular chambers, increase in the heart to body weight ratio and increase in atrial natriuretic factor and skeletal α-actin expression. Electron microscopy showed increased numbers of mitochondria and vacuoles in cardiomyocytes. Apoptosis as measured by TUNEL staining was increased in ErbB2 conditional knockout mice. Aortic stenosis caused more severe cardiac dysfunction in mutant mice. In addition, cardiomyocytes isolated from these mice were more susceptible to doxorubicin. Collectively, these data demonstrate that the ErbB2 receptor is essential for maintaining normal cardiac physiological function and morphology.

Mouse models		Cardiac phenotype	References
Neuregulin1 knockout (NRG1 KO)	EGF-like domain (pan NRG1 KO)	Homozygous die around E10.5 Absence of ventricular trabeculae; defect of endocardial cushion. Heart failure	(Meyer and Birchmeier, 1995)
	Ig-like domain (Type I and II NRG1 KO)	Homozygous die around E10.5 Lack ventricular trabeculae. Heart failure	(Kramer et al., 1996b)
	Cytoplasmic tail (Type I NRG1 KO)	Homozygous die around E10.5 Lack ventricular trabeculae. Heart failure	(Liu et al., 1998a)
	Endothelial specific conditional NRG1 KO	Normal cardiac function at baseline. Increased infarct area and apoptosis after ischemia-reperfusion	(Hedhli et al., 2011)
ErbB2 KO	Constitutive ErbB2 KO	Homozygous die around E10.5. Defect of ventricular trabeculae	(Lee et al., 1995)
	Cardiomyocyte-specific conditional KO	Survived to adulthood. Mice progressively developed dilated cardiomyopathy at the age of 3-6 months.	(Crone et al., 2002; Ozcelik et al., 2002)
ErbB4 KO		Homozygous die around E10.5. Defect of ventricular trabeculae	(Gassmann et al., 1995)
ErbB3 KO		Homozygous die around E13.5. Defect of cardiac cushions and valves.	(Erickson et al., 1997)

Table 1. Cardiac phenotypes in transgenic mouse models with disruption of the Neuregulin1 gene or the ErbB receptor genes

4. Neuregulin1-ErbB signaling protects the heart from doxorubicin cardiotoxicity

Studies in animal models show that Neuregulin1 injections alleviate doxorubicin-induced cardiac dysfunction in mice. Further, studies show that the Neuregulin1-ErbB signaling protects the heart from doxorubicin cardiotoxicity via several mechanisms which include inhibition of doxorubicin-induced apoptosis, loss of mitochondrial integrity, loss of myofibrils, and impaired calcium homeostasis.

4.1 Neuregulin1 protects the heart from doxorubicin-induced cardiac dysfunction: Studies in animal models

Studies from our laboratory show that doxorubicin induces a worsened cardiac dysfunction in Neuregulin1 knockout mice (Liu et al., 2005). We used heterozygous mice with Neuregulin1 EGF-like domain deletion (Meyer and Birchmeier, 1995). The RNA expression of Neuregulin1α and β isoforms was decreased in the hearts of knockout mice (unpublished data). These mice were fertile and no abnormalities were found in cardiac function and morphology at the baseline. When mice were injected with doxorubicin (20 mg/kg, i.p. once), however, survival was decreased in doxorubicin-treated knockout mice compared to wild type mice (two week survival: 13 vs. 33 %). Cardiac function as assessed by echocardiography and left ventricular catheterization showed worsened cardiac systolic function in doxorubicin-treated knockout mice. We further showed that the activation of ErbB2 and downstream signaling molecules Akt, mTOR and MAPK in the heart was more depressed in doxorubicin-treated knockout mice vs. wild type mice. These results suggest that Neuregulin1 is necessary for protecting the heart from doxorubicin.

Our laboratory and Liu et al. further demonstrated that injections of recombinant human Neuregulin1 proteins improve cardiac function in doxorubicin-treated animals (Liu et al., 2005; Liu et al., 2006; Bian et al., 2009). Comparing the two studies, we used recombinant human glial growth factor 2 (GGF2), and a subacute doxorubicin cardiotoxicity mouse model (doxorubicin, 20 mg/kg, i.p. once). GGF2 was injected subcutanously daily using the dosage of 0.75 mg/kg/day (Bian et al., 2009); while Liu et al. used a recombinant EGF-like domain (β_{2a} isoform) of Neuregulin1 proteins, and a chronic doxorubicin rat model (3.3 mg/kg/week, i.v. for 4 weeks). Recombinant Neuregulin1 was injected i.v. daily for the first 7 days using the dosage of 20μg/kg/day (Liu et al., 2006). Despite the different isoforms of Neuregulin1, the dosage, the route of drug administration and the animal models used, both studies showed that injections of recombinant Neuregulin1 significantly improved survival and cardiac systolic function in doxorubicin-injured mice and rats. These studies demonstrate that Neureuglin1 injections can protect the heart from doxorubicin-induced heart failure.

4.2 Neuregulin1-ErbB signaling inhibits doxorubicin-induced cardiomyocyte apoptosis

The anti-apoptotic effects of the Neureuglin1-ErbB signaling pathway activation were assessed in doxorubicin-treated neonatal rat cardiomyocytes and adult rat cardiomyocytes in culture, in Neuregulin1 EGF-like domain knockout mice and in ErbB2 conditional knockout mice.

In cultured neonatal rat cardiomyocytes, Fukazawa et al showed that daunorubicin (anthracycline drug) significantly increased apoptosis as assessed by three different methods which were TUNEL staining, flow cytometric quantification of subG1 cell fraction and caspase3 activation. Co-incubation of recombinant Neuregulin1 (GGF2) with daunorubicin significantly reduced apoptosis. This effect of Neuregulin1 was associated with the activation of Akt. Adenoviral infection of a dominant negative Akt abolished this effect of Neuregulin1, suggesting Akt is necessary for neuregulin1's anti-apoptotic effects. In addition, activation of Akt by neuregulin1 was abolished by the ErbB4, but not ErbB2, inhibitor. Together, these observations suggest that Neuregulin1 protects cardiomyocytes from daunorubicin-induced apoptosis via activations of ErbB4 and Akt (Fukazawa et al., 2003). Another study by Rohrbach et al. also showed that Neuregulin1 inhibited daunorubicin-induced cytochrome c release, and caspase3 activation. In addition, Neuregulin1 inhibited daunorubicin-induced increase in the ratio of pro-apoptotic protein Bcl-xS to anti-apoptotic protein Bcl-xL (Rohrbach et al., 2005a).

In doxorubicin-treated mice, we observed increases of caspase3, 6, 9 and caspase8 activations in the heart, suggesting both intrinsic and extrinsic apoptosis pathways were activated in these hearts. Concomitant Neureuglin1 injections significantly reduced the activations of these caspases (Bian et al., 2009). However, decreased activation of the Neuregulin-ErbB signaling does not further increase anthracycline drug doxorubicin or daunorubicin-induced apoptosis as measured by TUNEL staining. In mice with heterozygous knockout of the Neuregulin1 EGF-like domain, the number of TUNEL-positive cardiomyocytes was increased in doxorubicin-treated mouse hearts; however, there were no significant differences between doxorubicin-treated wild type and knockout mice (Liu et al., 2005). Similarly, in neonatal and adult rat cardiomyocytes, neither the anti-ErbB2 antibody nor the ErbB2 inhibitor further increased doxorubicin or daunorubicin-induced TUNEL staining (Fukazawa et al., 2003; Pentassuglia et al., 2009). These results, however, may be caused by the TUNEL staining method, which is relatively insensitive. In ErbB2 conditional knockout mouse hearts, very low levels of apoptotic cells was detected by TUNEL assay, while a more sensitive ligation-mediated PCR DNA fragmentation assay was able to detect the increase of apoptotic cells in ErbB2 knockout hearts (Crone et al., 2002).

Studies have also demonstrated that ErbB2 inhibition itself can induce mitochondrial dysfunction and increase apoptotic signals in cardiomyocytes as well as in adult hearts (Crone et al., 2002; Grazette et al., 2004). In cultured neonatal and adult rat cardiomyocytes, anti-ErbB2 antibody increased the ratio of Bcl-xS/Bcl-xL, translocation of BAX to mitochondria, cytochrome c release and caspase activation. These changes caused a loss of mitochondrial membrane potential and a decrease of ATP levels. Restoration of Bcl-xL levels prevented mitochondrial dysfunction (Grazette et al., 2004). In ErbB2 conditional knockout mice, apoptosis was increased in the heart. *In vivo* expression of the anti-apoptotic gene Bcl-xL partially reduced chamber dilation and restored contractility in the ErbB2 knockout mice. Cardiomyocytes isolated from the ErbB2 knockout mice were more sensitive to doxorubicin-induced cell death (Crone et al., 2002).

4.3 Neuregulin1-ErbB signaling prevents doxorubicin-induced cardiac myofibrillar disarray and loss

One of the pathological features of doxorubicin-induced cardiotoxicity is myofibril loss and disarray in cardiomyocytes. In adult rat cardiomyocytes, doxorubicin treatment resulted in myofilament disarray (Sawyer et al., 2002; Pentassuglia et al., 2009). Simultaneous treatments with doxorubicin and an anti-ErbB2 antibody, or a dual inhibitor that targets both ErbB2 and ErbB1, caused an additive effect on myofibril damage. Conversely, recombinant Neuregulin1 reduced this effect of doxorubicin. Neuregulin1 activated both PI3K and MAPK pathways in cardiomyocytes. Inhibition of ErbB2 prevented activations of these pathways by Neuregulin1. In addition, inhibition of MAPK, but not PI3K, induced myofrilament damage in adult rat cardiomyocytes similar to that observed in ErbB2 antibody or inhibitor treated cardiomyocytes (Pentassuglia et al., 2009). These results suggest that Neuregulin1 may prevent myofibril damage by activating ErbB2 and MAPK.

In addition to preventing doxorubicin-induced myofibrillar disarray, the Neuregulin1-ErbB signaling also reduces doxorubicin-induced loss of cardiac troponin proteins (Bian et al., 2009). In doxorubicin-treated mouse hearts, cardiac troponin proteins (cTnI, cTnT and cTnC) were down-regulated. These were associated with a moderate increase in serum cTnI, but not cTnT, suggesting mechanisms other than releasing troponin proteins to serum may exist. Concurrent Neuregulin1 injections significantly prevented doxorubicin-induced loss of cardiac troponin proteins in the heart.

These phenotypes were again observed in cultured neonatal rat cardiomyocytes. Neuregulin1 co-treatment prevented doxorubicin-induced down-regulation of cTnI and cTnT proteins in cultured cardiomyocytes. These effects of Neuregulin1 were abolished by ErbB2, but not ErbB4, inhibition. These effects were also prevented by PI3K, Akt and mTOR inhibitors (Bian et al., 2009).

Further studies showed that doxorubicin reduced RNA expression of cTnI and cTnT in cardiomyocytes, while Neuregulin1 treatment reversed these effects of doxorubicin. The effect of Neuregulin1 on maintaining cTnI and cTnT proteins in doxorubicin-treated cardiomyocytes was reduced by cycloheximide (Bian et al., 2009). These results suggest that Neuregulin1 may maintain cTnI and cTnT levels by increasing transcription and translation of these proteins.

Neuregulin1 may also maintain cardiac troponins by decreasing doxorubicin-induced degradation of these proteins. Doxorubicin-activated caspases directly degraded cTnT. Doxorubicin also increased ubiquitination of cTnI. Neuregulin1 inhibited these effects of doxorubicin (Bian et al., 2009).

Results from Neuregulin1 treated normal cardiomyocytes provided clues on how it may protect cardiomyocytes from stresses, such as doxorubicin. In cultured adult rat cardiomyocytes, Neuregulin1 induced lamellipodia formation and elongation of cardiomyocytes, which restored the cell-to-cell contact of cultured cardiomyocytes. This was associated with Neuregulin1 activation of focal adhesion kinase (FAK) and formation of a complex which includes ErbB2, FAK, $p130^{CAS}$ and paxillin. FAK is pivotal for formation of the focal adhesion complex, cell spreading and motility. Neuregulin1-induced activation of FAK was inhibited by an anti-ErbB2 antibody.

In cultured adult rat cardiomyocytes, Neuregulin1 also increased the phosphorylation of GATA4, a transcriptional factor that regulates genes encoding cardiac sarcomeric proteins and important for cardiac development. Inhibition of the ErbB2 receptor or the MAPK pathway prevented phosphorylation of GATA4 by Neuregulin1. Further studies are needed to demonstrate whether these mechanisms are involved in the cardioprotective effects of Neuregulin1 in doxorubicin-injured cardiomyocytes or hearts.

4.4 Neuregulin1-ErbB signaling maintains calcium homeostasis in doxorubicin-treated cardiomyocytes

Doxorubicin disturbs calcium homeostasis and contractile function of the heart. In the acute phase, doxorubicin increases cardiac systolic and diastolic functions; while in the later stage, it causes heart failure in patients (Brown et al., 1989a).

Timolati et al. established a model in cultured cardiomyocytes which mimics this change (Timolati et al., 2006). When adult rat cardiomyocytes were treated with 1μM doxorubicin for 18 hours, cardiomyocytes calcium amplitude and fractional shortening were significantly increased. Intracellular diastolic calcium and time to 50% relaxation were modestly increased, suggesting increased cardiomyocyte systolic function in these cardiomyocytes. On the other hand, treatment of cardiomyocytes with 10μM doxorubicin for 18 hours caused significant decreases in calcium amplitude and fractional shortening as well as increases in intracellular diastolic calcium and time to 50% relaxation, suggesting systolic and diastolic function were decreased in these cardiomyocytes. In addition, doxorubicin (10μM) induced a down-regulation of SERCA proteins and SR calcium content.

Neuregulin1 treatment 3 hours prior to doxorubicin attenuated doxorubicin-induced alterations of contractility in cardiomyocytes (Timolati et al., 2006). Neuregulin1 decreased calcium amplitude and fractional shortening in 1μM doxorubicin-treated cardiomyocytes while increased these indices in 10μM doxorubicin-treated cells. Neuregulin1 also normalized the diastolic calcium and time to 50% relaxation in both 1 and 10μM doxorubicin-treated cardiomyocytes. In addition, Neuregulin1 increased SERCA proteins in 10μM doxorubicin-treated cardiomyocytes.

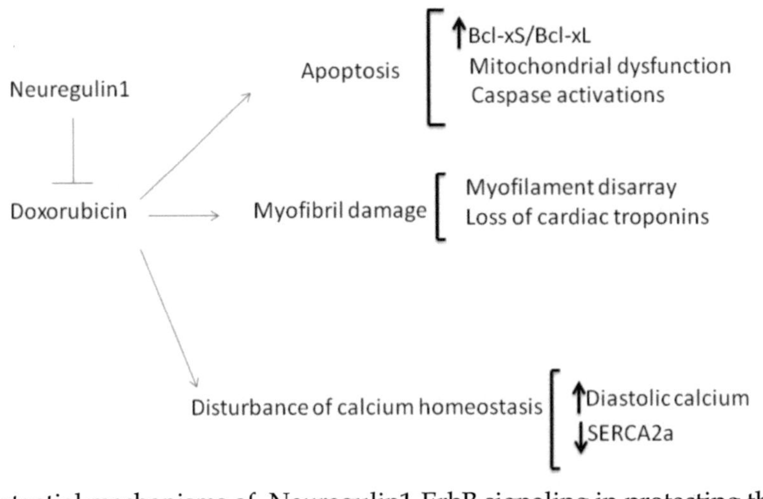

Fig. 2. The potential mechanisms of Neuregulin1-ErbB signaling in protecting the heart from doxorubicin-induced cardiotoxicity. The Neuregulin1-ErbB signaling protects cardiomyocytes from doxorubicin-induced apoptosis which include mitochondrial dysfunction, caspase activation and increase in the Bcl-xS/Bcl-xL ratio, myofibril damage which includes myofilament disarray and loss of cardiac troponins, and disturbance of calcium homeostasis which includes the increase of intracellular diastolic calcium and the decrease of SERCA2a.

In another study, Pentassuglia et al. showed that ErbB2 receptor inhibition aggravated doxorubicin-induced decrease in cardiomyocyte fractional shortening (Pentassuglia et al., 2009).

Taken together, these studies demonstrated that Neuregulin1-ErbB signaling is pivotal for inhibiting doxorubicin-induced mitochondrial dysfunction, apoptosis, myofibril disarray and loss, as well as disturbance of calcium homeostasis in the heart. They have provided mechanisms of Neuregulin1's protective effects in doxorubicin-injured hearts, as well as Trastuzumab-induced cardiotoxicity (Figure 2).

5. Conclusions

Doxorubicin-induced cardiotoxicity is a severe side effect of, and therefore, a major clinical obstacle to, cancer therapy by using this drug. The discovery of the cardiac protective role of the Neuregulin1-ErbB signaling pathway in doxorubicin-injured hearts has opened a new area for developing methods to prevent or cure doxorubicin-induced heart failure. The Neuregulin-ErbB signaling is an evolutionally conserved signaling pathway which plays critical roles in the development of multiple organ systems, including the heart. In addition to the cardiac protective effects in heart failure, this signaling pathway is one of the most mutated pathways in cancer. Understanding how this pathway protects the heart from doxorubicin injury is a first and necessary step towards using Neuregulin1 and potentially other ErbB ligands in cancer survivors.

During the past 10 years, the cardioprotective effects of the Neuregulin-ErbB signaling have been tested in other cardiovascular diseases. Studies have demonstrated that in addition to doxorubicin-induced heart failure, Neuregulin1 also improves cardiac function in ischemia-reperfusion, viral infection, and pacing induced heart failure (Liu et al., 2006; Bersell et al., 2009; Hedhli et al., 2011). In addition, Neuregulin1 promotes cell cycle reentry of differentiated adult cardiomyocytes, improves angiogenesis in the heart (Bersell et al., 2009; Hedhli et al., 2011), and promotes embryonic stem cell differentiation into the cardiac lineage (Sun et al., 2011). Clinical trials are ongoing using Neureuglin1 for the treatment of heart failure in patients (Gao et al., 2010). It is conceivable that Neuregulin1 may become a new drug for heart failure, including doxorubicin-induced cardiotoxicity.

6. Acknowledgements

This work is supported by NASA (Goukassian, NNX11AD22G) and American Heart Association Grant-In-Aid (Yan, 10GRNT4710003).

7. References

Alimandi, M., Romano, A., Curia, M. C., Muraro, R., Fedi, P., Aaronson, S. A., Di Fiore, P. P. and Kraus, M. H. (1995) 'Cooperative signaling of ErbB3 and ErbB2 in neoplastic transformation and human mammary carcinomas', *Oncogene* 10(9): 1813-21.

Anderson, B. and Sawyer, D. B. (2008) 'Predicting and preventing the cardiotoxicity of cancer therapy', *Expert Rev Cardiovasc Ther* 6(7): 1023-33.

Appelbaum, F., Strauchen, J. A., Graw, R. G., Jr., Savage, D. D., Kent, K. M., Ferrans, V. J. and Herzig, G. P. (1976) 'Acute lethal carditis caused by high-dose combination chemotherapy. A unique clinical and pathological entity', *Lancet* 1(7950): 58-62.

Aries, A., Paradis, P., Lefebvre, C., Schwartz, R. J. and Nemer, M. (2004) 'Essential role of GATA-4 in cell survival and drug-induced cardiotoxicity', *Proc Natl Acad Sci U S A* 101(18): 6975-80.

Aroian, R. V., Koga, M., Mendel, J. E., Ohshima, Y. and Sternberg, P. W. (1990) 'The let-23 gene necessary for Caenorhabditis elegans vulval induction encodes a tyrosine kinase of the EGF receptor subfamily', *Nature* 348(6303): 693-9.

Barry, E., Alvarez, J. A., Scully, R. E., Miller, T. L. and Lipshultz, S. E. (2007a) 'Anthracycline-induced cardiotoxicity: course, pathophysiology, prevention and management', *Expert Opin Pharmacother* 8(8): 1039-58.

Barry, E., Alvarez, J. A., Scully, R. E., Miller, T. L. and Lipshultz, S. E. (2007b) 'Anthracycline-induced cardiotoxicity: course, pathophysiology, prevention and management', *Expert opinion on pharmacotherapy* 8(8): 1039-58.

Bersell, K., Arab, S., Haring, B. and Kuhn, B. (2009) 'Neuregulin1/ErbB4 signaling induces cardiomyocyte proliferation and repair of heart injury', *Cell* 138(2): 257-70.

Berthiaume, J. M. and Wallace, K. B. (2007) 'Adriamycin-induced oxidative mitochondrial cardiotoxicity', *Cell biology and toxicology* 23(1): 15-25.

Bian, Y., Sun, M., Silver, M., Ho, K. K., Marchionni, M. A., Caggiano, A. O., Stone, J. R., Amende, I., Hampton, T. G., Morgan, J. P. et al. (2009) 'Neuregulin-1 attenuated doxorubicin-induced decrease in cardiac troponins', *Am J Physiol Heart Circ Physiol* 297(6): H1974-83.

Billingham, M. E., Mason, J. W., Bristow, M. R. and Daniels, J. R. (1978) 'Anthracycline cardiomyopathy monitored by morphologic changes', *Cancer Treat Rep* 62(6): 865-72.

Boucek, R. J., Jr., Miracle, A., Anderson, M., Engelman, R., Atkinson, J. and Dodd, D. A. (1999) 'Persistent effects of doxorubicin on cardiac gene expression', *J Mol Cell Cardiol* 31(8): 1435-46.

Brown, K. A., Blow, A. J., Weiss, R. M. and Stewart, J. A. (1989a) 'Acute effects of doxorubicin on human left ventricular systolic and diastolic function', *American heart journal* 118(5 Pt 1): 979-82.

Brown, K. A., Blow, A. J., Weiss, R. M. and Stewart, J. A. (1989b) 'Acute effects of doxorubicin on human left ventricular systolic and diastolic function', *Am Heart J* 118(5 Pt 1): 979-82.

Bryant, J., Picot, J., Baxter, L., Levitt, G., Sullivan, I. and Clegg, A. (2007) 'Use of cardiac markers to assess the toxic effects of anthracyclines given to children with cancer: a systematic review', *Eur J Cancer* 43(13): 1959-66.

Burden, S. and Yarden, Y. (1997) 'Neuregulins and their receptors: a versatile signaling module in organogenesis and oncogenesis', *Neuron* 18(6): 847-55.

Burke, B. E., Olson, R. D., Cusack, B. J., Gambliel, H. A. and Dillmann, W. H. (2003) 'Anthracycline cardiotoxicity in transgenic mice overexpressing SR Ca2+-ATPase', *Biochem Biophys Res Commun* 303(2): 504-7.

Camenisch, T. D., Schroeder, J. A., Bradley, J., Klewer, S. E. and McDonald, J. A. (2002) 'Heart-valve mesenchyme formation is dependent on hyaluronan-augmented activation of ErbB2-ErbB3 receptors', *Nat Med* 8(8): 850-5.

Camprecios, G., Lorita, J., Pardina, E., Peinado-Onsurbe, J., Soley, M. and Ramirez, I. (2011) 'Expression, localization, and regulation of the neuregulin receptor ErbB3 in mouse heart', *J Cell Physiol* 226(2): 450-5.

Carraway, K. L., 3rd, Weber, J. L., Unger, M. J., Ledesma, J., Yu, N., Gassmann, M. and Lai, C. (1997) 'Neuregulin-2, a new ligand of ErbB3/ErbB4-receptor tyrosine kinases', *Nature* 387(6632): 512-6.

Childs, A. C., Phaneuf, S. L., Dirks, A. J., Phillips, T. and Leeuwenburgh, C. (2002a) 'Doxorubicin treatment in vivo causes cytochrome C release and cardiomyocyte apoptosis, as well as increased mitochondrial efficiency, superoxide dismutase activity, and Bcl-2:Bax ratio', *Cancer research* 62(16): 4592-8.

Childs, A. C., Phaneuf, S. L., Dirks, A. J., Phillips, T. and Leeuwenburgh, C. (2002b) 'Doxorubicin treatment in vivo causes cytochrome C release and cardiomyocyte apoptosis, as well as increased mitochondrial efficiency, superoxide dismutase activity, and Bcl-2:Bax ratio', *Cancer Res* 62(16): 4592-8.

Chugun, A., Temma, K., Oyamada, T., Suzuki, N., Kamiya, Y., Hara, Y., Sasaki, T., Kondo, H. and Akera, T. (2000) 'Doxorubicin-induced late cardiotoxicity: delayed impairment of Ca2+-handling mechanisms in the sarcoplasmic reticulum in the rat', *Can J Physiol Pharmacol* 78(4): 329-38.

Citri, A., Skaria, K. B. and Yarden, Y. (2003) 'The deaf and the dumb: the biology of ErbB-2 and ErbB-3', *Experimental cell research* 284(1): 54-65.

Citri, A. and Yarden, Y. (2006) 'EGF-ERBB signalling: towards the systems level', *Nature reviews. Molecular cell biology* 7(7): 505-16.

Crone, S. A., Zhao, Y. Y., Fan, L., Gu, Y., Minamisawa, S., Liu, Y., Peterson, K. L., Chen, J., Kahn, R., Condorelli, G. et al. (2002) 'ErbB2 is essential in the prevention of dilated cardiomyopathy', *Nat Med* 8(5): 459-65.

Curry, H. L., Parkes, S. E., Powell, J. E. and Mann, J. R. (2006) 'Caring for survivors of childhood cancers: the size of the problem', *Eur J Cancer* 42(4): 501-8.

d'Anglemont de Tassigny, A., Souktani, R., Henry, P., Ghaleh, B. and Berdeaux, A. (2004) 'Volume-sensitive chloride channels (ICl,vol) mediate doxorubicin-induced apoptosis through apoptotic volume decrease in cardiomyocytes', *Fundam Clin Pharmacol* 18(5): 531-8.

De Beer, E. L., Bottone, A. E. and Voest, E. E. (2001) 'Doxorubicin and mechanical performance of cardiac trabeculae after acute and chronic treatment: a review', *Eur J Pharmacol* 415(1): 1-11.

De Keulenaer, G. W., Doggen, K. and Lemmens, K. (2010) 'The vulnerability of the heart as a pluricellular paracrine organ: lessons from unexpected triggers of heart failure in targeted ErbB2 anticancer therapy', *Circ Res* 106(1): 35-46.

del Monte, F., Harding, S. E., Schmidt, U., Matsui, T., Kang, Z. B., Dec, G. W., Gwathmey, J. K., Rosenzweig, A. and Hajjar, R. J. (1999) 'Restoration of contractile function in isolated cardiomyocytes from failing human hearts by gene transfer of SERCA2a', *Circulation* 100(23): 2308-11.

Dikic, I., Tokiwa, G., Lev, S., Courtneidge, S. A. and Schlessinger, J. (1996) 'A role for Pyk2 and Src in linking G-protein-coupled receptors with MAP kinase activation', *Nature* 383(6600): 547-50.

Dodd, D. A., Atkinson, J. B., Olson, R. D., Buck, S., Cusack, B. J., Fleischer, S. and Boucek, R. J., Jr. (1993) 'Doxorubicin cardiomyopathy is associated with a decrease in calcium release channel of the sarcoplasmic reticulum in a chronic rabbit model', *J Clin Invest* 91(4): 1697-705.

Erickson, S. L., O'Shea, K. S., Ghaboosi, N., Loverro, L., Frantz, G., Bauer, M., Lu, L. H. and Moore, M. W. (1997) 'ErbB3 is required for normal cerebellar and cardiac development: a comparison with ErbB2-and heregulin-deficient mice', *Development* 124(24): 4999-5011.

Ewer, M. S. and Lippman, S. M. (2005) 'Type II chemotherapy-related cardiac dysfunction: time to recognize a new entity', *J Clin Oncol* 23(13): 2900-2.

Falls, D. L. (2003) 'Neuregulins: functions, forms, and signaling strategies', *Exp Cell Res* 284(1): 14-30.

Falls, D. L., Rosen, K. M., Corfas, G., Lane, W. S. and Fischbach, G. D. (1993) 'ARIA, a protein that stimulates acetylcholine receptor synthesis, is a member of the neu ligand family', *Cell* 72(5): 801-15.

Freeman, M. (1998) 'Complexity of EGF receptor signalling revealed in Drosophila', *Current opinion in genetics & development* 8(4): 407-11.

Fu, P. and Arcasoy, M. O. (2007) 'Erythropoietin protects cardiac myocytes against anthracycline-induced apoptosis', *Biochemical and biophysical research communications* 354(2): 372-8.

Fukazawa, R., Miller, T. A., Kuramochi, Y., Frantz, S., Kim, Y. D., Marchionni, M. A., Kelly, R. A. and Sawyer, D. B. (2003) 'Neuregulin-1 protects ventricular myocytes from anthracycline-induced apoptosis via erbB4-dependent activation of PI3-kinase/Akt', *Journal of molecular and cellular cardiology* 35(12): 1473-9.

Fuller, S. J., Sivarajah, K. and Sugden, P. H. (2008) 'ErbB receptors, their ligands, and the consequences of their activation and inhibition in the myocardium', *Journal of molecular and cellular cardiology* 44(5): 831-54.

Gambliel, H. A., Burke, B. E., Cusack, B. J., Walsh, G. M., Zhang, Y. L., Mushlin, P. S. and Olson, R. D. (2002) 'Doxorubicin and C-13 deoxydoxorubicin effects on ryanodine receptor gene expression', *Biochem Biophys Res Commun* 291(3): 433-8.

Gao, R., Zhang, J., Cheng, L., Wu, X., Dong, W., Yang, X., Li, T., Liu, X., Xu, Y., Li, X. et al. (2010) 'A Phase II, randomized, double-blind, multicenter, based on standard therapy, placebo-controlled study of the efficacy and safety of recombinant human neuregulin-1 in patients with chronic heart failure', *Journal of the American College of Cardiology* 55(18): 1907-14.

Gassmann, M., Casagranda, F., Orioli, D., Simon, H., Lai, C., Klein, R. and Lemke, G. (1995) 'Aberrant neural and cardiac development in mice lacking the ErbB4 neuregulin receptor', *Nature* 378(6555): 390-4.

Graus-Porta, D., Beerli, R. R., Daly, J. M. and Hynes, N. E. (1997) 'ErbB-2, the preferred heterodimerization partner of all ErbB receptors, is a mediator of lateral signaling', *The EMBO journal* 16(7): 1647-55.

Grazette, L. P., Boecker, W., Matsui, T., Semigran, M., Force, T. L., Hajjar, R. J. and Rosenzweig, A. (2004) 'Inhibition of ErbB2 causes mitochondrial dysfunction in cardiomyocytes: implications for herceptin-induced cardiomyopathy', *J Am Coll Cardiol* 44(11): 2231-8.

Green, P. S. and Leeuwenburgh, C. (2002) 'Mitochondrial dysfunction is an early indicator of doxorubicin-induced apoptosis', *Biochim Biophys Acta* 1588(1): 94-101.

Guy, P. M., Platko, J. V., Cantley, L. C., Cerione, R. A. and Carraway, K. L., 3rd (1994) 'Insect cell-expressed p180erbB3 possesses an impaired tyrosine kinase activity', *Proceedings of the National Academy of Sciences of the United States of America* 91(17): 8132-6.

Harari, D., Tzahar, E., Romano, J., Shelly, M., Pierce, J. H., Andrews, G. C. and Yarden, Y. (1999) 'Neuregulin-4: a novel growth factor that acts through the ErbB-4 receptor tyrosine kinase', *Oncogene* 18(17): 2681-9.

Hayes, N. V. and Gullick, W. J. (2008) 'The neuregulin family of genes and their multiple splice variants in breast cancer', *J Mammary Gland Biol Neoplasia* 13(2): 205-14.

Hedhli, N., Huang, Q., Kalinowski, A., Palmeri, M., Hu, X., Russell, R. R. and Russell, K. S. (2011) 'Endothelium-derived neuregulin protects the heart against ischemic injury', *Circulation* 123(20): 2254-62.

Helmes, M., Lim, C. C., Liao, R., Bharti, A., Cui, L. and Sawyer, D. B. (2003) 'Titin determines the Frank-Starling relation in early diastole', *The Journal of general physiology* 121(2): 97-110.

Hengartner, M. O. (2000) 'The biochemistry of apoptosis', *Nature* 407(6805): 770-6.

Holmes, W. E., Sliwkowski, M. X., Akita, R. W., Henzel, W. J., Lee, J., Park, J. W., Yansura, D., Abadi, N., Raab, H., Lewis, G. D. et al. (1992) 'Identification of heregulin, a specific activator of p185erbB2', *Science* 256(5060): 1205-10.

Ito, H., Miller, S. C., Billingham, M. E., Akimoto, H., Torti, S. V., Wade, R., Gahlmann, R., Lyons, G., Kedes, L. and Torti, F. M. (1990) 'Doxorubicin selectively inhibits muscle gene expression in cardiac muscle cells in vivo and in vitro', *Proc Natl Acad Sci U S A* 87(11): 4275-9.

Jemal, A., Siegel, R., Ward, E., Murray, T., Xu, J., Smigal, C. and Thun, M. J. (2006) 'Cancer statistics, 2006', *CA: a cancer journal for clinicians* 56(2): 106-30.

Kalinowski, A., Plowes, N. J., Huang, Q., Berdejo-Izquierdo, C., Russell, R. R. and Russell, K. S. (2010) 'Metalloproteinase-dependent cleavage of neuregulin and autocrine stimulation of vascular endothelial cells', *FASEB J* 24(7): 2567-75.

Kalivendi, S. V., Konorev, E. A., Cunningham, S., Vanamala, S. K., Kaji, E. H., Joseph, J. and Kalyanaraman, B. (2005a) 'Doxorubicin activates nuclear factor of activated T-lymphocytes and Fas ligand transcription: role of mitochondrial reactive oxygen species and calcium', *Biochem J.*

Kalivendi, S. V., Konorev, E. A., Cunningham, S., Vanamala, S. K., Kaji, E. H., Joseph, J. and Kalyanaraman, B. (2005b) 'Doxorubicin activates nuclear factor of activated T-lymphocytes and Fas ligand transcription: role of mitochondrial reactive oxygen species and calcium', *Biochem J* 389(Pt 2): 527-39.

Kang, Y. J., Chen, Y. and Epstein, P. N. (1996) 'Suppression of doxorubicin cardiotoxicity by overexpression of catalase in the heart of transgenic mice', *J Biol Chem* 271(21): 12610-6.

Kang, Y. J., Chen, Y., Yu, A., Voss-McCowan, M. and Epstein, P. N. (1997) 'Overexpression of metallothionein in the heart of transgenic mice suppresses doxorubicin cardiotoxicity', *J Clin Invest* 100(6): 1501-6.

Kapelko, V. I., Williams, C. P., Gutstein, D. E. and Morgan, J. P. (1996) 'Abnormal myocardial calcium handling in the early stage of adriamycin cardiomyopathy', *Arch Physiol Biochem* 104(2): 185-91.

Kario, E., Marmor, M. D., Adamsky, K., Citri, A., Amit, I., Amariglio, N., Rechavi, G. and Yarden, Y. (2005) 'Suppressors of cytokine signaling 4 and 5 regulate epidermal growth factor receptor signaling', *The Journal of biological chemistry* 280(8): 7038-48.

Kim, D. H., Landry, A. B., 3rd, Lee, Y. S. and Katz, A. M. (1989) 'Doxorubicin-induced calcium release from cardiac sarcoplasmic reticulum vesicles', *J Mol Cell Cardiol* 21(5): 433-6.

Klapper, L. N., Glathe, S., Vaisman, N., Hynes, N. E., Andrews, G. C., Sela, M. and Yarden, Y. (1999) 'The ErbB-2/HER2 oncoprotein of human carcinomas may function solely as a shared coreceptor for multiple stroma-derived growth factors', *Proceedings of the National Academy of Sciences of the United States of America* 96(9): 4995-5000.

Kobayashi, S., Lackey, T., Huang, Y., Bisping, E., Pu, W. T., Boxer, L. M. and Liang, Q. (2006) 'Transcription factor gata4 regulates cardiac BCL2 gene expression in vitro and in vivo', *Faseb J* 20(6): 800-2.

Kramer, R., Bucay, N., Kane, D. J., Martin, L. E., Tarpley, J. E. and Theill, L. E. (1996a) 'Neuregulins with an Ig-like domain are essential for mouse myocardial and neuronal development', *Proceedings of the National Academy of Sciences of the United States of America* 93(10): 4833-8.

Kramer, R., Bucay, N., Kane, D. J., Martin, L. E., Tarpley, J. E. and Theill, L. E. (1996b) 'Neuregulins with an Ig-like domain are essential for mouse myocardial and neuronal development', *Proc Natl Acad Sci U S A* 93(10): 4833-8.

Kurabayashi, M., Jeyaseelan, R. and Kedes, L. (1994) 'Doxorubicin represses the function of the myogenic helix-loop-helix transcription factor MyoD. Involvement of Id gene induction', *J Biol Chem* 269(8): 6031-9.

Kuramochi, Y., Cote, G. M., Guo, X., Lebrasseur, N. K., Cui, L., Liao, R. and Sawyer, D. B. (2004) 'Cardiac endothelial cells regulate reactive oxygen species-induced cardiomyocyte apoptosis through neuregulin-1beta/erbB4 signaling', *J Biol Chem* 279(49): 51141-7.

L'Ecuyer, T., Sanjeev, S., Thomas, R., Novak, R., Das, L., Campbell, W. and Vander Heide, R. S. (2006) 'DNA damage is an early event in doxorubicin-induced cardiac myocyte death', *Am J Physiol Heart Circ Physiol.*

Lee, K. F., Simon, H., Chen, H., Bates, B., Hung, M. C. and Hauser, C. (1995) 'Requirement for neuregulin receptor erbB2 in neural and cardiac development', *Nature* 378(6555): 394-8.

Lemmens, K., Segers, V. F., Demolder, M. and De Keulenaer, G. W. (2006) 'Role of neuregulin-1/ErbB2 signaling in endothelium-cardiomyocyte cross-talk', *J Biol Chem* 281(28): 19469-77.

Lewis, W. and Gonzalez, B. (1987) 'Actin isoform synthesis by cultured cardiac myocytes. Effects of doxorubicin', *Lab Invest* 56(3): 295-301.

Lim, C. C., Zuppinger, C., Guo, X., Kuster, G. M., Helmes, M., Eppenberger, H. M., Suter, T. M., Liao, R. and Sawyer, D. B. (2004a) 'Anthracyclines induce calpain-dependent titin proteolysis and necrosis in cardiomyocytes', *The Journal of biological chemistry* 279(9): 8290-9.

Lim, C. C., Zuppinger, C., Guo, X., Kuster, G. M., Helmes, M., Eppenberger, H. M., Suter, T. M., Liao, R. and Sawyer, D. B. (2004b) 'Anthracyclines induce calpain-dependent titin proteolysis and necrosis in cardiomyocytes', *J Biol Chem* 279(9): 8290-9.

Lipshultz, S. E., Colan, S. D., Gelber, R. D., Perez-Atayde, A. R., Sallan, S. E. and Sanders, S. P. (1991) 'Late cardiac effects of doxorubicin therapy for acute lymphoblastic leukemia in childhood', *The New England journal of medicine* 324(12): 808-15.

Lipshultz, S. E., Lipsitz, S. R., Sallan, S. E., Dalton, V. M., Mone, S. M., Gelber, R. D. and Colan, S. D. (2005) 'Chronic progressive cardiac dysfunction years after doxorubicin therapy for childhood acute lymphoblastic leukemia', *Journal of clinical oncology : official journal of the American Society of Clinical Oncology* 23(12): 2629-36.

Liu, F. F., Stone, J. R., Schuldt, A. J., Okoshi, K., Okoshi, M. P., Nakayama, M., Ho, K. K., Manning, W. J., Marchionni, M. A., Lorell, B. H. et al. (2005) 'Heterozygous knockout of neuregulin-1 gene in mice exacerbates doxorubicin-induced heart failure', *Am J Physiol Heart Circ Physiol* 289(2): H660-6.

Liu, X., Chua, C. C., Gao, J., Chen, Z., Landy, C. L., Hamdy, R. and Chua, B. H. (2004) 'Pifithrin-alpha protects against doxorubicin-induced apoptosis and acute cardiotoxicity in mice', *Am J Physiol Heart Circ Physiol* 286(3): H933-9.

Liu, X., Gu, X., Li, Z., Li, X., Li, H., Chang, J., Chen, P., Jin, J., Xi, B., Chen, D. et al. (2006) 'Neuregulin-1/erbB-activation improves cardiac function and survival in models of ischemic, dilated, and viral cardiomyopathy', *J Am Coll Cardiol* 48(7): 1438-47.

Liu, X., Hwang, H., Cao, L., Buckland, M., Cunningham, A., Chen, J., Chien, K. R., Graham, R. M. and Zhou, M. (1998a) 'Domain-specific gene disruption reveals critical regulation of neuregulin signaling by its cytoplasmic tail', *Proc Natl Acad Sci U S A* 95(22): 13024-9.

Liu, X., Hwang, H., Cao, L., Buckland, M., Cunningham, A., Chen, J., Chien, K. R., Graham, R. M. and Zhou, M. (1998b) 'Domain-specific gene disruption reveals critical regulation of neuregulin signaling by its cytoplasmic tail', *Proceedings of the National Academy of Sciences of the United States of America* 95(22): 13024-9.

LoPiccolo, J., Blumenthal, G. M., Bernstein, W. B. and Dennis, P. A. (2008) 'Targeting the PI3K/Akt/mTOR pathway: effective combinations and clinical considerations', *Drug Resist Updat* 11(1-2): 32-50.

Mackay, B., Ewer, M. S., Carrasco, C. H. and Benjamin, R. S. (1994) 'Assessment of anthracycline cardiomyopathy by endomyocardial biopsy', *Ultrastructural pathology* 18(1-2): 203-11.

Maeda, A., Honda, M., Kuramochi, T. and Takabatake, T. (1998) 'Doxorubicin cardiotoxicity: diastolic cardiac myocyte dysfunction as a result of impaired calcium handling in isolated cardiac myocytes', *Jpn Circ J* 62(7): 505-11.

Marchionni, M. A. (1995) 'Cell-cell signalling. neu tack on neuregulin', *Nature* 378(6555): 334-5.

Marchionni, M. A., Goodearl, A. D., Chen, M. S., Bermingham-McDonogh, O., Kirk, C., Hendricks, M., Danehy, F., Misumi, D., Sudhalter, J., Kobayashi, K. et al. (1993) 'Glial growth factors are alternatively spliced erbB2 ligands expressed in the nervous system', *Nature* 362(6418): 312-8.

Meyer, D. and Birchmeier, C. (1995) 'Multiple essential functions of neuregulin in development', *Nature* 378(6555): 386-90.

Meyer, D., Yamaai, T., Garratt, A., Riethmacher-Sonnenberg, E., Kane, D., Theill, L. E. and Birchmeier, C. (1997) 'Isoform-specific expression and function of neuregulin', *Development* 124(18): 3575-86.

Moasser, M. M. (2007) 'The oncogene HER2: its signaling and transforming functions and its role in human cancer pathogenesis', *Oncogene* 26(45): 6469-87.

Monvoisin, A., Alva, J. A., Hofmann, J. J., Zovein, A. C., Lane, T. F. and Iruela-Arispe, M. L. (2006) 'VE-cadherin-CreERT2 transgenic mouse: a model for inducible recombination in the endothelium', *Developmental dynamics : an official publication of the American Association of Anatomists* 235(12): 3413-22.

Moretti, E., Oakman, C. and Di Leo, A. (2009) 'Predicting anthracycline benefit: have we made any progress?', *Curr Opin Oncol* 21(6): 507-15.

Morris, J. K., Lin, W., Hauser, C., Marchuk, Y., Getman, D. and Lee, K. F. (1999) 'Rescue of the cardiac defect in ErbB2 mutant mice reveals essential roles of ErbB2 in peripheral nervous system development', *Neuron* 23(2): 273-83.

Mortensen, S. A., Olsen, H. S. and Baandrup, U. (1986) 'Chronic anthracycline cardiotoxicity: haemodynamic and histopathological manifestations suggesting a restrictive endomyocardial disease', *British heart journal* 55(3): 274-82.

Nakamura, T., Ueda, Y., Juan, Y., Katsuda, S., Takahashi, H. and Koh, E. (2000) 'Fas-mediated apoptosis in adriamycin-induced cardiomyopathy in rats: In vivo study', *Circulation* 102(5): 572-8.

Negro, A., Brar, B. K., Gu, Y., Peterson, K. L., Vale, W. and Lee, K. F. (2006) 'erbB2 is required for G protein-coupled receptor signaling in the heart', *Proc Natl Acad Sci U S A* 103(43): 15889-93.

Oeffinger, K. C., Mertens, A. C., Sklar, C. A., Kawashima, T., Hudson, M. M., Meadows, A. T., Friedman, D. L., Marina, N., Hobbie, W., Kadan-Lottick, N. S. et al. (2006) 'Chronic health conditions in adult survivors of childhood cancer', *The New England journal of medicine* 355(15): 1572-82.

Ondrias, K., Borgatta, L., Kim, D. H. and Ehrlich, B. E. (1990) 'Biphasic effects of doxorubicin on the calcium release channel from sarcoplasmic reticulum of cardiac muscle', *Circ Res* 67(5): 1167-74.

Outomuro, D., Grana, D. R., Azzato, F. and Milei, J. (2007a) 'Adriamycin-induced myocardial toxicity: new solutions for an old problem?', *Int J Cardiol* 117(1): 6-15.

Outomuro, D., Grana, D. R., Azzato, F. and Milei, J. (2007b) 'Adriamycin-induced myocardial toxicity: new solutions for an old problem?', *International journal of cardiology* 117(1): 6-15.

Ozcelik, C., Erdmann, B., Pilz, B., Wettschureck, N., Britsch, S., Hubner, N., Chien, K. R., Birchmeier, C. and Garratt, A. N. (2002) 'Conditional mutation of the ErbB2 (HER2) receptor in cardiomyocytes leads to dilated cardiomyopathy', *Proc Natl Acad Sci U S A* 99(13): 8880-5.

Paik, S., Bryant, J., Tan-Chiu, E., Yothers, G., Park, C., Wickerham, D. L. and Wolmark, N. (2000) 'HER2 and choice of adjuvant chemotherapy for invasive breast cancer: National Surgical Adjuvant Breast and Bowel Project Protocol B-15', *J Natl Cancer Inst* 92(24): 1991-8.

Peles, E., Bacus, S. S., Koski, R. A., Lu, H. S., Wen, D., Ogden, S. G., Levy, R. B. and Yarden, Y. (1992) 'Isolation of the neu/HER-2 stimulatory ligand: a 44 kd glycoprotein that induces differentiation of mammary tumor cells', *Cell* 69(1): 205-16.

Pentassuglia, L., Graf, M., Lane, H., Kuramochi, Y., Cote, G., Timolati, F., Sawyer, D. B., Zuppinger, C. and Suter, T. M. (2009) 'Inhibition of ErbB2 by receptor tyrosine kinase inhibitors causes myofibrillar structural damage without cell death in adult rat cardiomyocytes', *Exp Cell Res* 315(7): 1302-12.

Pentassuglia, L. and Sawyer, D. B. (2009) 'The role of Neuregulin-1beta/ErbB signaling in the heart', *Exp Cell Res* 315(4): 627-37.

Poizat, C., Puri, P. L., Bai, Y. and Kedes, L. (2005) 'Phosphorylation-dependent degradation of p300 by doxorubicin-activated p38 mitogen-activated protein kinase in cardiac cells', *Mol Cell Biol* 25(7): 2673-87.

Poizat, C., Sartorelli, V., Chung, G., Kloner, R. A. and Kedes, L. (2000) 'Proteasome-mediated degradation of the coactivator p300 impairs cardiac transcription', *Mol Cell Biol* 20(23): 8643-54.

Pritchard, K. I., Shepherd, L. E., O'Malley, F. P., Andrulis, I. L., Tu, D., Bramwell, V. H. and Levine, M. N. (2006) 'HER2 and responsiveness of breast cancer to adjuvant chemotherapy', *N Engl J Med* 354(20): 2103-11.

Rohrbach, S., Muller-Werdan, U., Werdan, K., Koch, S., Gellerich, N. F. and Holtz, J. (2005a) 'Apoptosis-modulating interaction of the neuregulin/erbB pathway with anthracyclines in regulating Bcl-xS and Bcl-xL in cardiomyocytes', *Journal of molecular and cellular cardiology* 38(3): 485-93.

Rohrbach, S., Muller-Werdan, U., Werdan, K., Koch, S., Gellerich, N. F. and Holtz, J. (2005b) 'Apoptosis-modulating interaction of the neuregulin/erbB pathway with antracyclines in regulating Bcl-xS and Bcl-xL in cardiomyocytes', *J Mol Cell Cardiol* 38(3): 485-93.

Rowan, R. A., Masek, M. A. and Billingham, M. E. (1988) 'Ultrastructural morphometric analysis of endomyocardial biopsies. Idiopathic dilated cardiomyopathy, anthracycline cardiotoxicity, and normal myocardium', *The American journal of cardiovascular pathology* 2(2): 137-44.

Safra, T. (2003) 'Cardiac safety of liposomal anthracyclines', *The oncologist* 8 Suppl 2: 17-24.

Sawyer, D. B., Zuppinger, C., Miller, T. A., Eppenberger, H. M. and Suter, T. M. (2002) 'Modulation of anthracycline-induced myofibrillar disarray in rat ventricular myocytes by neuregulin-1beta and anti-erbB2: potential mechanism for trastuzumab-induced cardiotoxicity', *Circulation* 105(13): 1551-4.

Schmidt, U., Hajjar, R. J., Helm, P. A., Kim, C. S., Doye, A. A. and Gwathmey, J. K. (1998) 'Contribution of abnormal sarcoplasmic reticulum ATPase activity to systolic and diastolic dysfunction in human heart failure', *J Mol Cell Cardiol* 30(10): 1929-37.

Schmidt, U., Hajjar, R. J., Kim, C. S., Lebeche, D., Doye, A. A. and Gwathmey, J. K. (1999) 'Human heart failure: cAMP stimulation of SR Ca(2+)-ATPase activity and phosphorylation level of phospholamban', *Am J Physiol* 277(2 Pt 2): H474-80.

Schulze, A., Lehmann, K., Jefferies, H. B., McMahon, M. and Downward, J. (2001) 'Analysis of the transcriptional program induced by Raf in epithelial cells', *Genes & development* 15(8): 981-94.

Schulze, W. X., Deng, L. and Mann, M. (2005) 'Phosphotyrosine interactome of the ErbB-receptor kinase family', *Molecular systems biology* 1: 2005 0008.

Simsir, S. A., Lin, S. S., Blue, L. J., Gockerman, J. P., Russell, S. D. and Milano, C. A. (2005) 'Left ventricular assist device as destination therapy in doxorubicin-induced cardiomyopathy', *The Annals of thoracic surgery* 80(2): 717-9.

Simunek, T., Sterba, M., Popelova, O., Adamcova, M., Hrdina, R. and Gersl, V. (2009) 'Anthracycline-induced cardiotoxicity: overview of studies examining the roles of oxidative stress and free cellular iron', *Pharmacological reports : PR* 61(1): 154-71.

Singal, P. K., Li, T., Kumar, D., Danelisen, I. and Iliskovic, N. (2000) 'Adriamycin-induced heart failure: mechanism and modulation', *Molecular and cellular biochemistry* 207(1-2): 77-86.

Slamon, D. J., Leyland-Jones, B., Shak, S., Fuchs, H., Paton, V., Bajamonde, A., Fleming, T., Eiermann, W., Wolter, J., Pegram, M. et al. (2001) 'Use of chemotherapy plus a monoclonal antibody against HER2 for metastatic breast cancer that overexpresses HER2', *The New England journal of medicine* 344(11): 783-92.

Stefansson, H., Sigurdsson, E., Steinthorsdottir, V., Bjornsdottir, S., Sigmundsson, T., Ghosh, S., Brynjolfsson, J., Gunnarsdottir, S., Ivarsson, O., Chou, T. T. et al. (2002) 'Neuregulin 1 and susceptibility to schizophrenia', *Am J Hum Genet* 71(4): 877-92.

Sun, M., Yan, X., Bian, Y., Caggiano, A. O. and Morgan, J. P. (2011) 'Improving murine embryonic stem cell differentiation into cardiomyocytes with neuregulin-1: differential expression of microRNA', *American journal of physiology. Cell physiology* 301(1): C21-30.

Swain, S. M., Whaley, F. S. and Ewer, M. S. (2003) 'Congestive heart failure in patients treated with doxorubicin: a retrospective analysis of three trials', *Cancer* 97(11): 2869-79.

Timolati, F., Ott, D., Pentassuglia, L., Giraud, M. N., Perriard, J. C., Suter, T. M. and Zuppinger, C. (2006) 'Neuregulin-1 beta attenuates doxorubicin-induced alterations of excitation-contraction coupling and reduces oxidative stress in adult rat cardiomyocytes', *Journal of molecular and cellular cardiology* 41(5): 845-54.

Toyoda, Y., Okada, M. and Kashem, M. A. (1998) 'A canine model of dilated cardiomyopathy induced by repetitive intracoronary doxorubicin administration', *J Thorac Cardiovasc Surg* 115(6): 1367-73.

van Dalen, E. C., van den Brug, M., Caron, H. N. and Kremer, L. C. (2006) 'Anthracycline-induced cardiotoxicity: comparison of recommendations for monitoring cardiac function during therapy in paediatric oncology trials', *Eur J Cancer* 42(18): 3199-205.
Von Hoff, D. D., Layard, M. W., Basa, P., Davis, H. L., Jr., Von Hoff, A. L., Rozencweig, M. and Muggia, F. M. (1979) 'Risk factors for doxorubicin-induced congestive heart failure', *Annals of internal medicine* 91(5): 710-7.
Wallace, K. B. (2003) 'Doxorubicin-induced cardiac mitochondrionopathy', *Pharmacol Toxicol* 93(3): 105-15.
Wehrens, X. H. and Marks, A. R. (2004) 'Novel therapeutic approaches for heart failure by normalizing calcium cycling', *Nat Rev Drug Discov* 3(7): 565-73.
Wen, D., Peles, E., Cupples, R., Suggs, S. V., Bacus, S. S., Luo, Y., Trail, G., Hu, S., Silbiger, S. M., Levy, R. B. et al. (1992) 'Neu differentiation factor: a transmembrane glycoprotein containing an EGF domain and an immunoglobulin homology unit', *Cell* 69(3): 559-72.
Wolpowitz, D., Mason, T. B., Dietrich, P., Mendelsohn, M., Talmage, D. A. and Role, L. W. (2000) 'Cysteine-rich domain isoforms of the neuregulin-1 gene are required for maintenance of peripheral synapses', *Neuron* 25(1): 79-91.
Yang, X., Arber, S., William, C., Li, L., Tanabe, Y., Jessell, T. M., Birchmeier, C. and Burden, S. J. (2001) 'Patterning of muscle acetylcholine receptor gene expression in the absence of motor innervation', *Neuron* 30(2): 399-410.
Yarden, Y. and Sliwkowski, M. X. (2001a) 'Untangling the ErbB signalling network', *Nat Rev Mol Cell Biol* 2(2): 127-37.
Yarden, Y. and Sliwkowski, M. X. (2001b) 'Untangling the ErbB signalling network', *Nature reviews. Molecular cell biology* 2(2): 127-37.
Yen, H. C., Oberley, T. D., Vichitbandha, S., Ho, Y. S. and St Clair, D. K. (1996) 'The protective role of manganese superoxide dismutase against adriamycin-induced acute cardiac toxicity in transgenic mice', *J Clin Invest* 98(5): 1253-60.
Youn, H. J., Kim, H. S., Jeon, M. H., Lee, J. H., Seo, Y. J. and Lee, Y. J. (2005) 'Induction of caspase-independent apoptosis in H9c2 cardiomyocytes by adriamycin treatment', *Molecular and cellular biochemistry* 270(1-2): 13-9.
Zhang, D., Sliwkowski, M. X., Mark, M., Frantz, G., Akita, R., Sun, Y., Hillan, K., Crowley, C., Brush, J. and Godowski, P. J. (1997) 'Neuregulin-3 (NRG3): a novel neural tissue-enriched protein that binds and activates ErbB4', *Proceedings of the National Academy of Sciences of the United States of America* 94(18): 9562-7.
Zhao, Y. Y., Sawyer, D. R., Baliga, R. R., Opel, D. J., Han, X., Marchionni, M. A. and Kelly, R. A. (1998) 'Neuregulins promote survival and growth of cardiac myocytes. Persistence of ErbB2 and ErbB4 expression in neonatal and adult ventricular myocytes', *J Biol Chem* 273(17): 10261-9.

5

Doxorubicin-Induced Oxidative Injury of Cardiomyocytes – Do We Have Right Strategies for Prevention?

Vukosava Milic Torres[1] and Viktorija Dragojevic Simic[2]
[1]Laboratory of Proteomics, Department of Genetics, National Institute of Health Dr Ricardo Jorge, Lisbon,
[2]Center for Clinical Pharmacology, Military Medical Academy, Belgrade,
[1]Portugal
[2]Serbia

1. Introduction

Anthracyclines are among the most utilised antitumour drugs ever developed. The discovery of one of the leading compounds, doxorubicin (DOX) in early 1960s was a major advance in the fight against cancer. According to the WHO, it belongs to the group of 17 essential drugs that are used to treat curable cancers or cancers for which the cost-benefit ratio clearly favours drug treatment (Sikora et al., 1999). It is used, often with other antineoplastic, in the treatment of Hodgkin's disease, non-Hodgkin's lymphomas, acute leukaemias, bone and soft-tissue sarcoma, neuroblastoma, Wilm's tumour, and malignant neoplasms of the bladder, breast, lung, ovary, and stomach. The mechanisms of cytotoxicity of DOX in cancer cells is complex including: inhibition of both DNA replication and RNA transcription; free radicals generation, leading to DNA damage or lipid peroxidation; DNA cross-linking; DNA alkylation; direct membrane damage due to lipid oxidation and inhibition of topoisomerase II (Gewirtz, 1999; Minotti et al., 2004). Today, topoisomarase II is generally recognized to be the cellular target of DOX, which act by stabilizing a reaction intermediate in which DNA strands are cut and covalently linked to this enzyme (Simunek et al., 2009). It blocks subsequent DNA resealing. Failure to relax the supercoiled DNA blocks DNA replication and transcription. Furthermore, DNA strand breaks may trigger apoptosis of cancer cells. However, as with all traditional antineoplastic drugs, DOX administration is accompanied by adverse drug reactions arising from the limited selectivity of their anticancer action (Aronson et al., 2006; McEvoy et al., 2010). Particularly common are bone marrow depression, which may be dose-limiting. White cell count reaches a nadir 10 to 15 days after a dose and usually recovers by about 21 days. Gastrointestinal disturbances include moderate or sometimes severe nausea and vomiting; stomatitis and oesophagitis may progress to ulceration. Alopecia occurs in the majority of patients. Occasional hypersensitivity reactions may also occur. However, a cumulative-dose dependent cardiac toxicity has been a major limitation of DOX use.

2. Doxorubicin-induced cardiotoxicity

Cardiac toxic effects were first documented during early clinical evaluations of DOX, and in the late 1970s, first retrospective clinical studies showed convincingly that the observed cardiac disturbances could be directly attributable to repeated DOX administration. At the same time, these studies established the cumulative DOX dose received as the main risk factor of cardiotoxicity (Green et al., 2001; Lefrak et al., 1973; Von Hoff et al., 1979). Considering that more than 50% of long term-survivors of childhood cancer alone were treated with DOX or another anthracycline, anthracycline-induced cardiotoxicity is a widely prevalent problem that cannot be ignored. Namely, long-term survivors of childhood cancer are 8 times more likely than the general population to die from cardiovascular-related disease and, compared to sibling controls, they are 15 times as likely to suffer from heart failure (HF)(Lipshultz & Adams, 2010; Lipshultz et al., 1991). Despite very large numbers of new anthracycline compounds synthesized and tested, only few ones have been approved for clinical use, and none of them has fulfilled expectations of substantially improved cardiac safety. Therefore, a growing need to develop effective and cardioprotective strategies remains, in order to find a balance between the risks of cardiotoxicity and the benefits of oncologic therapy with DOX.

2.1 Clinical presentation and risk factors of doxorubicin-induced cardiotoxicity

DOX-induced cardiotoxicity is most often divided into 3 categories: acute changes, early-onset chronic progressive cardiotoxicity and late-onset chronic progressive cardiotoxicity (Aronson et al., 2006; Schimmel et al., 2004; Wouters et al., 2005) Acute DOX-induced cardiotoxicity occurs during DOX administration or immediately afterwards. It typically involves transient electrocardiographic abnormalities such as non-specific ST-T changes and QT prolongation, vasodilatation and hypotension. Pericarditis-myocarditis syndrome and ventricular dysfunction which manifest 1 to 3 days after the DOX treatment are extremely rare, and were more frequently seen in early trials using very high doses of DOX. Most often, all of the disturbances attenuate after discontinuation of the therapy. Early-onset chronic cardiotoxicity, such as cardiomyopathy which progresses to congestive heart failure (CHF) usually occurs within 1 year after discontinuance of DOX therapy. CHF may occur as total cumulative dosage of DOX approaches or exceeds 550 mg/m^2. Chronic cardiotoxicity reflects a progressive injury and loss of cardiac myocytes, with increasing cumulative DOX dose resulting in thinning of ventricular wall and decreased systolic performance. It is characterised by dilated (less often restrictive, mostly in children) cardiomyopathy, with subsequent development of left ventricular contractile dysfunction and congestive heart failure. Histopathological changes are quite unique and consist of distension of the sarcoplasmic reticulum of myocytes, cytoplasmic vacuolization, swelling of mitochondria and myofibrillar disarray and loss (Ferrans et al., 1997). Symptoms of the CHF include tachycardia, tachypnea, dilatation of the heart, exercise intolerance, pulmonary oedema, peripheral oedema and needs for treatment with diuretics and cardiac glycosides. These manifestations may respond to cardiac supportive therapy and may be self limiting, or may be irreversible and unresponsive to therapy and fatal (Aronson et al., 2006; Singal & Iliskovic, 1998; Sweetman, 2011; Wouters et al., 2005). Finally, late-onset chronic progressive DOX-induced cardiotoxicity occurs at least 1 year after the completion of therapy, sometimes even after decades of a prolonged asymptomatic interval. It has been suggested that myocyte damage and ventricular dysfunction progress after the initial myocardial insult and may lead to late-onset cardiac decompensation. Although the DOX dose of 550 mg/m^2 was suggested to be relatively safe, CHF was found to begin at a lower cumulative dose in the presence of other risk factors, such as age above 70 years, combination therapy (cyclophosphamide, dacarbazine etc.), previous or concomitant mediastinal radiotherapy, history of pre-existing cardiac disease, or liver disease (Ludke et al., 2009; Singal & Iliskovic, 1998; Sweetman, 2011). Although sensitivity to DOX-induced cardiotoxicity exhibit large interindividual variation, the risk of developing impairment in myocardial function increases with increasing cumulative dose, occurring in 3-5, 5-8, and 6-20% in those receiving cumulative doses of 400, 450, or 500 mg/m^2, respectively, in schedules of rapid IV doses given every 3 weeks. The strong association between cumulative DOX dose and cardiotoxicity obviously is more important with increasing time after treatment (Lipshultz & Adams, 2010). Some clinicians suggest that late-onset cardiotoxicity can be clinically manifest in response to stressful situations (e.g. surgery, pregnancy), exercise and viral infection. Late-onset doxorubicin toxicity can be expected to be observed more frequently with the growing number of long-time survivors (survivors of childhood cancers) who have received DOX. Long term follow up shows that overt cardiac failure occurs from 0 to 16% of patients receiving anthracycline therapy. It depends on the cumulative dose, well recognized risk factor for late cardiotoxicity, radiation therapy involving the heart, age at diagnosis, greater length of follow up, higher dose rate and previous exposure to anthracycline (Kremer et al., 2002; McEvoy et al., 2010; Wouters et al., 2005). Therefore, recommendations for screening and management of late effects of therapeutic exposure used during treatment for pediatric malignancies are very important in every day practice.

2.2 Monitoring and markers of doxorubicin-induced cardiotoxicity

Clinical manifestations found on physical examination, and/or changes found on electrocardiographic (ECG) monitoring are not specific enough to diagnose DOX-induced cardiotoxicity. However, a persistent reduction in the voltage of the QRS wave is generally indicative of the need to perform further tests. Non-invasive cardiac monitoring, by means of serial echocardiography studies or radionuclide angiography, is useful in predicting the development of cardiomyopathy. However, since it may give normal results until damage is quite advanced, sensitivity may be improved with exercise stress tests (Singal & Iliskovic, 1998; Steinherz et al., 1992). Endomyocardial biopsy is the most sensitive indicator of cardiomyopathy, but it is limited by its invasiveness, need for histologic expertise, and costs. Therefore, there is need for simple methods, like serum and plasma markers to identify patients at risk. There is some preliminary evidence to suggest that concentrations of cardiac troponins and natriuretic peptides could be used as predictive markers of myocardial damage (Ludke et al., 2009; Schimmel et al., 2004). Anyway, according to the Childrens' Cancer Study Group (Steinherz et al., 1992), standard echocardiogram should be performed before the beginning of the treatment and at the third, sixth and 12th month after its completion. Subsequent exam should be repeated every 2 years for the rest of the life.

2.3 Prognosis and treatment

Historically, DOX-induced cardiomyopathies have a poor prognosis and mortality rate as high as 61% (Allen, 1992; Von Hoff et al., 1979; Wouters et al., 2005). It is refractory to conventional therapy, therefore cardiac transplantation is the only solution associated with improved survival (Aronson et al., 2006; Sweetman, 2011). Just recent study reports that the response of DOX-induced cardiomyopathy to the current standard medical therapy is better, especially in patients treated with β-blockers. Nowadays, in the treatment of CHF, including DOX-induced cardiomyopathy, β-blockers and angiotensin-converting enzyme (ACE) inhibitors, are proven Class I medications according to the American College of Cardiology/American Heart Association and Canadian Cardiovascular Society guidelines (Hunt, 2005; Malcom et al., 2008).

2.4 Mechanisms of doxorubicin induced cardiac Injury

Two important characteristics of doxorubicin induced cardiomyopathy are that is dose dependent and it is refractory to the commonly used therapeutic procedures (Lefrak et al., 1973; Singal & Iliskovic, 1998). Pathogenesis of cardiac injury caused by doxorubicin is multifactorial and it is in direct relationship with metabolism and antitumor activity of the drug (Figure. 1). Free radical stress, calcium overloading and mitochondrial dysfunction are main triggers in doxorubicin-induced cardiotoxicity. Subsequent gene expression changes and activation of the ubiquitin-proteasome system, cell death, as well as innate immunity activation all contribute to the toxicity (Shi et al., 2011). The level of the doxorubicin-induced oxidative stress is up to 10 times greater in the heart than in the other tissues (liver, kidney, spleen) (Davies & Doroshow, 1986; Doroshow & Davies, 1986; Gaetani et al., 1989; Lenzhofer et al., 1983; Milei et al., 1986; Mukherjee et al., 2003; Siveski-Iliskovic et al., 1995), and therefore oxidative injury of the heart is widely accepted theory presumed as a primary mechanism of the DOX-induced cardiotoxicity.

2.4.1 Role of iron and free radicals

Although doxorubicin-induced cardiotoxicity is multifactorial, formation of reactive oxygen species (ROS) has a leading role in promoting the oxidative myocardial damage. The high level of oxidative stress generated by anthracyclines is accounted to the molecular characteristics which allows drug to easily undergo redox reaction and subsequently free radical cascade.

Doxorubicin is belonging to the group of anthracycline antibiotics consist of naphthacenequinone nucleus linked through a glycosidic bond to an amino sugar, daunosamine (Figure. 2a). One-electron addition to the quinone moiety in ring C of DOX result in formation of a semiquinone that quickly regenerates its parent quinone by reducing oxygen to reactive oxygen species, like superoxide anion radical ($O_2^{\bullet-}$) and hydrogen peroxide (H_2O_2) (Figure. 2b).

This futile cycle is supported by a number of NAD(P)H-oxidoreductases [cytochrome P450 or -b5 reductases, mitochondrial NADH dehydrogenase, xanthine dehydrogenase, endothelial nitric oxide synthase (reductase domain) (Halliwell & Gutteridge, 2007; Minotti et al., 1999; Vasquez-Vivar et al., 1997). The dismutation of the $O_2^{\cdot-}$ is catalyzed by superoxide dismutase enzyme or it may occur spontaneously in the acidic environment - ($pH<7$). Hydrogen peroxide is low toxic molecule, which is eliminated from the body by enzymatic antioxidative defence system (catalase -CAT and glutathione peroxidase - GPx). However, in the presence of the transition metals, especially iron, H_2O_2 and $O_2^{\bullet-}$ can

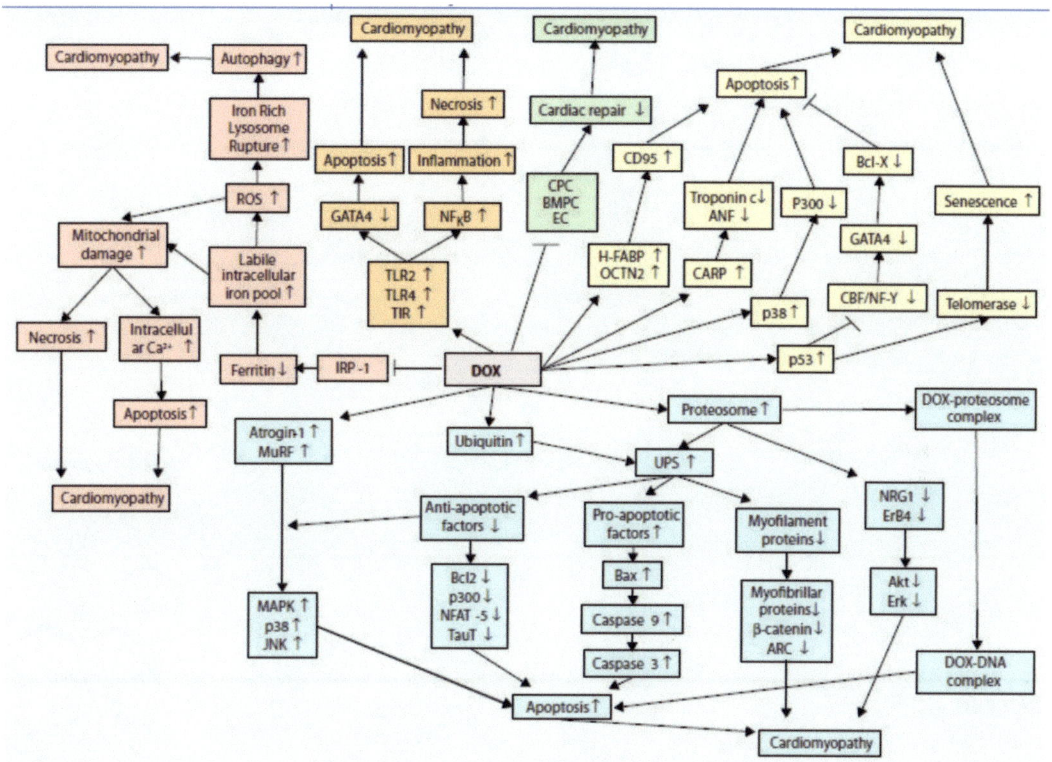

Fig. 1. A summary of potential mechanisms involved in doxorubicin (Dox)-induced cardiomyopathy as described in the text. The major mechanisms involve ROS and iron (red). Meanwhile, Dox-induced cell death (necrosis, apoptosis, and autophagy) and activation of innate immunity (brown), gene changes that reduce cardiac-specific gene expression or trigger apoptosis, induction of cardiac premature senescence in cardiomyocytes (yellow), activation of the ubiquitin-proteasome system (UPS) causing the balance of the protein system to shift toward pro-apoptosis, downregulation of prosurvival gene (NRG1 and ErB4) expression (blue), and impaired cardiac repair by inhibiting bone marrow, cardiac progenitor cell, and/or endothelial cell function (green) all emerge as potential mechanisms contributing to Dox cardiotoxicity. ROS reactive oxygen species, IRP iron regulatory protein, TLR toll-like receptor, TIR toll-interleukin-1 receptor, CARP cardiac Adriamycin-responsive protein, H-FABP heart fatty acid binding protein, OCTN organic cation/carnitine transporter, ARC apoptosis repressor with caspase recruitment domain, NFAT nuclear factors of activated T-cell, TauT taurine transporter, NRG neuregulin, ErbB epidermal growth factor receptor B, BMPC bone marrow cardiac progenitor cell, CPC cardiac progenitor cell, EC endothelial cell, arrows pointing up or down (inside text boxes) indicate increases or decreases in function or expression, horizontal arrows indicate positive regulatory sequence, blocks represent inhibition (Shi et al., 2011).

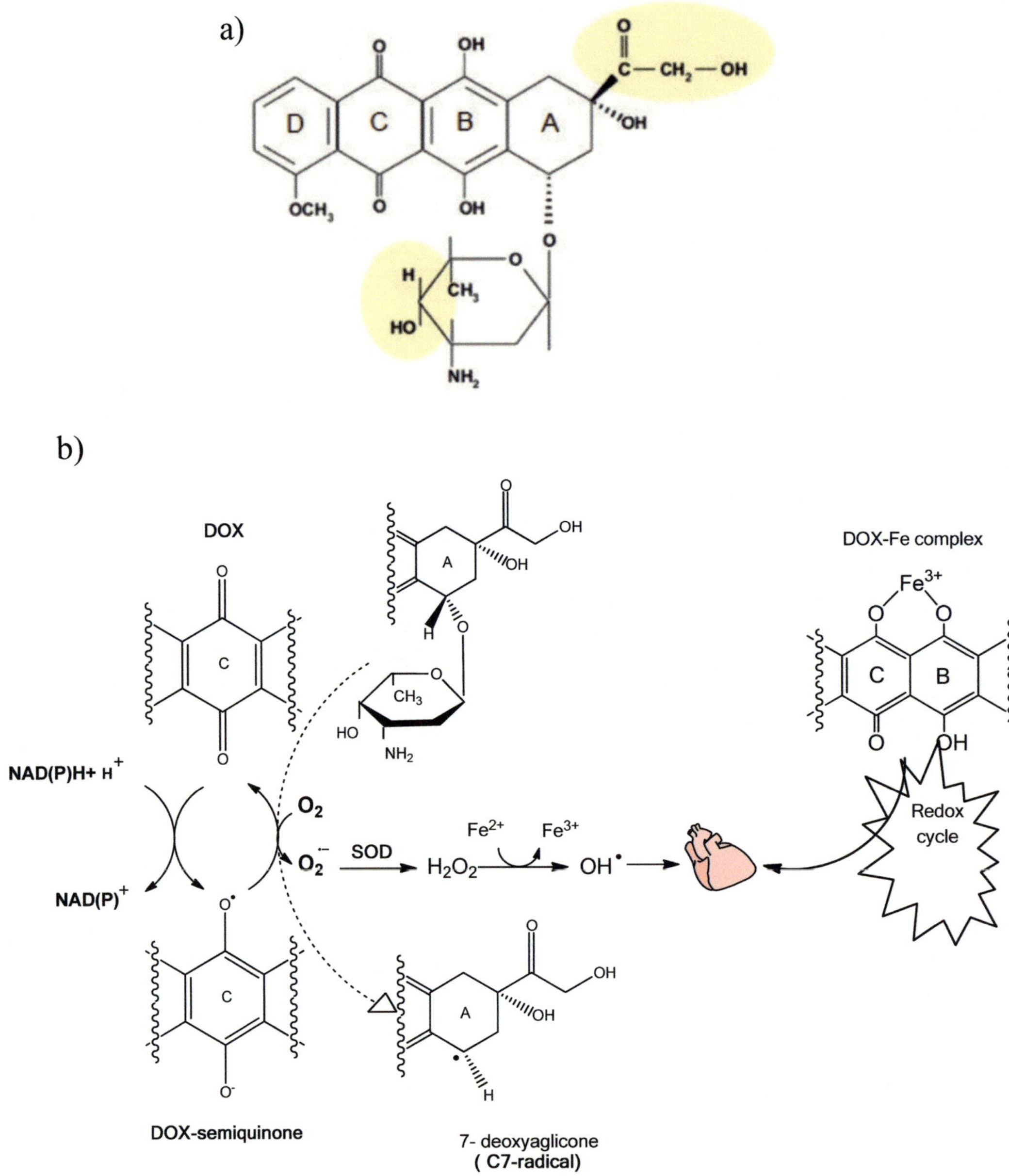

Fig. 2. Doxorubicin mediated redox cycling and free radical production

$$O_2^{\bullet-} + H_2O_2 \longrightarrow O_2 + OH^- + OH^{\bullet} \qquad (1)$$

$$O_2^{\bullet-} + Fe^{3+} \longrightarrow O_2 + Fe^{2+} \qquad (2)$$

$$H_2O_2 + Fe^{2+} \longrightarrow OH^- + OH^{\bullet} + Fe^{3+} \qquad (3)$$

generate highly toxic hydroxyl radical ($OH^{\bullet}$). This process is occurring during the Haber-Weiss reaction (1) which is actually quite slow. Presence of iron strongly catalyzes formation of $OH^{\bullet}$, in two step process. In the first step ferric ion (Fe^{3+}) is reduced in to ferrous ion (Fe^{2+}) by $O_2^{\bullet-}$ (2). Ferrous ion than reacts with hydrogen peroxide (generated during DOX reduction) resulting with formation of hydroxyl radicals (Fenton reaction) (3).

Unlike hydrogen peroxide and superoxide anion radical, hydroxyl radical is extremely reactive and cannot be neutralized by antioxidative enzymes. Instead, $OH^{\bullet}$ reacts with polyunsaturated fatty acids forming lipid peroxides, conjugated dienes and malonyl dialdeyde. As a consequence, the structure of lipid bilayer is modified resulting in cell membrane damage followed by cell dysfunction. In addition ROS can seriously affected proteins and nucleic acids, particularly ion channels and ion transporters (Halliwell & Gutteridge, 2007). Zhu et al. proved involvement of ROS in apoptosis in cardiac myocytes through p38 MAP kinase which is inhibited by CAT and SOD scavengers (Zhu et al., 1999). Cells have very little or no free iron available for catalyzing free radical reactions. However, studies have shown that redox cycling of doxorubicin directly increases the intracellular iron pool (Minotti et al., 1999; Xu et al., 2005; Xu et al., 2008). Formation of DOX semiquinone followed by $O_2^{\bullet-}$ generation is accompanied by iron releasing from ferritine. Ferritines are sphere shaped complex of 24 protein subunits with central cavity which can store up to 4500 atoms of iron. Eight channels through the sphere are lined by hydrophilic amino acid residues and six more are lined by hydrophobic residues. These transprotein channels provide the route for iron entry and exit from ferritin shell (Harrison et al., 1986; Theil, 1987). Anthracycline semiquinone is too large for entering the ferritin. However, superoxide anion is small enough to penetrate the shell and has reduction potential lower than that of polynuclear ferric oxohydroxide stored in the ferritin core. Combination of steric and thermodynamic factors thus enables $O_2^{\bullet-}$ to reach and reduce the iron pool of ferritin promoting the release of iron in its Fe(II) form through transprotein channels (Minotti, 1993; Minotti et al., 1999).

Furthermore, intracellular iron enrichment is mediated by doxorubicin and its metabolites. Cellular iron homeostasis is regulated by transferring receptor (TfR) and ferritin. Both TfR and ferritin are mainly regulated at a post-transcriptional level involving interactions of iron regulatory protein (IRP-1) and iron responsive elements (IRE) in target genes (Xu et al., 2005; Xu et al., 2008). Namely, DOX can disrupt the Fe-S cluster of cytoplasmatic aconitase and inhibit IRP-1 whose role is to adapt levels of cellular iron according to metabolic needs.

The second mechanism by which Fe promotes oxidative injury involves generation of doxorubicin-iron complexes (DOX-Fe). Anthracyclines chelate Fe(III) forming the 1:1, 2:1 or 3:1 iron complex with association constant of 10^{33} (Figure. 2b) (Beraldo et al., 1985; May et al., 1980). In the presence of reducing agents (as NADPH cytochrome P450 reductase, glutathione or cysteine) DOX-Fe (III) complex are converting into DOX-Fe (II). This reaction come along with the formation of $O_2^{\bullet-}$and conversion of quinone form of DOX to semiquinone free radical. Products of this reaction are further involving in the iron catalyzed Haber-Weiss reaction resulting in production of highly aggressive hydroxyl radicals (eq. 1-3). The semiquinone radical can be transform into C7 deoxydaglicone which is the potent alkylating agent.

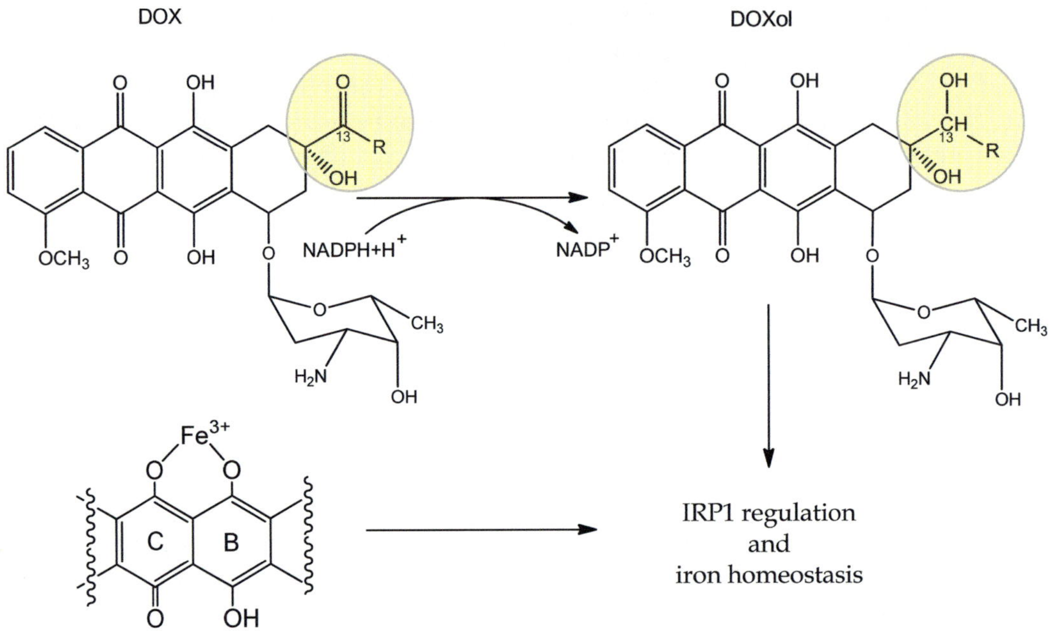

Fig. 3. Hypothesized mechanism of chronic cardiotoxicity mediated by DOXol and/or DOX-Fe complex

Different pathway of doxorubicin toxicity, other than oxidative injury, is involved in cardiac toxicity of the drug. Doxorubicinol (DOXol) is hydroxy metabolite of DOX formed upon two electron reduction on the C-13 carbonyl group of doxorubicin (Figure. 3). This reaction is catalyzed by NADPH dependent carbonyl reducatses (Forrest et al., 1991). DOXol is redox inactive and therefore not involved in free radical production. Notwithstanding, DOXol is involved in iron homeostasis (Licata et al., 2000; Minotti et al., 2001), myocardial energy metabolism, ionic gradients and calcium movements, impairing cardiac contraction and relaxation (Boucek et al., 1987; Olson, R. D. et al., 1988). Moreover, conversation of doxorubicin into DOXol significantly increases polarity of the parent drug molecule, thus favouring its retention within the cell. Considering the all aforesaid mechanisms of DOXol acting, it is logical conclusion that alcohol metabolite of doxorubicin is most likely responsible for the DOX induced chronic cardiomyopathy (Figure. 3), while iron mediated free radical injury promote acute cardiotoxicity This hypothesis is supported by findings of Miranda and co-workers which found that patients harbouring gene mutations in hereditary hemochromatosis show increased susceptibility to doxorubicin cardiotoxicity and exacerbated iron metabolism (Miranda et al., 2003). Numerous studies on transgenic mice with overexpressed antioxidants like catalase (Kang et al., 1996), superoxide dismutase (Abou El Hassan et al., 2003; Loch et al., 2009; Yen et al., 1996) and metallothionene (Kang, 1999; Kang et al., 1997; Merten et al., 2005; Sun & Kang, 2002; Sun et al., 2001) have shown beneficial against DOX induced cardiotoxicity, confirming strong involvement of free radicals in oxidative injury of the heart.

The high oxidative metabolism and the poor antioxidative defence, compared with other organs, most likely explains why the doxorubicin is selectively toxic to the heart. Compared to the liver, the cardiac antioxidant defense system is moderate. There is 150 times less catalase and four times less superoxide dismutase in the heart (Doroshow & Davies, 1986; Doroshow et al., 1980). In addition, the unique structure of cardiomyocytes, in which 50% of the cell organelles are mitochondria, serving both as a source and target for ROS, may explain why anthracycline antibiotics are selectively toxic to the heart (Berthiaume & Wallace, 2007). Cardiac mitochondria possess a NADH dehydrogenase on the outer surface of the inner mitochondrial membrane. Reduction of an anthracycline to the corresponding semiquinone by this enzyme produces an extremely high level of oxidative stress because the anthracycline transfers an electron to molecular oxygen and forms superoxide radicals. In relation to oxidative reactions, it must be emphasized that doxorubicin possess high affinity for cardiolipin, cardiospecific phospholipid that is reach in polyunsaturated fatty acids also placed in inner mitochondrial membrane. This high affinity, besides accumulation of DOX in interior of cardiomyocytes, also enables formation of DOX-cardiolipin complexes which can act as the substrate for the initiation of lipid peroxidation (Goormaghtigh & Ruysschaert, 1984). Once initiated, peroxidation continues autocatalytically, and has a progressive course that results in structural and functional changes in the heart tissue. The ultimate damage to mitochondria is oxidative damage of the mitochondrial DNA, which interferes with the regenerative capacity of the organelle. Once this irreversible damage occurs, the cardiomyocytes are destined to undergo apoptosis or necrosis, an event that may not occur until months or years after chemotherapy is completed (Davies & Doroshow, 1986; Doroshow et al., 1980). Therefore, the most significant pathological changes appear in the heart.

It is evident that there are still unknowns about exact mechanisms of the toxic effects of doxorubicin and its metabolites. In spite numerous investigations at the molecular level, iron mediated free radical injury and alteration in intracellular iron homeostasis have a key role in cardiotoxicity of anthracycline antibiotics and therefore considered classical mechanism underlying cardiac impairment induced by DOX.

2.5 Strategies for cardioprotection

Today's oncologists must be fully aware of cardiovascular risks to avoid or prevent adverse cardiovascular effects. The primary goal in the prevention is to minimise cardiac toxicities and to maximise oncological efficacy (Dorr, 1991; Schimmel et al., 2004). Currently, several preventive measures, such as: limiting cumulative dose of DOX, altering its administration, using new anthracycline analogues; combination with protective drugs and nutritional supplements are used.

2.5.1 Limiting cumulative dose of doxorubicin

Before the association between higher cumulative dose of DOX and the greater risk of cardiotoxicity was established, cumulative DOX doses greater than 400 mg/m^2 were administered to children with acute lymphoblastic leukaemia (ALL). Unfortunately, progressive cardiotoxic effects, clinically important, continued years after the DOX treatment completion (Lipshultz et al., 1991; Lipshultz et al., 2005). As a result, cumulative doses of DOX given to high-risk children and adolescent with ALL were reduced to a cumulative dose no more than 360 mg/m^2. Later on, after median follow up of 8.1 year, on the basis of obtained results, the cumulative DOX dose for high-risk ALL patients were further reduced to 300 mg/m^2 (Nysom et al., 1998). However, patients vary widely in sensitivity and these values represent relatively arbitrary choices on a continuum of risk: there is no single safe dose (Shan et al., 1996; Von Hoff et al., 1979). Studies of late-onset anthracycline cardiotoxicity in childhood cancer survivors indicate that doses of DOX as low as 100 mg/m^2 increase the risk of reduced fractional shortening and higher afterload, whereas a cumulative dose of 270 mg/m^2 increases the risk of such abnormalities 4.5-fold. Even at doses that produce no symptoms, subclinical myocardial damage may occur, and in children this may result in diminished cardiac reserve and heart disease in later life (Hale & Lewis, 1994; Lipshultz et al., 1991).

2.5.2 Altering doxorubicin administration

Alteration of the dosage schedule to weekly rather than three-weekly dosage, or the use of continuous infusion, has also been advocated as a way of reducing doxorubicin cardiotoxicity (Legha et al., 1982a; Lum et al., 1985; Torti et al., 1983). At the same time, it was believed that continuous infusion might provide some cardioprotective benefits, because long-term exposures to drugs at modest concentrations would be safer than a pulsed supply of the drug at higher concentrations. Therefore, it was incorporated in many pediatric protocols although the comparative efficacy of these dosage schedules in various cancers and long-term effects on the development of DOX-induced cardiotoxicity have not been established tz (Lipshultz et al., 2005; Lipshultz et al., 2010). However, recently published meta-analysis performed to clarify the risk of early and late cardiotoxicity of anthracycline agents in patients treated for breast or ovarian cancer, lymphoma, myeloma or sarcoma showed that DOX given as bolus significantly increased the risk of clinical and subclinical cardiotoxicity compared with continuous infusion.

2.5.3 Use of doxorubicin-analogues

Several anthracycline derivatives have been developed with the aim of reducing the inherent cardiotoxicity of this class of compounds, including esorubicin, quelamycin, rodorubicin, and detorubicin. However, although this strategy has had some success, it turned out that almost all these compounds exhibit some degree of cardiotoxicity (Aronson et al., 2006; Sweetman, 2011; Weiss, 1992; Wouters et al., 2005). Epirubicin, idarubicin and mitoxantrone are the most promising ones. In the recently performed meta-analysis epirubicin significantly decreased the risk of clinical cardiotoxicity OR 0.39 (0.16, 0.57; $p<0.008$; $I^2 = 0.5\%$), as well as any cardiotoxic event compared with DOX (Smith et al., 2010).

2.5.4 New drug-delivery systems and doxorubicin application

A promising approach to increase the efficacy and decrease the side-effects of DOX is its binding to drug delivery system, such as liposomes, nanoparticles and different cancer-targeting systems. Among the structural modifications of DOX, the liposome-encapsulated, is the one of the most promising cardioprotectants (Ludke et al., 2009). Liposomes are preferentially taken up by tissues enriched in phagocytic reticuloendothelial cells and with a sinusoidal capillary system like the liver and spleen. The continuous capillaries containing tissues, like heart muscle hardly take up liposomes, but it is not the case with the leaky capillary system of tumor site. Thus, the changes in tissue distribution of liposomal DOX lead to less drug exposure in sensitive organs. The ability to reduce the plasma levels of free DOX is probably the source of the reduced cardiotoxicity provided by its liposomal formulation (Fulbright et al., 2010). Also, the release of drug is slow, which may avoid high peak plasma concentrations. It exists both in pegylated lyposomal and, at the moment, these two formulations are approved for clinical use by the US Food and Drug Administration (Ludke et al., 2009; Sweetman, 2011). Several randomized clinical trial in adults have examined the activity and cardiotoxicity of liposomal DOX. Most of them indicated that the activity of liposomal DOX is similar to that of conventional, whether given alone or in combination with other drugs. At the same time, the risk of cardiotoxicity is markedly lower with liposomal DOX (Gianni et al., 2008; McEvoy et al., 2010; Safra, 2003; Smith et al., 2010). However, although clinically approved, conventional DOX continues to be the major drug in antineoplastic combinations used in the management of most solid tumors. Nanoparticles made of biodegradable polymers are particles with sizes in range from 20 to 200 nm that can encapsulate hydrophilic or hydrophobic drugs. Drugs delivered by nanotechnology delivery systems have a prolonged time in the circulation (Ferrari, 2005). Although carbon nanotubes and gold nanoparticles have demonstrated potential as a new drug delivery system, clinical use has been restricted due to concerns regarding their biodegradability (Liu et al., 2008). These particles should link with tumor-targeting ligands, such as peptides and small molecules. At the moment, DOX nanoparticles shows great promise in improving the oral bioavailability and reducing cardiotoxicity, but so many issues wait to be resolved in the future (Kalaria et al., 2009).

2.5.5 Combination with protective drugs

Apart from cumulative dose limitations, several attempts have been made to develop chemoprotectants to prevent the cardiotoxicity of DOX, without attenuating its antitumor effect. Following the aforementioned free radical hypothesis, antioxidants used as free radical scavengers have been examined both in experiments, and in clinical trials. On the other hand, considering a very important role of iron and the DOX-iron complex, iron chelators have also been used for prevention of DOX-induced cardiotoxicity (Dorr, 1991; Links & Lewis, 1999; Simunek et al., 2009).

3. Dexrazoxane

One of the most examined protectors against DOX cardiotoxicity is dexrazoxane (DEX). Activity of DEX against DOX-induced cardiotoxicity may be attributable to the intracellular conversion of DEX to an open-ring derivative ADR-925 which chelates iron, since one means of generating oxygen-free radicals may involve intramolecular reduction of DOX-iron conjugate. The cardioprotective activity of DEX is thought to result primarily from chelation of free and/or DOX-bound ferric ions in the myocardium by ADR-925 and some other hydrolysis products of DEX (Dorr, 1996; Hasinoff, 1989). As a result, the pool of free iron in the myocardium is reduced and bound iron is displaced from its potentially damaging complexes with DOX, thus preventing the formation of superoxide radicals after redox recycling. DEX has been shown experimentally to reduce DOX-induced cardiotoxicity in mice (Alderton et al., 1990); in rats (Della Torre et al., 1999; Herman et al., 1994; Villani et al., 1990); in beagle dogs (Herman et al., 1988) and in miniature swine (Herman & Ferrans,

1983). Treatment with DEX not only significantly reduced the incidence of cardiac lesions, but also increased the survival rate in animals treated with anthracyclines compared with anthracycline-only treated controls. Actually, DEX allowed administration of significantly larger cumulative doses of DOX, that otherwise would have been lethal in these animal models (Wiseman & Spencer, 1998). Studies in rats and beagle dogs have shown that DEX is generally more effective when administered shortly before or simultaneously with, rather than after DOX. In randomized, controlled trials, DEX provided effective cardioprotection in both adults and children receiving DOX chemotherapy for various malignancies (Lipshultz et al., 2004; Lopez et al., 1998; Speyer et al., 1992; Swain et al., 1997; Venturini et al., 1996; Wexler et al., 1996). In recent meta - analysis, data on clinical heart failure from eight trials with a total of 1561 patients were collected (van Dalen et al., 2011a). There were 11 cases of clinical heart failure among 769 patients randomised to DEX and 69 among 792 randomised to the control group. The meta-analysis showed a benefit in favour of DEX use (RR 0.18, 95% CI 0.10 to 0.32, $P < 0.00001$). In another 6 randomized clinical trials which evaluated cardioprotective agent DEX, four on women with advanced breast cancer, one with young people with sarcoma and one with breast cancer or sarcoma DEX given with DOX significantly reduced the risk of clinical cardiotoxicity, subclinical cardiotoxicity and any cardiotoxic event compared with DOX with no cardioprotective agent (Smith et al., 2010). Data on response rate (defined as the number of patients in complete and partial remission) could be extracted from six trials with a total of 1021 patients. These trials used comparable criteria to assess tumour response. There were 223 complete and partial responses among 503 patients randomised to DEX and 260 among 518 randomised to the control group. Meta-analysis showed no significant difference between the treatment groups. However, an important question regarding any cardioprotective intervention during DOX therapy is whether the cardioprotective drug could decrease the heart damage by anthracyclines without reducing the anti-tumour efficacy and without negative effects on toxicities other than cardiac damage. At the moment, despite its clear cardioprotective effects, DEX is not routinely used in clinical practice. This might be explained by the suspicion of interference with anti-tumour efficacy (that is response rate and survival) and by the occurrence of secondary malignant disease. However, meta-analyses of DOX anti-tumour efficacy and the appearance of secondary malignant diseases showed no significant difference between patients who were treated with or without DEX (van Dalen et al., 2011a). This latter finding was also identified in a recent publication (van Dalen et al., 2011b). A meta-analysis including three of the four randomised trials available on secondary malignancies after DEX, did not show a significant difference in the occurrence of secondary malignancies between children treated with or without DEX (RR 1.16, 95% CI 0.06 to 22.17, P = 0.92). The protective effects of DEX against DOX-induced cardiotoxicity are further supported by studies in children with leukemias and lymphomas, as well as with other malignancies (Lipshultz et al., 2010; Testore et al., 2008). However, further research is needed to fully understand the subtle risks associated with the use of DEX, as well as which methods of DEX administration are most efficient, and which doses are necessary to achieve adequate protection in children. At the moment, DEX is the only cardioprotective agent with proven efficacy in cancer patients receiving DOX. DEX is approved in many countries, including the United States, Canada, and a number of European countries. Current guidelines support the use of DEX for patients with metastatic breast cancer who have received more than 300

mg/m^2 of DOX in metastatic setting and who may benefit from continued DOX-containing therapy; treatment of patients who received more than 300 mg/m^2 in the adjuvant setting should be individualized, with consideration given to the potential for DEX to decrease response rates as well as decreasing the risk of cardiac toxicity. It should not be used for patients with metastatic breast cancer receiving initial DOX-based chemotherapy (Hensley et al., 2009; McEvoy et al., 2010; Sweetman, 2011). There is insufficient evidence to make recommendation for the use of DEX in the treatment of pediatric malignancies. It can be considered in adult patients who have received more than 300 mg/m^2 of DOX-based therapy for patients with advanced or metastatic cancer who have previously received anthracyclines. However, since DEX may potentiate haematological toxicity induced by chemotherapy, or the results for these adverse effects are ambiguous, for each individual patient a physician should balance the cardioprotective effects of DEX against the possible risk of adverse side effects (Ludke et al., 2009; van Dalen et al., 2011a). In addition, DEX appears equally well tolerated when administered with DOX at either 10:1 or 20:1 dosage ratios (e.g. if 50 mg/m^2 of DOX is used, 500 mg/m^2 DEX should be given). A reconstituted DEX solution should be given intravenously by slow push or rapid-drip infusion from a bag, starting 15-30 minutes before DOX administration. The optimal treatment regimen and cost effectiveness of DEX, and its protective efficacy against late-onset cardiotoxicity in patients given DOX chemotherapy during childhood or adolescence, are yet to be determined (Cvetkovic & Scott, 2005). On September 6, 2007, the U.S. Food and Drug Administration approved Totect® 500 mg, (dexrazoxane hydrochloride for injection) for the treatment of extravasation resulting from i.v. anthracycline therapy, an uncommon but serious complication (Kane et al., 2008). From all these facts, it can be concluded that well-designed cardioprotective intervention, like usage of DEX, can be an effective option as a strategy for DOX-induced cardiotoxicity prevention. Moreover, our ability to develop drugs such as DEX depends on our understanding of the molecular mechanisms involved in both antineoplastic and cardiotoxic effects of DOX. As it has been already mentioned, the current prevailing hypothesis is that DEX exerts its cardioprotective effects by binding free Fe, loosely bound Fe and Fe complexed to DOX, thus enabling the prevention of site-specific oxygen radicals production that damages cellular components of the heart (Cvetkovic & Scott, 2005; Dorr, 1996; Hasinoff, 1989). However, none of the other Fe chelating agents examined (aroylhydrazone iron chelators, defepirone etc) has reached the high protective efficacy of DEX. On the other hand, ADR-925 has a lower affinity for Fe than other helators, so it can be concluded that the iron-chelating properties of a compound are not the main determinants of cardioprotective action (Kaiserova et al., 2007). In recent experimental study it was clearly shown that DEX exerted protective effect against chronic daunorubicin cardiotoxicity *in vivo* (rabbits). Its cardioprotectiveness was based on the rescue of cardiomyocytes not only from degenerative changes and non-programmed cell death, but also from programmed cell death (apoptosis), as well (Popelova et al., 2009). Actually, DEX was shown to block all the major apoptotic pathways, and, therefore, protection of cardiomyocytes did not seem to be primarily lipoperoxidation-dependent. Apart from all the aforementioned, it is already known that DEX binds directly to topoisomerase II and locks the enzyme in a stable and closed clamp conformation around DNA (Roca et al., 1994). Since, anthracyclines are, as already mentioned, topoisomerase II inhibitor, it has been proposed that DEX may have protective effects against such agents in this way (Lyu et al.,

2007). In addition, beta isoform of topoisomerase II is abundant in post-mitotic myocardium, including mitochondria (Wallace, 2007; Wang, 2002). It was also previously mentioned that DOX impairs calcium homeostasis in cardiomyocytes, not only affecting sarcoplasmic reticulum function, but also mitochondria (Minotti et al., 2004). The fact that anthracycline-induced calcium overload can be prevented with DEX, co-treatment gives one more explanation for its cardioprotective efficacy (Simunek et al., 2005). Namely, it was shown that systolic heart failure induced by chronic daunorubicin administration is primarily accompanied by persistent calcium overload of cardiac tissue and the protective action of DEX is associated with the restoration of normal myocardial Ca^{2+} content. Therefore, mechanisms other than the traditionally accepted "ROS and iron" hypothesis are involved in DOX-induced cardiotoxicity, and knowledge of them may be a better basis for designing approaches to achieve efficient and safe cardioprotection.

4. Amifostine

Amifostine is a simple aminothiol compound that is a product of a developmental program initiated in 1959 by the United States Army, in studies conducted at the Walter Reed Institute of Research to identify and synthesize drugs capable of conferring protection to individuals working in radioactive environments (Dragojevic-Simic & Dobric, 1996; van der Vijgh & Peters, 1994). As a result of this program, over 4,000 compounds were synthesized and tested. Amifostine, code named WR-2721, emerged as the lead compound. The drug was modeled after experimental studies, which showed reduced bone marrow toxicity when the sulfur-containing amino acid cysteine was administered before total body irradiation. It was the first cytoprotective agent to be identified as being capable of differentially protecting nonmalignant (normal) versus malignant cells from the cytotoxic effects of ionizing radiation and some antineoplastic agents (Yuhas, 1979; Yuhas et al., 1980; Yuhas & Storer, 1969). Amifostine itself is an organic phosphorothioate that is inactive until it is dephosporylated by alkaline phosphatase to yeald the active free thiol (SH) form, code named WR-1065 (Yuhas, 1980). Selectivity, in terms of cytoprotection of normal tissue, preferentially, is believed to be related to differential distribution and absorbption of the parent drug in better perfused normal tissues as well as greater alkaline phosphatase acitivity in normal tissues, related to the acidic pH values found in hypoxic tumor tissues (Calabro-Jones et al., 1988; Dragojevic-Simic & Dobric, 1996; Smoluk et al., 1988; Utley et al., 1984; Yuhas, 1980). Normal tissues, especially at the capillary level, have a higher specific activity of alkaline phosphatase which releases WR-1065 for rapid local uptake into normal tissues. In contrast, the activity of this enzyme in neoplastic capilaries is appreciable lower, a feature that contributes to this apparently selective uptake. It was also demonstrated that the rate constant for the uptake of WR-1065 across the cell membrane is accelerated with small differences in pH, favouring the pH of 7.4, which is found in normal tissues versus relative acidity in tumors (Calabro-Jones et al., 1988). Tissue distribution studies, performed in experimental animals, demonstrated the uptake of amifostine and its metabolite. Kidney, bladder, salivary gland and liver accumulate high level of drug; heart, small intestine and spleen accumulate it moderately, while the spinal cord, brain and tumours accumulate very little, if any (Utley et al., 1976; Washburn et al., 1976; Yuhas, 1980). The "ideal cytoprotector" should have: the ability to be administered before or concurrent with therapy, selectivity for normal versus cancer cells, ability to prevent/reduce toxicities of chemotherapies, no adverse effects on therapeutic efficacy, effectiveness against a variety of therapy-associated toxicities, a tolerable safety profile and simple way of administration (Capizzi, 1999b; Mabro et al., 1999; Spencer & Goa, 1995). The aforementioned findings concerning amifostine prompted numerous preclinical and clinical studies and led to the ultimate marketing approval many years later (Hensley et al., 2009). The American Society of Clinical Oncology recommends amifostine for prevention of cisplatin-associated nephrotoxicity, reduction of grade 3 and 4 neutropenia (alternative strategies are reasonable), and to decrease acute and late xerostomia with fractionated radiation therapy alone for head and neck cancer. The current US Food and Drug Administration-approved dose of amifostine is 910 mg/m^2 intravenously over 15 minutes, 30 minutes before chemotherapy. Common toxicities include acute hypotension, nausea, and fatigue. When given with radiation therapy, the recommended amifostine dose is 200 $mg/m^2/day$, as slow i.v. push over 3 minutes, 15 to 30 minutes before each fraction of radiation therapy. The hypotension associated with amifostine at this dose is less frequent, but still requires close monitoring (Hensley et al., 2009; McEvoy et al., 2010; Sweetman, 2011). As aforementioned, if administered before cytotoxic chemotherapy, amifostine provides cytoprotection of various normal tissues, with the exception of central nervous system, without attenuating its antitumor response (Capizzi, 1999a; Culy & Spencer, 2001; Dragojevic-Simic & Dobric, 1996; Kouvaris et al., 2007; Mabro et al., 1999; Spencer & Goa, 1995). It protects the bone marrow against both the harmful effects of ionizing radiation as well as cyclophosphamide, nitrogen mustard, melphalan, mitomicin C, carmustine, 5-fluorouracil, carboplatin and cisplatin. Protection from cisplatin nephrotoxicity and ototoxicity has been shown, as well as protection of peripheral neural tissue from cisplatin, paclitaxel, vincristine and vinblastine toxicity. However, data concerning amifostine efficacy in preventing the toxic effects of DOX are still insufficient (Bolaman et al., 2005; Dobric et al., 1998; Dragojevic-Simic et al., 2004; Nazeyrollas et al., 1999; Potemski et al., 2006). As previously mentioned, amifostine uptake has been documented to be relatively high in normal tissues compared with experimental tumors. Moreover, sixty minutes after amifostine injection, level in heart tissues was approximately sevenfold higher than in tumor and sixfold higher than in serum (Dorr, 1996; Yuhas, 1980). These tissue distribution studies suggest that apart from the bone marrow, salivary gland and kidneys, the heart might also benefit from cytoprotection provided by amifostine treatment prior to cardiotoxic radio- and chemotherapy. In our previous experiment in which general radioprotective efficacy of amifostine was examined in rats subjected to whole body irradiation (WBI, absolutely lethal dose of X-rays), it was shown that amifostine significantly protected rats and increased their survival comparing to the unprotected animals (Dobric et al., 2007; Trajkovic et al., 2007). Moreover, a mean cardiac damage (MCD) score, obtained by histopathological analysis, in amifostine-pretreated rats was significantly reduced compared with unprotected animals, on both days 7 and 28 after WBI. It has been supposed for a long time, according to data derived from the experiments with irradiated animals, that once inside the cell, protective effects of WR-1065 appear to be mediated by scavenging free radicals, hydrogen donation, induction of cellular hypoxia, the liberation of endogenous nonprotein sulfhydrils (mainly glutathione) from their bond with cell proteins, the formation of mixed disulphides to protect normal cells, etc (Brown, 1967; Grdina et al., 1995; Smoluk et al., 1988; Spencer & Goa, 1995). On the other hand, previous *in vitro* studies demonstrated that amifostine, and especially WR-1065, was able to scavenge OH. and O_2.⁻, including DOX-derived O_2.⁻ generated by NADH respiration of heart mitochondria particles. Marzatico et al., (2000) showed that amifostine scavenging activity is exerted mainly against highly reactive OH. , the most dangerous reactive oxygen species from a biological point of view (Marzatico et al., 2000). It was also shown that both amifostine and WR-1065 protected cultured neonatal rat cardiac myocytes against DOX-induced loss of cell viability (Dorr et al., 1996). These results had clinical relevance since they showed that the exposure concentrations of amifostine and WR-1065 were limited to 2.0 µg/ml, which was 10% of the peak plasma level achieved in humans given intravenous amifostine 740 mg/m^2 (Shaw et al., 1988). Effects of amifostine on perfused isolated rat heart and on acute DOX-induced cardiotoxicity were also examined (Nazeyrollas et al., 1999). Amifostine induced coronary vazodilatation, and, when associated with cardiotoxic concentrations of DOX, displayed cardioprotective effects, but the mechanism of its action was not elucidated. Moreover, *in vivo* experiments demonstrated that selective cytoprotection against DOX-induced toxicity with amifostine and WR-1065 can be achieved without abrogating antitumor activity of DOX (Bhanumathi et al., 1994; Dorr, 1996; Spencer & Goa, 1995). In our own previous study (Dobric et al., 2003; Dragojevic-Simic et al., 2004) the efficacy of amifostine (75 mg/kg *ip*) in reducing the cardiotoxicity of DOX in Wistar rats given in a dose of 1.25 mg/kg *ip*, 4 times per week, for 4 weeks was examined. Amifostine was administered each time, 20 min. before DOX. Mortality, general condition and body weight of animals were observed, while evaluation of cardioprotective efficacy of amifostine was performed by analyzing the ECG parameters, response to pro-arrhythmic agent aconitine, as well as activity registration of the *in situ* rat heart preparations. The pretreatment with amifostine significantly reduced mortality of rats comparing with unprotected group and reversed the arrhythmogenic dose of aconitine to values not significantly different from the control ones. It also antagonized DOX depressive effects on heart contractility. Moreover, a MCD score, obtained by histopathological analysis, in amifostine-pretreated rats was significantly reduced compared with unprotected animals, 4 weeks after the last dose of treatment. Also, amifostine significantly decreased number of mast cells in the heart in DOX-treated rats. Although mast cells could also be seen everywhere in the myocardium, they were predominantly situated around the blood vessels, like in control. Some other investigations in which rats were subjected to relatively high, cumulative dose of DOX, also showed protective effects of amifostine (Herman et al., 2000; Nazeyrollas et al., 2003). Amifostin dose was in range from 7 to 200 mg/kg, depending on the experimental model employed. However, concerning the methodology used, it was not possible to give some solid evidence about the amifostine molecular mechanism of action. We supposed that amifostine protected cardiomyocytes plasmalemma owing to its scavenging activity, and influenced the duration of action potential, especially the recovery phase and Ca^{2+} movement across the cellular membrane (Dragojevic-Simic et al., 2004). This might have contributed to the reduction of subsequent signalling pathways caused by DOX, since its detrimental effect eventually led to myofibrillar degeneration. Although there are some other opinions, our own results, as well as results obtained by other authors, support the statement that acute and chronic toxicity of DOX share the same mechanisms and, accordingly, chronic toxicity arises from repeated episodes of acute exposure, inducing cumulative damage (Dragojevic-Simic et al., 2011a; Dragojevic-Simic et al., 2004; Jensen,

1986; Luo et al., 1997; Pelikan et al., 1986). Thus, not only formation of highly reactive oxygen species, especially OH. , should be blamed for acute, as well as chronic DOX cardiotoxicity, but also their scavenging could be the main mechanisms of amifostine protection against both types of toxicities. According to Luo et al., (1997), reactive oxygen species, by inducing lipid peroxidation, after application of DOX produce cytotoxic aldehydes which result in inflamatory reactions (Luo et al., 1997). This eventually leads to increased synthesis of cytokines, infiltration of mononuclear cells and death of heart cells. In accordance with that, in our already described experiment (Dragojevic-Simic et al., 2004), the presence of mononuclear cells and fibroblasts was decreased in amifostine-protected rats compared with DOX-only treated group, and the necrotic cardiomyocytes were very rare. It has already been demonstrated that reactive oxygen species are increasingly produced by inflammatory cells in response to stimulation by cytokines such as TNF-α, IL-1, IL-6 and IL-17 and play an important role as messengers of the intracellular signaling pathways (Babbar & Casero, 2006; Jamaluddin et al., 2007). It was suggested that ROS, in turn, activate inflammatory cells that have part in the progression of inflammation. Therefore, targeting ROS may have a therapeutic value as a strategy to reduce the development of inflammation. It was already shown that amifostine, given in doses of 186 mg/kg *per os*, showed significant reduction of paw oedema in the carrageenan-induced paw inflammation in mice, comparable to that achieved by aspirin (Bhutia et al., 2010). Moreover, in our previous experiments amifostine reduced carrageenan-induced rat paw oedema achieving high degree of anti-inflammatory activity. Given in doses of 100, 200 and 300 mg/kg, *ip* 30 min before carrageenan challenge, it significantly reduced footpad swelling being the most effective in the highest dose tested (Dragojevic-Simic et al., 2011b). Therefore, anti-inflammatory effects of amifostine can contribute to its protective effects in DOX-induced cardiotoxicity. On the other hand, in our previous experiments amifostine provided significant protective effects against early toxic changes in rat heart induced by single high doses of DOX (6 and 10 mg/kg *iv*) (Dobric et al., 1998; Dragojevic-Simic et al., 2007; Dragojevic-Simic et al., 2011a). Amifostine (300 mg/kg *ip*, 30 min, before DOX) successfully prevented significantly increased activity of CK, AST, LDH and α-HBDH enzymes, as well as malondialdehyde (MDA) level in the serum of animals treated with DOX in a dose of 6mg/kg. In a similar experimental model Bolaman et al (2005) showed that MDA level was lower, and glutathione and catalase levels were higher in the hearts of amifostine-pretreated group of animals comparing to unprotected rats (Bolaman et al., 2005). In our experiment (Dragojevic-Simic et al., 2011a) the application of amifostine in rats treated with DOX dose of 10 mg/kg reduced MCD score to the value obtained in the group of rats treated with 6 mg/kg of DOX, only. The ultrastructural analysis (UA) showed that pretreatment with amifostine in rats which received 6mg/kg of DOX successfully protected sarcolemma of cardiomyocytes, while the mitochondria damage in the protected group was far less prominent. Capillaries were less morphologically changed and apoptosis of endothelial cells was extremely rare in comparison with non-treated animals. The UA of the rat heart 48 hours after administration of 6mg/kg of DOX in this experiment revealed cardiomyocyte alterations described as *oncosis*. This is in accordance with the results of other authors, who also showed that the earliest and most often changes in the rat heart after application of high doses of DOX were cellular oedema and swelling of the mitochondria in cardiomyocytes. On the other hand, low-dose DOX exposure induced apoptosis of these cells (L'Ecuyer et al., 2004; Olson, H. M. & Capen, 1977; Simunek et al., 2009; Zhang, Y. W. et al., 2009). Our findings concerning prominent protection of mitochondria with amifostine are in line with widely accepted hypothesis that mitochondria are a primary target of DOX-induced oxidative stress (Berthiaume & Wallace, 2007; Grdina et al., 2002). It is also known that amifostine is negative charged thiol and this protector accumulates within the mitochondria and around DNA, explaining higher protective amifostine potential for them than neutral or positive charged thiols, especially since some studies using perfused rat hearts showed that DOX is localized primarilly to the nucleus and mitochondria of the cell (Berthiaume & Wallace, 2007). It was also shown that both amifostine and WR-1065 significantly reduced DOX-induced heart cell toxicity, measured by ATP content normalised to total cellular protein (Marzatico et al., 2000). This finding can also be explained by effective protection of mitochondria, as in our study, since oxidative phosphorylation is one of the functions of this organelae which provides a substantial portion of the ATP needed to meet energy demands in the heart. On the other hand, as already mentioned, several lines of evidence suggest that amifostine is presumably modified into WR-1065 by membrane-bound alkaline phosphatase, highly expressed in the endothelium, It quickly penetrates into cells, where it acts as free-radicals scavengers and protects cells from oxidative damage (Calabro-Jones et al., 1988; Dragojevic-Simic & Dobric, 1996; Smoluk et al., 1988; Utley et al., 1984; Yuhas, 1980). Potent protective effects of amifostine pretreatment in the model of lipopolysaccharide (LPS) -induced lung injury *in vivo* and attenuation of pulmonary endothelial cell barrier dysfunction *in vitro via* attenuation of oxidative stress, inhibition of redox-sensitive MAP kinases, NF-κB inflammatory cascade, as well as attenuation of LPS-induced cytosceletal remodeling and disruption of endothelial cell adhesions leading to the preservation of endothelial cell monolayer integrity were shown (Fu et al., 2009). On the other hand, marked elevatation of the expression of antioxidant gene manganese superoxide dismutase (MnSOD) in human microvascular endothelial cells following their exposure to a WR-1065 can result in elevated resistance to the cytotoxic effects of ionizing radiation. Namely, MnSOD is nuclear-encoded mitochondrial enzyme that scavenges $O_2.^-$ in mitochondrial matrix, and has been shown to be highly protective against radiation-induced ROS (Murley et al., 2006). Based on the current data, we speculate that succesful amifostine protection of DOX-induced damage of heart capillaries, whose endothelium, as a rich source of oxidants, contributes a lot to the oxidant-rich environment at that locus in this model (Dobric et al., 1998; Dragojevic-Simic et al., 2007; Dragojevic-Simic et al., 2011a), may be mediated by its antioxidant properties resulting in downregulation of oxidative stress and redox-sensitive signalling cascades. It is obvious that mechanisms of amifostine protection against DOX-induced cardiotoxicity, different from traditionally emphasized "scavenging free radicals" are also involved in amifostine-induced cardioprotection. Therefore, not only further preclinical and clinical studies are needed in order to implement amifostine in everyday oncological practice more succesfully, but also they should enable further progress in elucidation of DOX cardiotoxicity mechanisms, which represent a perpetual enigma.

5. Fullerenol $C_{60}(OH)_{24}$

With discovery of fullerene, 25 years ago (Kroto et al., 1985), started new era in chemical sciences. Fullerene, the third carbon allotrope, is a classical engineered material with the potential application in biomedicine. Spherical fullerene C_{60}, known as backyball, is the most representative member of the fullerene family. With the shape of an icosahedron, containing 12 pentagons and 20 hexagons (Hirsch & Brettreich, 2005; Kratschmer et al.,

1990), C_{60} become symbol of symmetry in chemistry and important member of nanomaterials family (Figure. 4). Unique physical and chemical properties, made backyball to quickly find its application in the material science, electronics and nanotechnology.

The biological activities of fullerenes are considerably influenced by their chemical modifications and light treatment. The most relevant feature of fullerene C_{60} is the ability to act as a free radical scavenges. Properties attributed to the delocalized π double bond system of fullerene cage allow C_{60} to quench various free radicals more efficiently than conventional antioxidants. The chemical modification of fullerenes by adding the OH groups to their carbon surface yields a variety of polyhydroxylated structures $C_{60}(OH)_x$ exhibiting different degrees of solubility and antioxidant activity in the aqueous environment (Xing et al., 2004; Zhang, Jian-Min et al., 2004). Polyhydroxylated derivate of fullerene - fullerenol ($C_{60}(OH)_{24}$) was synthesized in alkaline media by complete substitution of bromine atoms of $C_{60}Br_{24}$, with hydroxyl groups (Figure. 5.). New polyhydroxylated derivate completely maintains symmetry of parent C_{60} molecule(Djordjevic et al., 2005). Combination of the moderate electron affinity of fullerenol and their allylic hydroxyl functional groups makes fullerenol a suitable candidate for water-soluble antioxidants in biological systems.

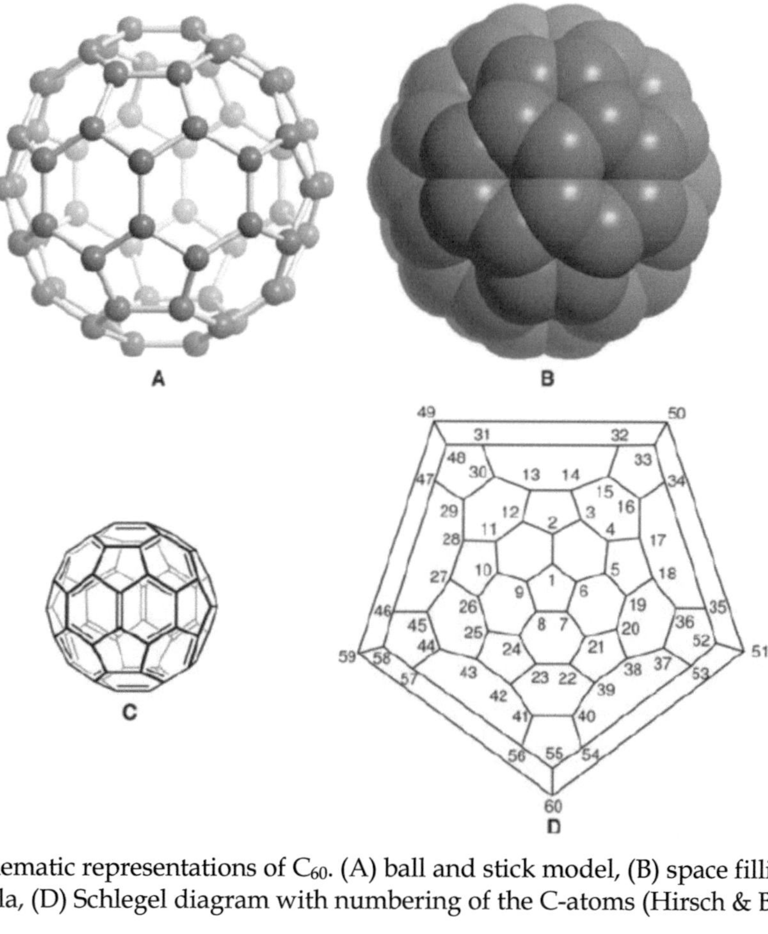

Fig. 4. Schematic representations of C_{60}. (A) ball and stick model, (B) space filling model, (C) VB formula, (D) Schlegel diagram with numbering of the C-atoms (Hirsch & Brettreich, 2005).

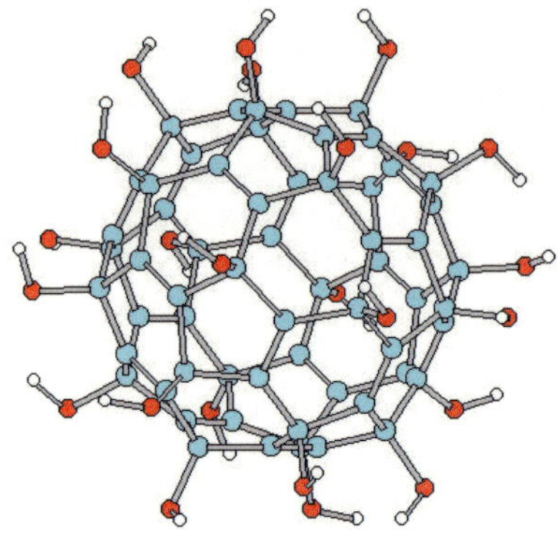

Fig. 5. Molecular structure of fullerenol

Fullerenol $C_{60}(OH)_{24}$ exhibited antioxidative activity in nanomolar concentrations in dose dependent manner against stable 2,2-diphenyl-1-picrylhydrzyl (DPPH) radical and hydroxyl radical ($OH^{\bullet}$) during the Fenton reaction using electron spin resonance (ESR) spectroscopy. Higher concentrations of fullerenol (0.71 - 0.88 mmol/L) stronger suppress production of hydroxyl radical than DPPH radical (Djordjevic et al., 2005). Authors suggested two possible mechanisms of antioxidative activity of fullerenol: (i) radical addition reaction of 2n ·OH radicals to remaining olefin double bonds of fullerenol core to yield $C_{60}(OH)_{24}$+2n·OH (n=1-12) and (ii) simultaneous hydrogen atom donation to DPPH and ·OH including the formation of relatively stable fullerenol radical $C_{60}(OH)_{23}O$ (Figure. 6.) (Djordjevic et al., 2005). These mechanisms are not mutually excluded. Studies of antioxidative activity of fullerenol, imply that fullerenol $C_{60}(OH)_{24}$ has the ability to act both as an iron chelator and as a direct free radical scavenger. Study with hydroxyfullerene and metal salts demonstrated that fullerenols react rapidly and irreversibly with variety of metal salts within the pH range of 3.0-8.5, forming insoluble metal-hydroxifullerene cross-linked polymers (Anderson & Barron, 2005).

Extensive *in vivo* studies on antioxidative protection of fullerenol against DOX induced toxicity were done. It was found that pretreatment with 100 mg/kg of fullerenol, succeed to abolish acute toxic effects on the heart, caused by single dose application of doxorubicin (10 mg/kg i.p.)(Milic Torres et al., 2010). Previous studies have shown that application of doxorubicin causes damage of the heart and baroreceptors, which is indicated by reflex alterations (Rabelo et al., 2001). Results of this study showed that in DOX treated animals the reflexes were maintained, but their appearance was delayed, which implies the presence of some heart damage. Fullerenol in both applied doses (50 and 100 mg/kg i.p.) almost completely annulated this DOX induced disturbance and the time for appearance of adrenaline-induced reflex bradicardia in ECG record was in the level of control values. The most intensive cardiac histopathological changes, induced by DOX, were noticeable by light microscopy on the 14th day after the treatment. Fullerenol applied as a pretreatment, in dosage of 100 mg/kg, exerted protection and sustained structural integrity of the cardiac cells in DOX treated animals (Figure. 7.). Fullerenol, applied alone, in dosage of 100 mg/kg caused mild vascular changes, which are likely to be reversible. Both applied dosages (50 and 100 mg/kg) used as a pretreatment, maintained the majority of investigated parameters (biochemical and parameters of oxidative stress) in the level of control values.

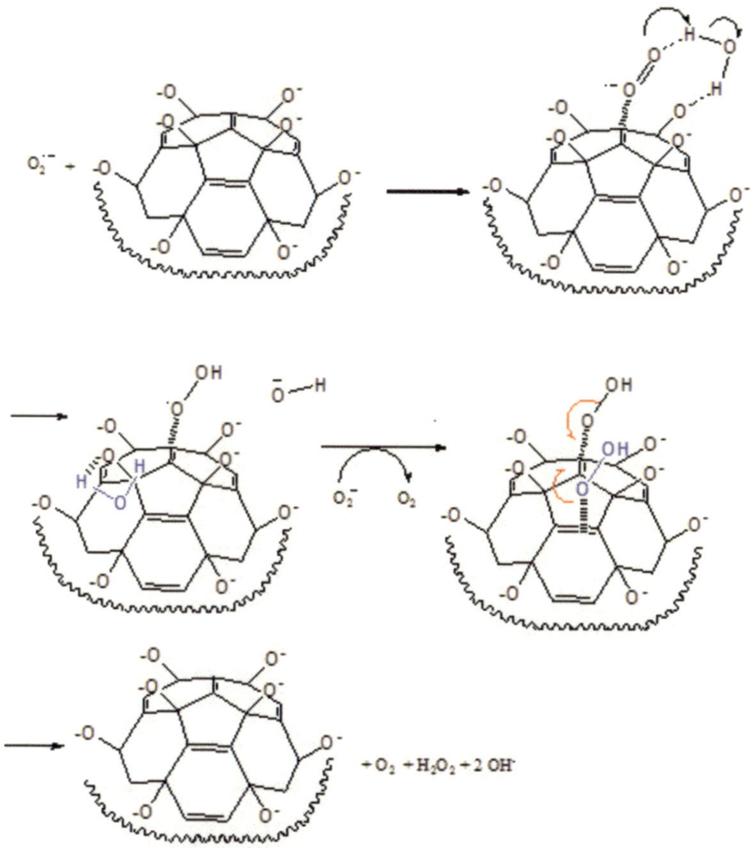

Fig. 6. Hypothesized mechanisms of fullerenol antioxidant activity

This indicates the protective effect of polyhydroxylated fullerene. Results of work Milic Torres et al., confirm the hypothesis and complete the previously conducted investigation that indicated that fullerenol possess high antioxidative and cytoprotective potential, without any recorded side effect. Considering mechanisms of DOX toxicity (predominantly based on free radical production), previous investigation and results obtained in our experiment, it can be concluded that protective role of fullerenol is established on its high antioxidative potential. Regarding to unique electrochemical features, fullerenol exerts its antioxidant effect acting as a free radical sponge and/or removing of free iron through formation of fullerenol-iron complex and therefore enable further reaction with cell damaging by ROS .

Protection against acute doxorubicin-induced toxicity was confirmed on other examinated parameters red blood cells (Djorjdevic-Milic et al., 2009), liver (Milic Torres V. et al. unpublished results), kidneys, lungs, and testicles, caused by administration of DOX in healthy Wistar rats (Srdjenovic et al., 2010).

Injac et al., evaluated protective effect of $C_{60}(OH)_{24}$ on acute tissue oxidative injury mediated by single application of doxorubicin (8 mg/kg, i.p.) on female Sprague-Dawley rats with chemically induced mammary carcinomas. In this study, ultrastructural analysis of

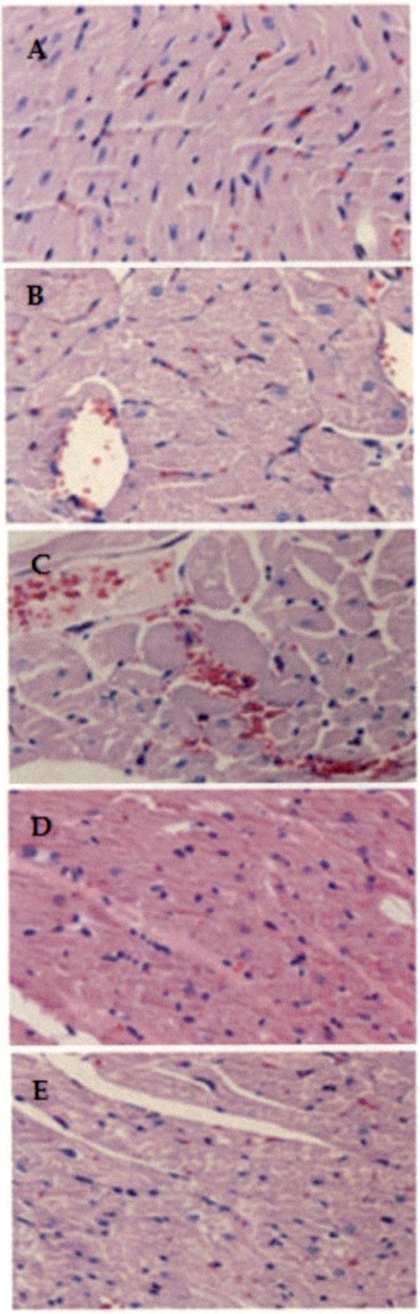

Fig. 7. Histological section of the heart (HE, 40x): A) control group - no histological lesions found; B) group treated with doxorubicin - appearance of numerous vacuoles, total degeneration of normal tissue structure C) group treated with 50mg/kg of fullerenol 30 min. prior doxorubicin - focal hemorraghia, total degeneration of myocytes ; D) group treated with 100mg/kg of fullerenol 30 min (Milic Torres et al., 2010).

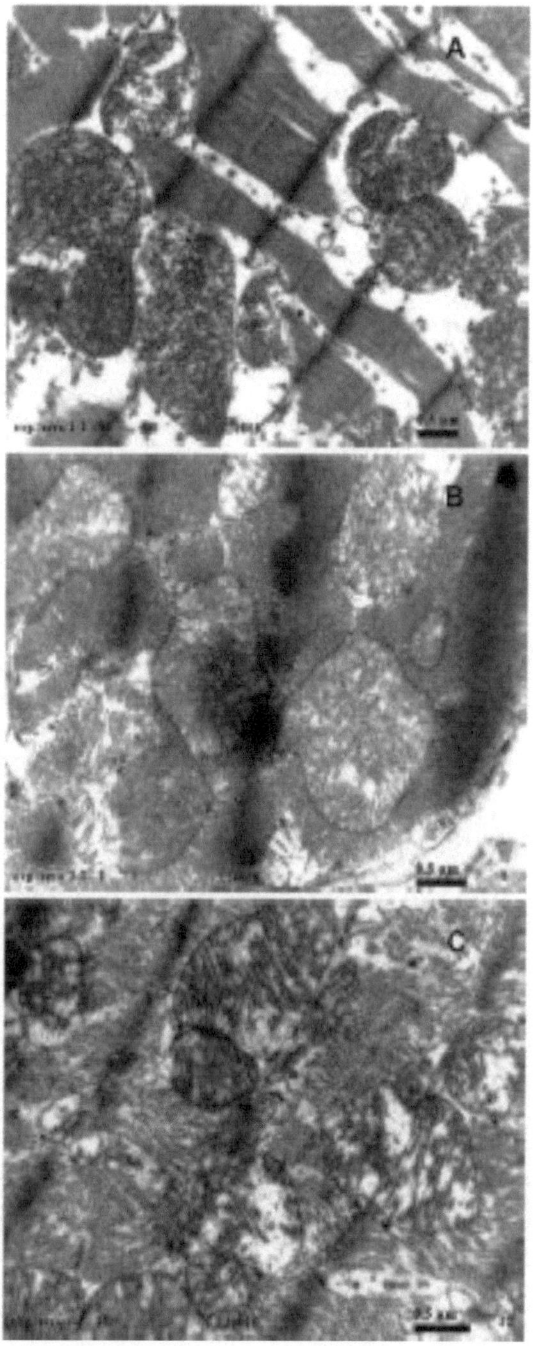

Fig. 8. Mitochondria showing (A) normal morphology, the double membrane envelope and lamellar cristae in the control rats; (B) irregular shape with lucent matrix and disorganised cristae in the Dox rats; and (C) amorphous material and rare disintegrated cristae in the Dox/Full rats (Injac, R. et al., 2008a).

ventricular tissues showed marked myocardial damage upon doxorubicin treatment. Ultrastructural analysis of the heart tissue from rats treated with doxorubicin and fullerenol indicated that hearts of the animals were protected from doxorubin-induced subcellular damage (Figure. 8.). Again, it was confirmed oxidative nature of cardiac injury caused by anthracycline application (elevated parameters of oxidative stress - SOD, MDA, GST, GSH, GR and TAS) and antioxidative capability of fullerenol, which maintain all examinated parameters at the basal level, when is applied as pretreatment to doxorubicin (Injac, R. et al., 2008a)

Protective effects of fullerenol $C_{60}(OH)_{24}$ on Wistar rats with colorectal carcinoma (chronic regimen of DOX administration - 1.5mg/kg/week, for 3 weeks)) was assessed by the same research group. They findings confirmed cardioprotective role of fullerenol, without modulation of antitumor activity of the drug. The myocardial lesions caused by doxorubicin administration were significantly reduced in animals received fullerenol. Functional and biochemical examination of the heart were in concordance with pathohystological findings. Moreover, fullerene exhibit significantly higher degree of protection over the well known antioxidant - vitamin C, which was used as a positive control (Injac, R. et al., 2009).

In favour to $C_{60}(OH)_{24}$ cardioprotectivity are going biodistribution studies of fullerene. Ji et al, found that the high concentration of the ^{125}I-$C_{60}(OH)_x$ in the heart was able to detect even three days after the administration (Ji et al., 2006)

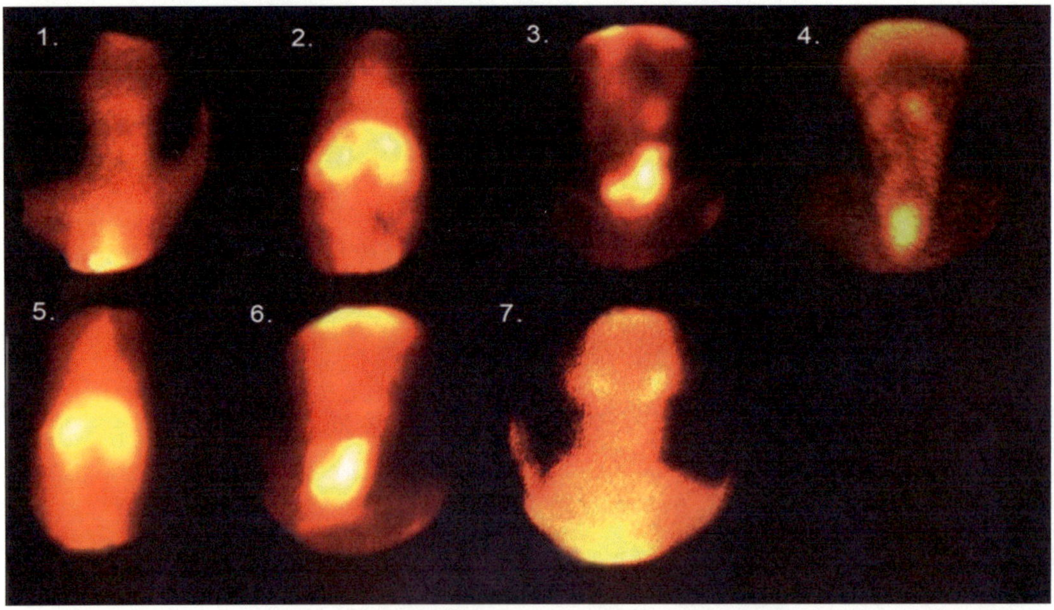

Fig. 9. Static scintigraphy analysis of dog: 1. heart activity after 1 hour; 2. liver activity after 1 hour; 3. kidney and urinary bladder activities after 24 hours; 4. kidney and urinary bladder activities after 21 hours; 5. liver, kidneys and urinary bladder activities after 24h; 6. salivary glands activity after 24 hours; 7. heart activity after 24 hours

Dynamic scintigraphy of the domestic dog, using $99mTcO_4$-tagged fullerenol ($[99mTc(CO)_3(H_2O)_3]$-$C_{60}(OH)_{22-24}$) discovered its presence in the heart, liver and spleen.

After administration of radiopharmaceutical, activity was first recorded on the heart, followed by liver and spleen (Figure. 9.). However, thirty minutes after, activity in all three organs was stabilized. The static scintigraphy reveals activity in the heart, liver, spleen and intestine after 1h, in salivary glands after 4 h and after 21 h the activity was detected in kidneys, urinary bladder and urinary tract. After 24 hours, the activity was detected in liver, spleen, kidneys and urinary bladder (Figure. 9.). These results suggest liver and urinary elimination mechanisms of tested xenobiotic with clearance of >24h (Djordjević et al., 2010).

Special interest for further investigation with fullerenol will be focused on its radioprotective activity in animal models, and on cardioprotective effects in doxorubicin-induced cardiotoxicity. However, main drawback for application of fullerenol as a system tissue protector is its water solubility of 0.44 mg/l, which is not satisfactory (Injac, Rade et al., 2008b). Enchasing of solubility using surfactants (Milic Torres et al., 2011) or co-solvent (Injac, Rade et al., 2008b), can facilitate fullerenol parenteral or oral application.

All these findings suggests that fullerenol $C_{60}(OH)_{24}$ have all properties of ideal cardioprotector against doxorubicin-induced cardiotoxicity - selectivity, ROS scavenger, iron chelator, low toxicity and no modulatory effect on antitumor activity of anthracyclines. Further *ex vivo* experiments as well as improvement of pharmaceutical formulations of the fullerene are strongly needed.

6. Natural products

The production of free radicals as a by product of DOX metabolism is the cardiotoxic mechanism with earliest recognition and widest attention. Therefore, searching for ideal protection against free radical injury was and still is a big scientific challenge. Application of natural antioxidants was first and logical path in this journey.

Numerous studies about protective effects of vitamin E against DOX-induced cardiotoxicity are quite controversial. *Vitamin E:* Protective effect vitamin E exerted against chronic DOX-induced toxicity on rabbit model when is administrated in high dosage as a pretreatment (170 mg/kg)(Van Vleet & Ferrans, 1980) or given in combination with vitamin A, reducing myocardial damage for 30% and maintained heart contractility (Milei et al., 1986). Berthiaume and co-workers found that alpha-tocopherol supplemented diet result in significant enrichment of cardiac mitochondrial membranes with vitamin E and diminished content of oxidized cardiac proteins associated with DOX treatment. However, vitamin E supplemented diet failed to protect against mitochondrial dysfunction and cardiac histopathology. These findings suggested that tocopherol enrichment is not sufficient to protect cardiac mitochondrial membranes from DOX induced toxicity (Berthiaume et al., 2005). In doxorubicin treated leukemic mice, free alpha tocopherol and tocopherol acetate cause potentiation of doxorubicin toxicity (Alberts et al., 1978). High dosage of vitamin E failed to protect the heart tissue of the rabbits received cumulative dose of 400 mg/sq m of DOX in chronic regimen. Notwithstanding, coadministration of vitamin E result in increasing life span (Breed et al., 1980). Vitamin E administrated in high dosage of 5000 IU/day, in chronic regimen (17 days) just cause mild amelioration of DOX-induced cardiotoxicity in miniature swine(Herman & Ferrans, 1983). Alpha-tocopherol in oral dose of $2g/m^2$ applied daily enriches human serum with vitamin E from six to eight fold. However, coadministrated with DOX in cumulative dose level of $550\ mg/m^2$ did not offered substantial protection against congestive heart failure which appeared in tested human individuals (Legha et al., 1982b). *Vitamin A*: Pretreatment of rats in dosage of 25 IU/kg of vitamin A, two days before single dose administration of DOX (10mg/kg *i.v.*) substantially reduced the peroxidative damage of the heart lipids and proteins, and markedly lowered serum values of lactate dehydrogenase and creatine kinase. This applied regimen sustained structural integration of the heart and prolonged life span of tested animals pointing on protective role of vitamin A in DOX-induced cardiotoxicity (Tesoriere et al., 1994). Lu and co-workers suggests strong cardioprotective activity of *beta-carotene*, when is given as a pretreatment to DOX (Lu et al., 1996). *L-carnitine* appared to be cardioprotective in doxorubicin treated rats, due to improved cardiac energy metabolism and reduced lipid peroxidation (Luo et al., 1999). Pretreatment of isolated rat cardiac myocytes with L-carnitine (200 μg/ml) found to inhibit the doxorubicin induced sphingomyelin hydrolysis, ceramide generation and cell death in dose dependent manner (Andrieu-Abadie et al., 1999). Aplication of *alpha-lipoic* acid exerted cytoprotective activity against free radical injury induced by doxorubicin. It succeed to maintain biochemical parameters of oxidative stress of treated rats and to sustain structural integrity of the rat heart as well (Al-Majed et al., 2002; Balachandar et al., 2003). Extensive review was made about *coenzyme Q-10* in prevention of anthracycline-induced cardiotoxicity. Both, preclinical and clinical studies suggest its cardioprotective role without compromising antitumor activity of the DOX. Applied in daily dose range between 50 and 120 mg/day coenzyme Q-10 can ameliorate majority of side effects associated with anthracycline administration including heart failure (Conklin, 2005). Wistar rats were treated with doxorubicin (4mg/kg) and *lycopene* (5 mg/kg body weight a day) during seven week period. Morphologic examination revealed that doxorubicin-induced myocyte damage was significantly suppressed in rats treated with lycopene. Lycopene supplementation provided myocyte protection without preventing interstitial collagen accumulation increase, although cardiac dysfunction was not preserved (Anjos Ferreira et al., 2007). Lycopene may reduce or prevent the side effects of chemotherapy due its antioxidative and anti-inflammatory properties (Sahin et al., 2010). *Probucol*, a lipid-lowering agent with known antioxidative properties, coadministrated with DOX to the male Sprague-Dawley in dosage of 10 mg/kg during four weeks with pretreatment of additional two weeks, completely abolished increase in oxidative stress, glutathione peroxidase (GSH-Px) inactivation and Mn dependent SOD downregulation during DOX cardiomyopathy. Li et al. suggested that rather oxidative stress mediated changes at the enzyme protein level playing role in toxicity of DOX than downregulation of the GSH-Px gene transcription or translation (Li, T. et al., 2000; Li, T. & Singal, 2000). *Low molecular weight heparin* (LMWH) administration to DOX-induced rats prevented the rise in serum and tissue levels of LDH, aminotransferases and ALP, while these parameters were significantly elevated in the DOX group in comparison with the control group. Cardiotoxicity indicated by rise in serum CPK in the DOX group was attenuated by LMWH treatment. LMWH decreased the cardiac lipid peroxidation induced by DOX. Histologic examination revealed that the DOX-induced deleterious changes in the heart were offset by LMWH treatment (Deepa & Varalakshmi, 2003). Chlopcikova and co-workers were tested chemoprotective effects of caffeic (CA), chlorogenic (CHA) and rosmarinic (RA) acids the toxicity of doxorubicin in neonatal rat cardiomyocytes and the iron-dependent DOX induced lipid peroxidation of heart membranes, mitochondria and microsomes. The test compounds protected cardiomyocytes against DOX induced oxidative stress (RA > CHA > or = CA) on all monitored parameters. Substantial preservation of monolayer integrity of the cardiomyocytes by test compounds was also found microscopically. All the acids were more effective in the assays used than dexrazoxan. RA showed the most effective cytoprotectivity. All the acids significantly reduced the iron-dependent DOX induced lipid peroxidation of heart membranes, although CHA from the all tested compounds was found to be the most effective (Chlopcikova et al., 2004). Efficacy of the aqueous extract of the *Centella asiatica* was evaluated on the mitochondrial enzymes; mitochondrial antioxidant status in adriamycin induced myocardial injury. Pretreatment of the Wistar rats during three weeks with aqueous extract of Centella asiatica (orally 200 mg/kg body wt/ day) followed by co-treatment with DOX (2.5 mg/kg, i.p. two weeks) effectively counteracted the alterations in mitochondrial enzymes and mitochondrial defence system. In addition, transmission electron microscopy study confirms the restoration of cellular normalcy and accredits the cytoprotective role of Centella asiatica against adriamycin induced myocardial injury. Results of Gnanapragasam et al. suggest that the aqueous extract of Centella asiatica not only possesses antioxidant properties but it may also reduce the extent of mitochondrial damage (Gnanapragasam et al., 2007). Oral administration of *Aloe barbadensis gel* - aloe vera (100 and 200 mg/kg), to the albino rats during 10 days, produced a significant protection against cardiotoxicity induced by DOX (single dose 7.5 mg/kg *i.v.*). Aloe vera gel kept serum levels of LDH, CPK, cardiac lipid peroxides, tissue catalase and tissue SOD along with the blood and tissue GSH on the basal values. The results revealed that aloe vera gel exhibit a dose dependent protection against DOX induced cardiotoxicity (Kaithwas et al., 2011). Effect of methanolic extract of fruits of *Piper longum* (PLM) on the biochemical changes, tissue peroxidative damage and abnormal antioxidant levels in DOX induced cardiotoxicity in Wistar rats was investigated by Wakade and co-workers. Piper longum extract was administered to the Wistar rats in two different doses, by gastric gavage (250 mg/kg and 500 mg/kg) during three weeks followed by unidose of DOX (15 mg/kg, i.p.) at the 21st day. Activities of myocardial antioxidant enzymes (CAT, SOD, GSH-Px, GR and GSSG) were significantly lowered due to cardiotoxicity in rats administered with DOX. PLM pretreatment maintain of these endogenous antioxidants on the level of control. Structural examination of the heart revealed degenerative changes and cellular infiltrations in rats administered with DOX and pretreatment with PLM reduced the intensity of such lesions. The results indicate that PLM administration offers significant protection against DOX induced oxidative stress and reduces the cardiotoxicity of the administrated antineoplastic drug (Wakade et al., 2008). Flavonoid scavenging activity of *propolis* has been investigated against oxidative injury of the heart, induced by single dose administration of DOX (20 mg/kg, *i.p.*). Pretreatment of rats with propolis extract, given per os (100 mg/kg/day) during four days prior to DXR injection, substantially reduced the peroxidative damage of the heart mitochondria. It was evident significant reducing both mitochondrial MDA formation and production of superoxide anion. These data are demonstrated potent role of propolis extract counteracting doxorubicin caused cardiotoxicity (Alyane et al., 2008). Strong cardioprotection based on ROS scavenging activity against acute DOX induced toxicity was exhibited by: *hesperetin* - hypocholesterolemic citrus flavonoid (50 and 100 mg/kg) (Trivedi et al., 2011); *melatonin* (2x 5mg/kg) (Aydemir et al., 2010); *resveratrol* (10 mg/kg)(Danz et al., 2009; Olukman et al., 2009; Tatlidede et al., 2009); *procyanidins* from grape seeds (15 mg/kg)(Li, W. et al., 2009); *silymarin*, flavonolignans extracted from *Silybum marianum* (50 mg/kg) (El-Shitany et al., 2008) and *salvianolic acid* from *Salvia miltiorrhiza* (3 x 40mg/kg before DOX)(Jiang et al., 2008).

It is obvious that diverse natural products have powerful ability to counteract the toxicity of doxorubicin and other anthracycline antibiotics. Unfortunately, the results from the studies conducted so far, are from pre clinical phase, rarely some of them reach clinical trials, and none is defined as a commercial protector. Use of natural antioxidants, against DOX induced cardiotoxicity, according to our knowledge, are recommended by a physician as a supplement to the treatment protocols in oncology. There are no scientific and clear evidences of their beneficial effects in large cohorts.

7. Conclusion

Cardiac complications induced by doxorubicin therapy are of considerable importance today as when was appeared 30 years ago. Furthermore, the number of the patients surviving cancer and chemotherapy is bigger nowdays and appearance of subclinical cardiac dysfunction is even more frequent. Mechanisms underlying cardiotoxicity of DOX are complex. In spite of multitude hypothesises involving gene expression changes, activation of ubiquitin-proteasome system, cell death as well as innate immunity activation, oxidative injury of the heart and alteration in iron homeostasis most likely to have primary role in cardiotoxicity developed by doxorubicin. No single drug will be able to prevent cardiotoxicity. Therefore, more clinical studies are needed to elucidate the mechanism and develop strategies in prevention against DOX-induced cardiotoxicity.

8. Acknowledgement

This work is supported by Fundação para a Ciência e Tecnologia, Portugal (Grant no. SFRH/BPD/43365/2008)

9. References

Abou El Hassan, M. A., Heijn, M., Rabelink, M. J., van der Vijgh, W. J., Bast, A. & Hoeben, R. C. (2003). The protective effect of cardiac gene transfer of CuZn-sod in comparison with the cardioprotector monohydroxyethylrutoside against doxorubicin-induced cardiotoxicity in cultured cells. *Cancer Gene Ther*. Vol. 10, No. 4, (Apr), pp. 270-277, ISSN 0929-1903

Al-Majed, A. A., Gdo, A. M., Al-Shabanah, O. A. & Mansour, M. A. (2002). Alpha-lipoic acid ameliorates myocardial toxicity induced by doxorubicin. *Pharmacol Res*. Vol. 46, No. 6, (Dec), pp. 499-503, ISSN 1043-6618

Alberts, D. S., Peng, Y. M. & Moon, T. E. (1978). alpha-Tocopherol pretreatment increases adriamycin bone marrow toxicity. *Biomedicine*. Vol. 29, No. 6, (Oct), pp. 189-191, ISSN 0300-0893

Alderton, P., Gross, J. & Green, M. D. (1990). Role of (+-)-1,2-bis(3,5-dioxopiperazinyl-1-yl)propane (ICRF-187) in modulating free radical scavenging enzymes in doxorubicin-induced cardiomyopathy. *Cancer Res*. Vol. 50, No. 16, (Aug 15), pp. 5136-5142, ISSN 0008-5472

Allen, A. (1992). The cardiotoxicity of chemotherapeutic drugs. *Semin Oncol*. Vol. 19, No. 5, (Oct), pp. 529-542, ISSN 0093-7754

Alyane, M., Kebsa, L. B., Boussenane, H. N., Rouibah, H. & Lahouel, M. (2008). Cardioprotective effects and mechanism of action of polyphenols extracted from propolis against doxorubicin toxicity. *Pak J Pharm Sci.* Vol. 21, No. 3, (Jul), pp. 201-209, ISSN 1011-601X

Anderson, R. & Barron, A. R. (2005). Reaction of hydroxyfullerene with metal salts: a route to remediation and immobilization. *J Am Chem Soc.* Vol. 127, No. 30, (Aug 3), pp. 10458-10459, ISSN 0002-7863

Andrieu-Abadie, N., Jaffrezou, J. P., Hatem, S., Laurent, G., Levade, T. & Mercadier, J. J. (1999). L-carnitine prevents doxorubicin-induced apoptosis of cardiac myocytes: role of inhibition of ceramide generation. *FASEB J.* Vol. 13, No. 12, (Sep), pp. 1501-1510, ISSN 0892-6638

Anjos Ferreira, A. L., Russell, R. M., Rocha, N., Placido Ladeira, M. S., Favero Salvadori, D. M., Oliveira Nascimento, M. C., Matsui, M., Carvalho, F. A., Tang, G., Matsubara, L. S. & Matsubara, B. B. (2007). Effect of lycopene on doxorubicin-induced cardiotoxicity: an echocardiographic, histological and morphometrical assessment. *Basic Clin Pharmacol Toxicol.* Vol. 101, No. 1, (Jul), pp. 16-24, ISSN 1742-7835

Aronson, J. K., Dukes, M. N. G. & Meyler, L. (2006). *Anthracyclines and related compounds.* Meyler's Side Effects of Drugs: The International Encyclopedia of Adverse Drug Reactions and Interactions (Fifteenth Edition), J. K. Aronson, (Ed.), 245-255, Elsevier, ISBN 978-0-444-51005-1, Amsterdam, Holland

Aydemir, S., Ozdemir, I. & Kart, A. (2010). Role of exogenous melatonin on adriamycin-induced changes in the rat heart. *Eur Rev Med Pharmacol Sci.* Vol. 14, No. 5, (May), pp. 435-441, ISSN 1128-3602

Babbar, N. & Casero, R. A., Jr. (2006). Tumor necrosis factor-alpha increases reactive oxygen species by inducing spermine oxidase in human lung epithelial cells: a potential mechanism for inflammation-induced carcinogenesis. *Cancer Res.* Vol. 66, No. 23, (Dec 1), pp. 11125-11130, ISSN 0008-5472

Balachandar, A. V., Malarkodi, K. P. & Varalakshmi, P. (2003). Protective role of DLalpha-lipoic acid against adriamycin-induced cardiac lipid peroxidation. *Hum Exp Toxicol.* Vol. 22, No. 5, (May), pp. 249-254, ISSN 0960-3271

Beraldo, H., Garnier-Suillerot, A., Tosi, L. & Lavelle, F. (1985). Iron(III)-adriamycin and Iron(III)-daunorubicin complexes: physicochemical characteristics, interaction with DNA, and antitumor activity. *Biochemistry.* Vol. 24, No. 2, (Jan 15), pp. 284-289, ISSN 0006-2960

Berthiaume, J. M., Oliveira, P. J., Fariss, M. W. & Wallace, K. B. (2005). Dietary vitamin E decreases doxorubicin-induced oxidative stress without preventing mitochondrial dysfunction. *Cardiovasc Toxicol.* Vol. 5, No. 3, pp. 257-267, ISSN 1530-7905

Berthiaume, J. M. & Wallace, K. B. (2007). Adriamycin-induced oxidative mitochondrial cardiotoxicity. *Cell Biol Toxicol.* Vol. 23, No. 1, (Jan), pp. 15-25, ISSN 0742-2091

Bhanumathi, P., Saleesh, E. D. & Vasudevan, D. M. (1994). WR-1065 as a chemoprotector in Adriamycin chemotherapy. *Cancer Letters.* Vol. 81, No. 2, pp. 171-175, ISSN 0304-3835.

Bhutia, Y. D., Vijayaraghavan, R. & Pathak, U. (2010). Analgesic and anti-inflammatory activity of amifostine, DRDE-07, and their analogs, in mice. *Indian J Pharmacol.* Vol. 42, No. 1, (Feb), pp. 17-20, ISSN 1998-3751

Bolaman, Z., Cicek, C., Kadikoylu, G., Barutca, S., Serter, M., Yenisey, C. & Alper, G. (2005). The protective effects of amifostine on adriamycin-induced acute cardiotoxicity in rats. *Tohoku J Exp Med.* Vol. 207, No. 4, (Dec), pp. 249-253, ISSN 0040-8727

Boucek, R. J., Jr., Olson, R. D., Brenner, D. E., Ogunbunmi, E. M., Inui, M. & Fleischer, S. (1987). The major metabolite of doxorubicin is a potent inhibitor of membrane-associated ion pumps. A correlative study of cardiac muscle with isolated membrane fractions. *J Biol Chem*. Vol. 262, No. 33, (Nov 25), pp. 15851-15856, ISSN 0021-9258

Breed, J. G., Zimmerman, A. N., Dormans, J. A. & Pinedo, H. M. (1980). Failure of the antioxidant vitamin E to protect against adriamycin-induced cardiotoxicity in the rabbit. *Cancer Res*. Vol. 40, No. 6, (Jun), pp. 2033-2038, ISSN 0008-5472

Brown, P. E. (1967). Mechanism of action of aminothiol radioprotectors. *Nature*. Vol. 213, No. 5074, (Jan 28), pp. 363-364, ISSN 0028-0836

Calabro-Jones, P. M., Aguilera, J. A., Ward, J. F., Smoluk, G. D. & Fahey, R. C. (1988). Uptake of WR-2721 derivatives by cells in culture: identification of the transported form of the drug. *Cancer Res*. Vol. 48, No. 13, (Jul 1), pp. 3634-3640, ISSN 0008-5472

Capizzi, R. L. (1999a). The preclinical basis for broad-spectrum selective cytoprotection of normal tissues from cytotoxic therapies by amifostine. *Semin Oncol*. Vol. 26, No. 2 Suppl 7, (Apr), pp. 3-21, ISSN 0093-7754

Capizzi, R. L. (1999b). Recent developments and emerging options: the role of amifostine as a broad-spectrum cytoprotective agent. *Semin Oncol*. Vol. 26, No. 2 Suppl 7, (Apr), pp. 1-2, ISSN 0093-7754

Chlopcikova, S., Psotova, J., Miketova, P., Sousek, J., Lichnovsky, V. & Simanek, V. (2004). Chemoprotective effect of plant phenolics against anthracycline-induced toxicity on rat cardiomyocytes. Part II. caffeic, chlorogenic and rosmarinic acids. *Phytother Res*. Vol. 18, No. 5, (May), pp. 408-413, ISSN 0951-418X

Conklin, K. A. (2005). Coenzyme q10 for prevention of anthracycline-induced cardiotoxicity. *Integr Cancer Ther*. Vol. 4, No. 2, (Jun), pp. 110-130, ISSN 1534-7354

Culy, C. R. & Spencer, C. M. (2001). Amifostine: an update on its clinical status as a cytoprotectant in patients with cancer receiving chemotherapy or radiotherapy and its potential therapeutic application in myelodysplastic syndrome. *Drugs*. Vol. 61, No. 5, pp. 641-684, ISSN 0012-6667

Cvetkovic, R. S. & Scott, L. J. (2005). Dexrazoxane: a review of its use for cardioprotection during anthracycline chemotherapy. *Drugs*. Vol. 65, No. 7, pp. 1005-1024, ISSN 0012-6667

Danz, E. D., Skramsted, J., Henry, N., Bennett, J. A. & Keller, R. S. (2009). Resveratrol prevents doxorubicin cardiotoxicity through mitochondrial stabilization and the Sirt1 pathway. *Free Radic Biol Med*. Vol. 46, No. 12, (Jun 15), pp. 1589-1597, ISSN 1873-4596

Davies, K. J. & Doroshow, J. H. (1986). Redox cycling of anthracyclines by cardiac mitochondria. I. Anthracycline radical formation by NADH dehydrogenase. *J Biol Chem*. Vol. 261, No. 7, (Mar 5), pp. 3060-3067, ISSN 0021-9258

Deepa, P. R. & Varalakshmi, P. (2003). Protective effect of low molecular weight heparin on oxidative injury and cellular abnormalities in adriamycin-induced cardiac and hepatic toxicity. *Chem Biol Interact*. Vol. 146, No. 2, (Oct 25), pp. 201-210, ISSN 0009-2797

Della Torre, P., Mazue, G., Podesta, A., Moneta, D., Sammartini, U. & Imondi, A. R. (1999). Protection against doxorubicin-induced cardiotoxicity in weanling rats by dexrazoxane. *Cancer Chemother Pharmacol*. Vol. 43, No. 2, pp. 151-156, ISSN 0344-5704

Djordjević, A., Ajdinović, B., Dopudja, M., Trajković, S., Milovanovic, Z., Maksin, T., Nešković, O., Bogdanović, V., Trpkov, Đ. & Cvetićanin, J. (2010). Scintigraphy of the domestic dog using [99mTc(CO)$_3$(H$_2$O)$_3$]-C$_{60}$(OH)$_{22\text{-}24}$. *Digest Journal of Nanomaterials and Biostructures*. Vol. 6, No. January-March, pp. 99-106

Djordjevic, A., Canadanovic-Brunet, J., Vojnovic-Miloradov, M. & Bogdanovic, G. (2005). Antioxidant properties and hypothetical radical mechanism of fullerenol $C_{60}(OH)_{24}$. *Oxidation Communications* Vol. 27, No. pp. 806-812

Djorjdevic-Milic, V., Stankov, K., Injac, R., Djordjevic, A., Srdjenovic, B., Govedarica, B., Radic, N., Dragojevic-Simic, V. & Strukelj, B. (2009). Activity of antioxidative enzymes in erythrocytes after a single dose administration of doxorubicin in rats pretreated with fullerenol C(60)(OH)(24). *Toxicol Mech Methods*. Vol. 19, No. 1, (Jan), pp. 24-28, ISSN 1537-6524.

Dobric, S., Dragojevic-Simic, V., Bokonjic, D., Milovanovic, S., Marincic, D. & Jovic, P. (1998). The efficacy of selenium, WR-2721, and their combination in the prevention of adriamycin-induced cardiotoxicity in rats. *J Environ Pathol Toxicol Oncol*. Vol. 17, No. 3-4, pp. 291-299, ISSN 0731-8898

Dobric, S., Dragojevic-Simic, V., Jacevic, V., Bokonjic, D., Zolotarevski, L. & Jelic, K. (2003). 311 Amifostine protection against doxorubicin-induced rat heart mast cell accumulation. *Toxicology Letters*. Vol. 144, Supplement 1, No. 0, pp. s85-s86, ISSN 0378-4274.

Dobric, S., Dragojevic-Simic, V., Trajkovic, S., Jacevic, V., Aleksandar, D. & Bokonjic, D. (2007). General and cardioprotective efficacy of fullerenol C60(OH)24 in X-ray irradiated rats. *Basic & Clinical Pharmacology & Toxicology*. Vol. 101, No. pp. 70-71, ISSN 1742-7843.

Doroshow, J. H. & Davies, K. J. (1986). Redox cycling of anthracyclines by cardiac mitochondria. II. Formation of superoxide anion, hydrogen peroxide, and hydroxyl radical. *J Biol Chem*. Vol. 261, No. 7, (Mar 5), pp. 3068-3074, ISSN 0021-9258

Doroshow, J. H., Locker, G. Y. & Myers, C. E. (1980). Enzymatic defenses of the mouse heart against reactive oxygen metabolites: alterations produced by doxorubicin. *J Clin Invest*. Vol. 65, No. 1, (Jan), pp. 128-135, ISSN 0021-9738

Dorr, R. T. (1991). Chemoprotectants for cancer chemotherapy. *Semin Oncol*. Vol. 18, No. 1 Suppl 2, (Feb), pp. 48-58, ISSN 0093-7754

Dorr, R. T. (1996). Cytoprotective agents for anthracyclines. *Semin Oncol*. Vol. 23, No. 4 Suppl 8, (Aug), pp. 23-34, ISSN 0093-7754

Dorr, R. T., Lagel, K. & McLean, S. (1996). Cardioprotection of rat heart myocytes with amifostine (Ethyol) and its free thiol, WR-1065, in vitro. *Eur J Cancer*. Vol. 32A Suppl 4, No. pp. S21-25, ISSN 0959-8049

Dragojevic-Simic, V. & Dobric, S. (1996). [The cytoprotective agent amifostine (WR-2721): current clinical use and trends in its development]. *Vojnosanit Pregl*. Vol. 53, No. 4, (Jul-Aug), pp. 305-310, ISSN 0042-8450

Dragojevic-Simic, V., Dobrić, S., Jacevic, V. & Bokonjic, D. (2007). Amifostine protects against early toxic changes in rat heart induced by high dose of doxorubicin. *Basic & Clinical Pharmacology & Toxicology*. Vol. 101, No. pp. 118-119, ISSN 1742-7843.

Dragojevic-Simic, V., Dobrić, S., Jacevic, V., Bokonjic, D., Milosavljevic, I. & Kovacevic, A. (2011a). Efficacy of amifostine in protection against early toxic changes in rat heart induced by doxorubicin. *Vojnosanit Pregled. in press*

Dragojevic-Simic, V., Dobric, S. L., Bokonjic, D. R., Vucinic, Z. M., Sinovec, S. M., Jacevic, V. M. & Dogovic, N. P. (2004). Amifostine protection against doxorubicin cardiotoxicity in rats. *Anticancer Drugs*. Vol. 15, No. 2, (Feb), pp. 169-178, ISSN 0959-4973

Dragojevic-Simic, V., Jacevic, V., Dobric, S., Djordjevic, A., Bokonjic, D., Bajcetic, M. & Injac, R. (2011b). Anti-inflammatory activity of fullerenol $C_{60}(OH)_{24}$ nanoparticles in a model of acute inflammation in rats. *Digest Journal of Nanomaterials and Biostructures*. Vol. 6, No. 2, (April - June), pp. 819 - 827, ISSN

El-Shitany, N. A., El-Haggar, S. & El-desoky, K. (2008). Silymarin prevents adriamycin-induced cardiotoxicity and nephrotoxicity in rats. *Food Chem Toxicol*. Vol. 46, No. 7, (Jul), pp. 2422-2428, ISSN 0278-6915

Ferrans, V. J., Clark, J. R., Zhang, J., Yu, Z. X. & Herman, E. H. (1997). Pathogenesis and prevention of doxorubicin cardiomyopathy. *Tsitologiia*. Vol. 39, No. 10, pp. 928-937, ISSN 0041-3771

Ferrari, M. (2005). Cancer nanotechnology: opportunities and challenges. *Nat Rev Cancer*. Vol. 5, No. 3, (Mar), pp. 161-171, ISSN 1474-175X

Forrest, G. L., Akman, S., Doroshow, J., Rivera, H. & Kaplan, W. D. (1991). Genomic sequence and expression of a cloned human carbonyl reductase gene with daunorubicin reductase activity. *Mol Pharmacol*. Vol. 40, No. 4, (Oct), pp. 502-507, ISSN 0026-895X

Fu, P., Birukova, A. A., Xing, J., Sammani, S., Murley, J. S., Garcia, J. G., Grdina, D. J. & Birukov, K. G. (2009). Amifostine reduces lung vascular permeability via suppression of inflammatory signalling. *Eur Respir J*. Vol. 33, No. 3, (Mar), pp. 612-624, ISSN 1399-3003

Fulbright, J. M., Huh, W., Anderson, P. & Chandra, J. (2010). Can anthracycline therapy for pediatric malignancies be less cardiotoxic? *Curr Oncol Rep*. Vol. 12, No. 6, (Nov), pp. 411-419, ISSN 1534-6269

Gaetani, G. F., Galiano, S., Canepa, L., Ferraris, A. M. & Kirkman, H. N. (1989). Catalase and glutathione peroxidase are equally active in detoxification of hydrogen peroxide in human erythrocytes. *Blood*. Vol. 73, No. 1, (Jan), pp. 334-339, ISSN 0006-4971

Gewirtz, D. A. (1999). A critical evaluation of the mechanisms of action proposed for the antitumor effects of the anthracycline antibiotics adriamycin and daunorubicin. *Biochem Pharmacol*. Vol. 57, No. 7, (Apr 1), pp. 727-741, ISSN 0006-2952

Gianni, L., Herman, E. H., Lipshultz, S. E., Minotti, G., Sarvazyan, N. & Sawyer, D. B. (2008). Anthracycline cardiotoxicity: from bench to bedside. *J Clin Oncol*. Vol. 26, No. 22, (Aug 1), pp. 3777-3784, ISSN 1527-7755

Gnanapragasam, A., Yogeeta, S., Subhashini, R., Ebenezar, K. K., Sathish, V. & Devaki, T. (2007). Adriamycin induced myocardial failure in rats: protective role of Centella asiatica. *Mol Cell Biochem*. Vol. 294, No. 1-2, (Jan), pp. 55-63, ISSN 0300-8177

Goormaghtigh, E. & Ruysschaert, J. M. (1984). Anthracycline glycoside-membrane interactions. *Biochim Biophys Acta*. Vol. 779, No. 3, (Sep 3), pp. 271-288, ISSN 0006-3002

Grdina, D. J., Murley, J. S. & Kataoka, Y. (2002). Radioprotectants: current status and new directions. *Oncology*. Vol. 63 Suppl 2, No. pp. 2-10, ISSN 0030-2414

Grdina, D. J., Shigematsu, N., Dale, P., Newton, G. L., Aguilera, J. A. & Fahey, R. C. (1995). Thiol and disulfide metabolites of the radiation protector and potential chemopreventive agent WR-2721 are linked to both its anti-cytotoxic and anti-mutagenic mechanisms of action. *Carcinogenesis*. Vol. 16, No. 4, (Apr), pp. 767-774, ISSN 0143-

Green, D. M., Grigoriev, Y. A., Nan, B., Takashima, J. R., Norkool, P. A., D'Angio, G. J. & Breslow, N. E. (2001). Congestive heart failure after treatment for Wilms' tumor: a report from the National Wilms' Tumor Study group. *J Clin Oncol*. Vol. 19, No. 7, (Apr 1), pp. 1926-1934, ISSN 0732-183X

Hale, J. P. & Lewis, I. J. (1994). Anthracyclines: cardiotoxicity and its prevention. *Arch Dis Child*. Vol. 71, No. 5, (Nov), pp. 457-462, ISSN 1468-2044

Halliwell, B. & Gutteridge, J. (2007). *Free Radicals in Biology and Medicine*. Oxford University Press, ISBN 978-0-19-856869-8, London, U.K.

Harrison, P. M., Treffry, A. & Lilley, T. H. (1986). Ferritin as an iron-storage protein: mechanisms of iron uptake. *Journal of Inorganic Biochemistry*. Vol. 27, No. 4, pp. 287-293, ISSN 0162-0134.

Hasinoff, B. B. (1989). The interaction of the cardioprotective agent ICRF-187 [+)-1,2-bis(3,5-dioxopiperazinyl-1-yL)propane); its hydrolysis product (ICRF-198); and other chelating agents with the Fe(III) and Cu(II) complexes of adriamycin. *Agents Actions*. Vol. 26, No. 3-4, (Mar), pp. 378-385, ISSN 0065-4299

Hensley, M. L., Hagerty, K. L., Kewalramani, T., Green, D. M., Meropol, N. J., Wasserman, T. H., Cohen, G. I., Emami, B., Gradishar, W. J., Mitchell, R. B., Thigpen, J. T., Trotti, A., 3rd, von Hoff, D. & Schuchter, L. M. (2009). American Society of Clinical Oncology 2008 clinical practice guideline update: use of chemotherapy and radiation therapy protectants. *J Clin Oncol*. Vol. 27, No. 1, (Jan 1), pp. 127-145, ISSN 1527-7755

Herman, E. H. & Ferrans, V. J. (1983). Influence of vitamin E and ICRF-187 on chronic doxorubicin cardiotoxicity in miniature swine. *Lab Invest*. Vol. 49, No. 1, (Jul), pp. 69-77, ISSN 0023-6837

Herman, E. H., Ferrans, V. J., Young, R. S. & Hamlin, R. L. (1988). Pretreatment with ICRF-187 allows a marked increase in the total cumulative dose of doxorubicin tolerated by beagle dogs. *Drugs Exp Clin Res*. Vol. 14, No. 9, pp. 563-570, ISSN 0378-6501

Herman, E. H., Zhang, J., Chadwick, D. P. & Ferrans, V. J. (2000). Comparison of the protective effects of amifostine and dexrazoxane against the toxicity of doxorubicin in spontaneously hypertensive rats. *Cancer Chemother Pharmacol*. Vol. 45, No. 4, pp. 329-334, ISSN 0344-5704

Herman, E. H., Zhang, J. & Ferrans, V. J. (1994). Comparison of the protective effects of desferrioxamine and ICRF-187 against doxorubicin-induced toxicity in spontaneously hypertensive rats. *Cancer Chemother Pharmacol*. Vol. 35, No. 2, pp. 93-100, ISSN 0344-5704

Hirsch, A. & Brettreich, M. (2005). *Fullerenes: Chemistry and Reactions*. Wiley-VCH Verlag GmbH & Co. KGaA, ISBN 9783527603497, Weinheim, Germany.

Hunt, S. A. (2005). ACC/AHA 2005 guideline update for the diagnosis and management of chronic heart failure in the adult: a report of the American College of Cardiology/American Heart Association Task Force on Practice Guidelines (Writing Committee to Update the 2001 Guidelines for the Evaluation and Management of Heart Failure). *J Am Coll Cardiol*. Vol. 46, No. 6, (Sep 20), pp. e1-82, ISSN 1558-3597

Injac, R., Perse, M., Boskovic, M., Djordjevic-Milic, V., Djordjevic, A., Hvala, A., Cerar, A. & Strukelj, B. (2008a). Cardioprotective effects of fullerenol $C_{60}(OH)_{24}$ on a single dose doxorubicin-induced cardiotoxicity in rats with malignant neoplasm. *Technol Cancer Res Treat*. Vol. 7, No. 1, (Feb), pp. 15-25, ISSN 1533-0346.

Injac, R., Perse, M., Cerne, M., Potocnik, N., Radic, N., Govedarica, B., Djordjevic, A., Cerar, A. & Strukelj, B. (2009). Protective effects of fullerenol C60(OH)24 against doxorubicin-induced cardiotoxicity and hepatotoxicity in rats with colorectal cancer. *Biomaterials*. Vol. 30, No. 6, (Feb), pp. 1184-1196, ISSN 1878-5905

Injac, R., Radic, N., Govedarica, B., Djordjevic, A. & Strukelj, B. (2008b). Bioapplication and activity of fullerenol $C_{60}(OH)_{24}$. *African Journal of Biotechnology* Vol. 7, No. 25, (29 December 2008), pp. 4940-4950, ISSN 1684-5315.

Jamaluddin, M., Wang, S., Boldogh, I., Tian, B. & Brasier, A. R. (2007). TNF-alpha-induced NF-kappaB/RelA Ser(276) phosphorylation and enhanceosome formation is mediated by an ROS-dependent PKAc pathway. *Cell Signal*. Vol. 19, No. 7, (Jul), pp. 1419-1433, ISSN 0898-6568

Jensen, R. A. (1986). Doxorubicin cardiotoxicity: contractile changes after long-term treatment in the rat. *J Pharmacol Exp Ther*. Vol. 236, No. 1, (Jan), pp. 197-203, ISSN 0022-3565

Ji, Z. Q., Sun, H., Wang, H., Xie, Q., Liu, Y. & Wang, Z. (2006). Biodistribution and tumor uptake of C60(OH) x in mice. *Journal of Nanoparticle Research*. Vol. 8, No. 1, pp. 53-63, ISSN 1388-0764.

Jiang, B., Zhang, L., Li, M., Wu, W., Yang, M., Wang, J. & Guo, D. A. (2008). Salvianolic acids prevent acute doxorubicin cardiotoxicity in mice through suppression of oxidative stress. *Food Chem Toxicol*. Vol. 46, No. 5, (May), pp. 1510-1515, ISSN 0278-69150278-6915 (Linking).

Kaiserova, H., Simunek, T., Sterba, M., den Hartog, G. J., Schroterova, L., Popelova, O., Gersl, V., Kvasnickova, E. & Bast, A. (2007). New iron chelators in anthracycline-induced cardiotoxicity. *Cardiovasc Toxicol*. Vol. 7, No. 2, pp. 145-150, ISSN 1530-7905

Kaithwas, G., Dubey, K. & Pillai, K. K. (2011). Effect of aloe vera (Aloe barbadensis Miller) gel on doxorubicin-induced myocardial oxidative stress and calcium overload in albino rats. *Indian J Exp Biol*. Vol. 49, No. 4, (Apr), pp. 260-268, ISSN 0019-5189

Kalaria, D. R., Sharma, G., Beniwal, V. & Ravi Kumar, M. N. (2009). Design of biodegradable nanoparticles for oral delivery of doxorubicin: in vivo pharmacokinetics and toxicity studies in rats. *Pharm Res*. Vol. 26, No. 3, (Mar), pp. 492-501, ISSN 0724-8741

Kane, R. C., McGuinn, W. D., Jr., Dagher, R., Justice, R. & Pazdur, R. (2008). Dexrazoxane (Totect): FDA review and approval for the treatment of accidental extravasation following intravenous anthracycline chemotherapy. *Oncologist*. Vol. 13, No. 4, (Apr), pp. 445-450, ISSN 1083-7159

Kang, Y. J. (1999). The antioxidant function of metallothionein in the heart. *Proc Soc Exp Biol Med*. Vol. 222, No. 3, (Dec), pp. 263-273, ISSN 0037-9727

Kang, Y. J., Chen, Y. & Epstein, P. N. (1996). Suppression of doxorubicin cardiotoxicity by overexpression of catalase in the heart of transgenic mice. *J Biol Chem*. Vol. 271, No. 21, (May 24), pp. 12610-12616, ISSN 0021-9258

Kang, Y. J., Chen, Y., Yu, A., Voss-McCowan, M. & Epstein, P. N. (1997). Overexpression of metallothionein in the heart of transgenic mice suppresses doxorubicin cardiotoxicity. *J Clin Invest*. Vol. 100, No. 6, (Sep 15), pp. 1501-1506, ISSN 0021-9738

Kouvaris, J. R., Kouloulias, V. E. & Vlahos, L. J. (2007). Amifostine: the first selective-target and broad-spectrum radioprotector. *Oncologist*. Vol. 12, No. 6, (Jun), pp. 738-747, ISSN 1083-7159

Kratschmer, W., Lamb, L. D., Fostiropoulos, K. & Huffman, D. R. (1990). Solid C60: a new form of carbon. *Nature*. Vol. 347, No. pp. 354 - 358

Kremer, L. C., van Dalen, E. C., Offringa, M. & Voute, P. A. (2002). Frequency and risk factors of anthracycline-induced clinical heart failure in children: a systematic review. *Ann Oncol*. Vol. 13, No. 4, (Apr), pp. 503-512, ISSN 0923-7534

Kroto, H. W., Heath, J. R., O'Brien, S. C., Curl, R. F. & Smalley, R. E. (1985). C60: Buckminsterfullerene. *Nature*. Vol. 318, No. pp. 162-163

L'Ecuyer, T., Allebban, Z., Thomas, R. & Vander Heide, R. (2004). Glutathione S-transferase overexpression protects against anthracycline-induced H9C2 cell death. *Am J Physiol Heart Circ Physiol*. Vol. 286, No. 6, (Jun), pp. H2057-2064, ISSN 0363-6135

Lefrak, E. A., Pitha, J., Rosenheim, S. & Gottlieb, J. A. (1973). A clinicopathologic analysis of adriamycin cardiotoxicity. *Cancer*. Vol. 32, No. 2, (Aug), pp. 302-314, ISSN 0008-543X

Legha, S. S., Benjamin, R. S., Mackay, B., Ewer, M., Wallace, S., Valdivieso, M., Rasmussen, S. L., Blumenschein, G. R. & Freireich, E. J. (1982a). Reduction of doxorubicin cardiotoxicity by prolonged continuous intravenous infusion. *Ann Intern Med*. Vol. 96, No. 2, (Feb), pp. 133-139, ISSN 0003-4819

Legha, S. S., Wang, Y. M., Mackay, B., Ewer, M., Hortobagyi, G. N., Benjamin, R. S. & Ali, M. K. (1982b). Clinical and pharmacologic investigation of the effects of alpha-tocopherol on adriamycin cardiotoxicity. *Ann N Y Acad Sci*. Vol. 393, No. pp. 411-418, ISSN 0077-8923

Lenzhofer, R., Magometschnigg, D., Dudczak, R., Cerni, C., Bolebruch, C. & Moser, K. (1983). Indication of reduced doxorubicin-induced cardiac toxicity by additional treatment with antioxidative substances. *Experientia*. Vol. 39, No. 1, (Jan 15), pp. 62-64, ISSN 0014-4754

Li, T., Danelisen, I., Bello-Klein, A. & Singal, P. K. (2000). Effects of probucol on changes of antioxidant enzymes in adriamycin-induced cardiomyopathy in rats. *Cardiovasc Res*. Vol. 46, No. 3, (Jun), pp. 523-530, ISSN 0008-6363

Li, T. & Singal, P. K. (2000). Adriamycin-induced early changes in myocardial antioxidant enzymes and their modulation by probucol. *Circulation*. Vol. 102, No. 17, (Oct 24), pp. 2105-2110, ISSN 1524-4539

Li, W., Xu, B., Xu, J. & Wu, X. L. (2009). Procyanidins produce significant attenuation of doxorubicin-induced cardiotoxicity via suppression of oxidative stress. *Basic Clin Pharmacol Toxicol*. Vol. 104, No. 3, (Mar), pp. 192-197, ISSN 1742-7843

Licata, S., Saponiero, A., Mordente, A. & Minotti, G. (2000). Doxorubicin metabolism and toxicity in human myocardium: role of cytoplasmic deglycosidation and carbonyl reduction. *Chem Res Toxicol*. Vol. 13, No. 5, (May), pp. 414-420, ISSN 0893-228X

Links, M. & Lewis, C. (1999). Chemoprotectants: a review of their clinical pharmacology and therapeutic efficacy. *Drugs*. Vol. 57, No. 3, (Mar), pp. 293-308, ISSN 0012-6667

Lipshultz, S. E. & Adams, M. J. (2010). Cardiotoxicity after childhood cancer: beginning with the end in mind. *J Clin Oncol*. Vol. 28, No. 8, (Mar 10), pp. 1276-1281, ISSN 1527-7755

Lipshultz, S. E., Colan, S. D., Gelber, R. D., Perez-Atayde, A. R., Sallan, S. E. & Sanders, S. P. (1991). Late cardiac effects of doxorubicin therapy for acute lymphoblastic leukemia in childhood. *N Engl J Med*. Vol. 324, No. 12, (Mar 21), pp. 808-815, ISSN 0028-4793

Lipshultz, S. E., Lipsitz, S. R., Sallan, S. E., Dalton, V. M., Mone, S. M., Gelber, R. D. & Colan, S. D. (2005). Chronic progressive cardiac dysfunction years after doxorubicin therapy for childhood acute lymphoblastic leukemia. *J Clin Oncol*. Vol. 23, No. 12, (Apr 20), pp. 2629-2636, ISSN 0732-183X

Lipshultz, S. E., Rifai, N., Dalton, V. M., Levy, D. E., Silverman, L. B., Lipsitz, S. R., Colan, S. D., Asselin, B. L., Barr, R. D., Clavell, L. A., Hurwitz, C. A., Moghrabi, A., Samson, Y., Schorin, M. A., Gelber, R. D. & Sallan, S. E. (2004). The effect of dexrazoxane on myocardial injury in doxorubicin-treated children with acute lymphoblastic leukemia. *N Engl J Med*. Vol. 351, No. 2, (Jul 8), pp. 145-153, ISSN 1533-4406

Lipshultz, S. E., Scully, R. E., Lipsitz, S. R., Sallan, S. E., Silverman, L. B., Miller, T. L., Barry, E. V., Asselin, B. L., Athale, U., Clavell, L. A., Larsen, E., Moghrabi, A., Samson, Y., Michon, B., Schorin, M. A., Cohen, H. J., Neuberg, D. S., Orav, E. J. & Colan, S. D. (2010). Assessment of dexrazoxane as a cardioprotectant in doxorubicin-treated children with high-risk acute lymphoblastic leukaemia: long-term follow-up of a prospective, randomised, multicentre trial. *Lancet Oncol*. Vol. 11, No. 10, (Oct), pp. 950-961, ISSN 1474-5488

Liu, Z., Davis, C., Cai, W., He, L., Chen, X. & Dai, H. (2008). Circulation and long-term fate of functionalized, biocompatible single-walled carbon nanotubes in mice probed by Raman spectroscopy. *Proc Natl Acad Sci U S A*. Vol. 105, No. 5, (Feb 5), pp. 1410-1415, ISSN 1091-6490

Loch, T., Vakhrusheva, O., Piotrowska, I., Ziolkowski, W., Ebelt, H., Braun, T. & Bober, E. (2009). Different extent of cardiac malfunction and resistance to oxidative stress in heterozygous and homozygous manganese-dependent superoxide dismutase-mutant mice. *Cardiovasc Res*. Vol. 82, No. 3, (Jun 1), pp. 448-457, ISSN 1755-3245

Lopez, M., Vici, P., Di Lauro, K., Conti, F., Paoletti, G., Ferraironi, A., Sciuto, R., Giannarelli, D. & Maini, C. L. (1998). Randomized prospective clinical trial of high-dose epirubicin and dexrazoxane in patients with advanced breast cancer and soft tissue sarcomas. *J Clin Oncol*. Vol. 16, No. 1, (Jan), pp. 86-92, ISSN 0732-183X

Lu, H. Z., Geng, B. Q., Zhu, Y. L. & Yong, D. G. (1996). Effects of beta-carotene on doxorubicin-induced cardiotoxicity in rats. *Zhongguo Yao Li Xue Bao*. Vol. 17, No. 4, (Jul), pp. 317-320, ISSN 0253-9756

Ludke, A. R., Al-Shudiefat, A. A., Dhingra, S., Jassal, D. S. & Singal, P. K. (2009). A concise description of cardioprotective strategies in doxorubicin-induced cardiotoxicity. *Can J Physiol Pharmacol*. Vol. 87, No. 10, (Oct), pp. 756-763, ISSN 1205-7541

Lum, B. L., Svec, J. M. & Torti, F. M. (1985). Doxorubicin: alteration of dose scheduling as a means of reducing cardiotoxicity. *Drug Intell Clin Pharm*. Vol. 19, No. 4, (Apr), pp. 259-264, ISSN 0012-6578

Luo, X., Evrovsky, Y., Cole, D., Trines, J., Benson, L. N. & Lehotay, D. C. (1997). Doxorubicin-induced acute changes in cytotoxic aldehydes, antioxidant status and cardiac function in the rat. *Biochim Biophys Acta*. Vol. 1360, No. 1, (Feb 27), pp. 45-52, ISSN 0006-3002

Luo, X., Reichetzer, B., Trines, J., Benson, L. N. & Lehotay, D. C. (1999). L-carnitine attenuates doxorubicin-induced lipid peroxidation in rats. *Free Radic Biol Med*. Vol. 26, No. 9-10, (May), pp. 1158-1165, ISSN 0891-5849

Lyu, Y. L., Kerrigan, J. E., Lin, C. P., Azarova, A. M., Tsai, Y. C., Ban, Y. & Liu, L. F. (2007). Topoisomerase IIbeta mediated DNA double-strand breaks: implications in doxorubicin cardiotoxicity and prevention by dexrazoxane. *Cancer Res*. Vol. 67, No. 18, (Sep 15), pp. 8839-8846, ISSN 0008-5472

Mabro, M., Faivre, S. & Raymond, E. (1999). A risk-benefit assessment of amifostine in cytoprotection. *Drug Saf*. Vol. 21, No. 5, (Nov), pp. 367-387, ISSN 0114-5916

Malcom, J., Arnold, O., Howlett, J. G., Ducharme, A., Ezekowitz, J. A., Gardner, M. J., Giannetti, N., Haddad, H., Heckman, G. A., Isaac, D., Jong, P., Liu, P., Mann, E., McKelvie, R. S., Moe, G. W., Svendsen, A. M., Tsuyuki, R. T., O'Halloran, K., Ross, H. J., Sequeira, E. J. & White, M. (2008). Canadian Cardiovascular Society Consensus Conference guidelines on heart failure--2008 update: best practices for the transition of care of heart failure patients, and the recognition, investigation and treatment of cardiomyopathies. *Can J Cardiol*. Vol. 24, No. 1, (Jan), pp. 21-40, ISSN 1916-7075

Marzatico, F., Porta, C., Moroni, M., Bertorelli, L., Borasio, E., Finotti, N., Pansarasa, O. & Castagna, L. (2000). In vitro antioxidant properties of amifostine (WR-2721, Ethyol). *Cancer Chemother Pharmacol*. Vol. 45, No. 2, pp. 172-176, ISSN 0344-5704

May, P. M., Williams, G. K. & Williams, D. R. (1980). Solution chemistry studies of adriamycin--iron complexes present in vivo. *Eur J Cancer*. Vol. 16, No. 9, (Sep), pp. 1275-1276, ISSN 0014-2964

McEvoy, K. G., Snow, K. E., Miller, J., Kester, L. & Welsh, H. O. (2010). AHFS Drug Information 2010, K. G. McEvoy, (Ed.), American Society of Health-System Pharmacists, ISBN 1585282472, Bethesda, Maryland, U.S.

Merten, K. E., Feng, W., Zhang, L., Pierce, W., Cai, J., Klein, J. B. & Kang, Y. J. (2005). Modulation of cytochrome C oxidase-va is possibly involved in metallothionein protection from doxorubicin cardiotoxicity. *J Pharmacol Exp Ther*. Vol. 315, No. 3, (Dec), pp. 1314-1319, ISSN 0022-3565

Milei, J., Boveris, A., Llesuy, S., Molina, H. A., Storino, R., Ortega, D. & Milei, S. E. (1986). Amelioration of adriamycin-induced cardiotoxicity in rabbits by prenylamine and vitamins A and E. *Am Heart J*. Vol. 111, No. 1, (Jan), pp. 95-102, ISSN 0002-8703

Milic Torres, V., Posa, M., Srdjenovic, B. & Simplicio, A. L. (2011). Solubilization of fullerene C60 in micellar solutions of different solubilizers. *Colloids Surf B Biointerfaces*. Vol. 82, No. 1, (Jan 1), pp. 46-53, ISSN 1873-4367

Milic Torres, V., Srdjenovic, B., Jacevic, V., Dragojevic-Simic, V., Djordjevic, A. & Simplicio, A. L. (2010). Fullerenol $C_{60}(OH)_{24}$ prevents doxorubicin-induced acute cardiotoxicity in rats. *Pharmacol Rep*. Vol. 62, No. 4, pp. 707-718, ISSN 1734-1140

Minotti, G. (1993). Sources and role of iron in lipid peroxidation. *Chem Res Toxicol*. Vol. 6, No. 2, (Mar-Apr), pp. 134-146, ISSN 0893-228X

Minotti, G., Cairo, G. & Monti, E. (1999). Role of iron in anthracycline cardiotoxicity: new tunes for an old song? *FASEB J*. Vol. 13, No. 2, (Feb), pp. 199-212, ISSN 0892-6638

Minotti, G., Menna, P., Salvatorelli, E., Cairo, G. & Gianni, L. (2004). Anthracyclines: molecular advances and pharmacologic developments in antitumor activity and cardiotoxicity. *Pharmacol Rev*. Vol. 56, No. 2, (Jun), pp. 185-229, ISSN 0031-6997

Minotti, G., Ronchi, R., Salvatorelli, E., Menna, P. & Cairo, G. (2001). Doxorubicin irreversibly inactivates iron regulatory proteins 1 and 2 in cardiomyocytes: evidence for distinct metabolic pathways and implications for iron-mediated cardiotoxicity of antitumor therapy. *Cancer Res*. Vol. 61, No. 23, (Dec 1), pp. 8422-8428, ISSN 0008-5472

Miranda, C. J., Makui, H., Soares, R. J., Bilodeau, M., Mui, J., Vali, H., Bertrand, R., Andrews, N. C. & Santos, M. M. (2003). Hfe deficiency increases susceptibility to cardiotoxicity and exacerbates changes in iron metabolism induced by doxorubicin. *Blood*. Vol. 102, No. 7, (Oct 1), pp. 2574-2580, ISSN 0006-4971

Mukherjee, S., Banerjee, S. K., Maulik, M., Dinda, A. K., Talwar, K. K. & Maulik, S. K. (2003). Protection against acute adriamycin-induced cardiotoxicity by garlic: role of endogenous antioxidants and inhibition of TNF-alpha expression. *BMC Pharmacol*. Vol. 3, No. (Dec 20), pp. 16, ISSN 1471-2210

Murley, J. S., Kataoka, Y., Weydert, C. J., Oberley, L. W. & Grdina, D. J. (2006). Delayed radioprotection by nuclear transcription factor kappaB -mediated induction of manganese superoxide dismutase in human microvascular endothelial cells after exposure to the free radical scavenger WR1065. *Free Radic Biol Med*. Vol. 40, No. 6, (Mar 15), pp. 1004-1016, ISSN 0891-5849

Nazeyrollas, P., Frances, C., Prevost, A., Costa, B., Lorenzato, M., Kantelip, J. P., Elaerts, J. & Millart, H. (2003). Efficiency of amifostine as a protection against doxorubicin toxicity in rats during a 12-day treatment. *Anticancer Res*. Vol. 23, No. 1A, (Jan-Feb), pp. 405-409, ISSN 0250-7005

Nazeyrollas, P., Prevost, A., Baccard, N., Manot, L., Devillier, P. & Millart, H. (1999). Effects of amifostine on perfused isolated rat heart and on acute doxorubicin-induced cardiotoxicity. *Cancer Chemother Pharmacol*. Vol. 43, No. 3, pp. 227-232, ISSN 0344-5704

Nysom, K., Holm, K., Lipsitz, S. R., Mone, S. M., Colan, S. D., Orav, E. J., Sallan, S. E., Olsen, J. H., Hertz, H., Jacobsen, J. R. & Lipshultz, S. E. (1998). Relationship between cumulative anthracycline dose and late cardiotoxicity in childhood acute lymphoblastic leukemia. *J Clin Oncol*. Vol. 16, No. 2, (Feb), pp. 545-550, ISSN 0732-183X

Olson, H. M. & Capen, C. C. (1977). Subacute cardiotoxicity of adriamycin in the rat: biochemical and ultrastructural investigations. *Lab Invest*. Vol. 37, No. 4, (Oct), pp. 386-394, ISSN 0023-6837

Olson, R. D., Mushlin, P. S., Brenner, D. E., Fleischer, S., Cusack, B. J., Chang, B. K. & Boucek, R. J., Jr. (1988). Doxorubicin cardiotoxicity may be caused by its metabolite, doxorubicinol. *Proc Natl Acad Sci U S A*. Vol. 85, No. 10, (May), pp. 3585-3589, ISSN 0027-8424

Olukman, M., Can, C., Erol, A., Oktem, G., Oral, O. & Cinar, M. G. (2009). Reversal of doxorubicin-induced vascular dysfunction by resveratrol in rat thoracic aorta: Is there a possible role of nitric oxide synthase inhibition? *Anadolu Kardiyol Derg*. Vol. 9, No. 4, (Aug), pp. 260-266, ISSN 1308-0032

Pelikan, P. C., Weisfeldt, M. L., Jacobus, W. E., Miceli, M. V., Bulkley, B. H. & Gerstenblith, G. (1986). Acute doxorubicin cardiotoxicity: functional, metabolic, and morphologic alterations in the isolated, perfused rat heart. *J Cardiovasc Pharmacol*. Vol. 8, No. 5, (Sep-Oct), pp. 1058-1066, ISSN 0160-2446

Popelova, O., Sterba, M., Haskova, P., Simunek, T., Hroch, M., Guncova, I., Nachtigal, P., Adamcova, M., Gersl, V. & Mazurova, Y. (2009). Dexrazoxane-afforded protection against chronic anthracycline cardiotoxicity in vivo: effective rescue of cardiomyocytes from apoptotic cell death. *Br J Cancer*. Vol. 101, No. 5, (Sep 1), pp. 792-802, ISSN 1532-1827

Potemski, P., Polakowski, P., Wiktorowska-Owczarek, A. K., Owczarek, J., Pluzanska, A. & Orszulak-Michalak, D. (2006). Amifostine improves hemodynamic parameters in doxorubicin-pretreated rabbits. *Pharmacol Rep*. Vol. 58, No. 6, (Nov-Dec), pp. 966-972, ISSN 1734-1140

Rabelo, E., De Angelis, K., Bock, P., Gatelli Fernandes, T., Cervo, F., Bello Klein, A., Clausell, N. & Claudia Irigoyen, M. (2001). Baroreflex sensitivity and oxidative stress in adriamycin-induced heart failure. *Hypertension*. Vol. 38, No. 3 Pt 2, (Sep), pp. 576-580, ISSN 1524-4563

Roca, J., Ishida, R., Berger, J. M., Andoh, T. & Wang, J. C. (1994). Antitumor bisdioxopiperazines inhibit yeast DNA topoisomerase II by trapping the enzyme in the form of a closed protein clamp. *Proc Natl Acad Sci U S A*. Vol. 91, No. 5, (Mar 1), pp. 1781-1785, ISSN 0027-8424

Safra, T. (2003). Cardiac safety of liposomal anthracyclines. *Oncologist*. Vol. 8 Suppl 2, No. pp. 17-24, ISSN 1083-7159

Sahin, K., Sahin, N. & Kucuk, O. (2010). Lycopene and chemotherapy toxicity. *Nutr Cancer*. Vol. 62, No. 7, pp. 988-995, ISSN 1532-7914

Schimmel, K. J., Richel, D. J., van den Brink, R. B. & Guchelaar, H. J. (2004). Cardiotoxicity of cytotoxic drugs. *Cancer Treat Rev*. Vol. 30, No. 2, (Apr), pp. 181-191, ISSN 0305-7372

Shan, K., Lincoff, A. M. & Young, J. B. (1996). Anthracycline-induced cardiotoxicity. *Ann Intern Med*. Vol. 125, No. 1, (Jul 1), pp. 47-58, ISSN 0003-4819

Shaw, L. M., Glover, D., Turrisi, A., Brown, D. Q., Bonner, H. S., Norfleet, A. L., Weiler, C., Glick, J. H. & Kligerman, M. M. (1988). Pharmacokinetics of WR-2721. *Pharmacol Ther*. Vol. 39, No. 1-3, pp. 195-201, ISSN 0163-7258

Shi, Y., Moon, M., Dawood, S., McManus, B. & Liu, P. P. (2011). Mechanisms and management of doxorubicin cardiotoxicity. *Herz*. Vol. 36, No. 4, (Jun), pp. 296-305, ISSN 1615-6692

Sikora, K., Advani, S., Koroltchouk, V., Magrath, I., Levy, L., Pinedo, H., Schwartsmann, G., Tattersall, M. & Yan, S. (1999). Essential drugs for cancer therapy: a World Health Organization consultation. *Ann Oncol*. Vol. 10, No. 4, (Apr), pp. 385-390, ISSN 0923-7534

Simunek, T., Sterba, M., Holeckova, M., Kaplanova, J., Klimtova, I., Adamcova, M., Gersl, V. & Hrdina, R. (2005). Myocardial content of selected elements in experimental anthracycline-induced cardiomyopathy in rabbits. *Biometals*. Vol. 18, No. 2, (Apr), pp. 163-169, ISSN 0966-0844

Simunek, T., Sterba, M., Popelova, O., Adamcova, M., Hrdina, R. & Gersl, V. (2009). Anthracycline-induced cardiotoxicity: overview of studies examining the roles of oxidative stress and free cellular iron. *Pharmacol Rep*. Vol. 61, No. 1, (Jan-Feb), pp. 154-171, ISSN 1734-1140

Singal, P. K. & Iliskovic, N. (1998). Doxorubicin-induced cardiomyopathy. *N Engl J Med*. Vol. 339, No. 13, (Sep 24), pp. 900-905, ISSN 0028-4793

Siveski-Iliskovic, N., Hill, M., Chow, D. A. & Singal, P. K. (1995). Probucol Protects Against Adriamycin Cardiomyopathy Without Interfering With Its Antitumor Effect. *Circulation*. Vol. 91, No. 1, (January 1, 1995), pp. 10-15

Smith, L. A., Cornelius, V. R., Plummer, C. J., Levitt, G., Verrill, M., Canney, P. & Jones, A. (2010). Cardiotoxicity of anthracycline agents for the treatment of cancer: systematic review and meta-analysis of randomised controlled trials. *BMC Cancer*. Vol. 10, No. pp. 337, ISSN 1471-2407

Smoluk, G. D., Fahey, R. C., Calabro-Jones, P. M., Aguilera, J. A. & Ward, J. F. (1988). Radioprotection of cells in culture by WR-2721 and derivatives: form of the drug responsible for protection. *Cancer Res*. Vol. 48, No. 13, (Jul 1), pp. 3641-3647, ISSN 0008-5472

Spencer, C. M. & Goa, K. L. (1995). Amifostine. A review of its pharmacodynamic and pharmacokinetic properties, and therapeutic potential as a radioprotector and cytotoxic chemoprotector. *Drugs*. Vol. 50, No. 6, (Dec), pp. 1001-1031, ISSN 0012-6667

Speyer, J. L., Green, M. D., Zeleniuch-Jacquotte, A., Wernz, J. C., Rey, M., Sanger, J., Kramer, E., Ferrans, V., Hochster, H., Meyers, M. & et al. (1992). ICRF-187 permits longer treatment with doxorubicin in women with breast cancer. *J Clin Oncol*. Vol. 10, No. 1, (Jan), pp. 117-127, ISSN 0732-183X

Srdjenovic, B., Milic-Torres, V., Grujic, N., Stankov, K., Djordjevic, A. & Vasovic, V. (2010). Antioxidant properties of fullerenol C60(OH)24 in rat kidneys, testes, and lungs treated with doxorubicin. *Toxicol Mech Methods*. Vol. 20, No. 6, (Jul), pp. 298-305, ISSN 1537-6524

Steinherz, L. J., Graham, T., Hurwitz, R., Sondheimer, H. M., Schwartz, R. G., Shaffer, E. M., Sandor, G., Benson, L. & Williams, R. (1992). Guidelines for cardiac monitoring of children during and after anthracycline therapy: report of the Cardiology Committee of the Childrens Cancer Study Group. *Pediatrics*. Vol. 89, No. 5 Pt 1, (May), pp. 942-949, ISSN 0031-4005

Sun, X. & Kang, Y. J. (2002). Prior increase in metallothionein levels is required to prevent doxorubicin cardiotoxicity. *Exp Biol Med (Maywood)*. Vol. 227, No. 8, (Sep), pp. 652-657, ISSN 1535-3702

Sun, X., Zhou, Z. & Kang, Y. J. (2001). Attenuation of doxorubicin chronic toxicity in metallothionein-overexpressing transgenic mouse heart. *Cancer Res*. Vol. 61, No. 8, (Apr 15), pp. 3382-3387, ISSN 0008-5472

Swain, S. M., Whaley, F. S., Gerber, M. C., Weisberg, S., York, M., Spicer, D., Jones, S. E., Wadler, S., Desai, A., Vogel, C., Speyer, J., Mittelman, A., Reddy, S., Pendergrass, K., Velez-Garcia, E., Ewer, M. S., Bianchine, J. R. & Gams, R. A. (1997). Cardioprotection with dexrazoxane for doxorubicin-containing therapy in advanced breast cancer. *J Clin Oncol*. Vol. 15, No. 4, (Apr), pp. 1318-1332, ISSN 0732-183X

Sweetman, S. (2011). Martindale: The Complete Drug Reference, *International Journal of Pharmacy Practice*, S. Sweetman, (Ed.), Pharmaceutical Press, ISBN 978 0 85369 933 0, London, U.K.

Tatlidede, E., Sehirli, O., Velioglu-Ogunc, A., Cetinel, S., Yegen, B. C., Yarat, A., Suleymanoglu, S. & Sener, G. (2009). Resveratrol treatment protects against doxorubicin-induced cardiotoxicity by alleviating oxidative damage. *Free Radic Res*. Vol. 43, No. 3, (Mar), pp. 195-205, ISSN 1029-2470

Tesoriere, L., Ciaccio, M., Valenza, M., Bongiorno, A., Maresi, E., Albiero, R. & Livrea, M. A. (1994). Effect of vitamin A administration on resistance of rat heart against doxorubicin-induced cardiotoxicity and lethality. *J Pharmacol Exp Ther*. Vol. 269, No. 1, (Apr), pp. 430-436, ISSN 0022-3565

Testore, F., Milanese, S., Ceste, M., de Conciliis, E., Parello, G., Lanfranco, C., Manfredi, R., Ferrero, G., Simoni, C., Miglietta, L., Ferro, S., Giaretto, L. & Bosso, G. (2008). Cardioprotective effect of dexrazoxane in patients with breast cancer treated with anthracyclines in adjuvant setting: a 10-year single institution experience. *Am J Cardiovasc Drugs*. Vol. 8, No. 4, pp. 257-263, ISSN 1175-3277

Theil, E. C. (1987). Ferritin: structure, gene regulation, and cellular function in animals, plants, and microorganisms. *Annu Rev Biochem*. Vol. 56, No. pp. 289-315, ISSN 0066-4154

Torti, F. M., Bristow, M. R., Howes, A. E., Aston, D., Stockdale, F. E., Carter, S. K., Kohler, M., Brown, B. W., Jr. & Billingham, M. E. (1983). Reduced cardiotoxicity of doxorubicin delivered on a weekly schedule. Assessment by endomyocardial biopsy. *Ann Intern Med*. Vol. 99, No. 6, (Dec), pp. 745-749, ISSN 0003-4819

Trajkovic, S., Dobric, S., Jacevic, V., Dragojevic-Simic, V., Milovanovic, Z. & Dordevic, A. (2007). Tissue-protective effects of fullerenol C60(OH)24 and amifostine in irradiated rats. *Colloids Surf B Biointerfaces*. Vol. 58, No. 1, (Jul 1), pp. 39-43, ISSN 0927-7765

Trivedi, P. P., Kushwaha, S., Tripathi, D. N. & Jena, G. B. (2011). Cardioprotective Effects of Hesperetin against Doxorubicin-Induced Oxidative Stress and DNA Damage in Rat. *Cardiovasc Toxicol*. Vol. No. (May 7), pp. ISSN 1559-0259

Utley, J. F., Marlowe, C. & Waddell, W. J. (1976). Distribution of 35S-labeled WR-2721 in normal and malignant tissues of the mouse1,2. *Radiat Res*. Vol. 68, No. 2, (Nov), pp. 284-291, ISSN 0033-7587

Utley, J. F., Seaver, N., Newton, G. L. & Fahey, R. C. (1984). Pharmacokinetics of WR-1065 in mouse tissue following treatment with WR-2721. *Int J Radiat Oncol Biol Phys*. Vol. 10, No. 9, (Sep), pp. 1525-1528, ISSN 0360-3016

van Dalen, E. C., Caron, H. N., Dickinson, H. O. & Kremer, L. C. (2011a). Cardioprotective interventions for cancer patients receiving anthracyclines. *Cochrane Database Syst Rev*. Vol. No. 6, pp. CD003917, ISSN 1469-493X

van Dalen, E. C., van den Berg, H., Raphael, M. F., Caron, H. N. & Kremer, L. C. (2011b). Should anthracyclines and dexrazoxane be used for children with cancer? *Lancet Oncol*. Vol. 12, No. 1, (Jan), pp. 12-13, ISSN 1474-5488 van der Vijgh, W. J. & Peters, G. J. (1994). Protection of normal tissues from the cytotoxic effects of chemotherapy and radiation by amifostine (Ethyol): preclinical aspects. *Semin Oncol*. Vol. 21, No. 5 Suppl 11, (Oct), pp. 2-7, ISSN 0093-7754

Van Vleet, J. F. & Ferrans, V. J. (1980). Evaluation of vitamin E and selenium protection against chronic adriamycin toxicity in rabbits. *Cancer Treat Rep*. Vol. 64, No. 2-3, (Feb-Mar), pp. 315-317, ISSN 0361-5960

Vasquez-Vivar, J., Martasek, P., Hogg, N., Masters, B. S., Pritchard, K. A., Jr. & Kalyanaraman, B. (1997). Endothelial nitric oxide synthase-dependent superoxide generation from adriamycin. *Biochemistry*. Vol. 36, No. 38, (Sep 23), pp. 11293-11297, ISSN 0006-2960

Venturini, M., Michelotti, A., Del Mastro, L., Gallo, L., Carnino, F., Garrone, O., Tibaldi, C., Molea, N., Bellina, R. C., Pronzato, P., Cyrus, P., Vinke, J., Testore, F., Guelfi, M., Lionetto, R., Bruzzi, P., Conte, P. F. & Rosso, R. (1996). Multicenter randomized controlled clinical trial to evaluate cardioprotection of dexrazoxane versus no cardioprotection in women receiving epirubicin chemotherapy for advanced breast cancer. *J Clin Oncol*. Vol. 14, No. 12, (Dec), pp. 3112-3120, ISSN 0732-183X

Villani, F., Galimberti, M., Monti, E., Cova, D., Lanza, E., Rozza-Dionigi, A., Favalli, L. & Poggi, P. (1990). Effect of ICRF-187 pretreatment against doxorubicin-induced delayed cardiotoxicity in the rat. *Toxicol Appl Pharmacol*. Vol. 102, No. 2, (Feb), pp. 292-299, ISSN 0041-008X

Von Hoff, D. D., Layard, M. W., Basa, P., Davis, H. L., Jr., Von Hoff, A. L., Rozencweig, M. & Muggia, F. M. (1979). Risk factors for doxorubicin-induced congestive heart failure. *Ann Intern Med*. Vol. 91, No. 5, (Nov), pp. 710-717, ISSN 0003-4819

Wakade, A. S., Shah, A. S., Kulkarni, M. P. & Juvekar, A. R. (2008). Protective effect of Piper longum L. on oxidative stress induced injury and cellular abnormality in adriamycin induced cardiotoxicity in rats. *Indian J Exp Biol*. Vol. 46, No. 7, (Jul), pp. 528-533, ISSN 0019-5189

Wallace, K. B. (2007). Adriamycin-induced interference with cardiac mitochondrial calcium homeostasis. *Cardiovasc Toxicol*. Vol. 7, No. 2, pp. 101-107, ISSN 1530-7905

Wang, J. C. (2002). Cellular roles of DNA topoisomerases: a molecular perspective. *Nat Rev Mol Cell Biol*. Vol. 3, No. 6, (Jun), pp. 430-440, ISSN 1471-0072

Washburn, L. C., Rafter, J. J. & Hayes, R. L. (1976). Prediction of the effective radioprotective dose of WR-2721 in humans through an interspecies tissue distribution study. *Radiat Res*. Vol. 66, No. 1, (Apr), pp. 100-105, ISSN 0033-7587

Weiss, R. B. (1992). The anthracyclines: will we ever find a better doxorubicin? *Semin Oncol*. Vol. 19, No. 6, (Dec), pp. 670-686, ISSN 0093-7754

Wexler, L. H., Andrich, M. P., Venzon, D., Berg, S. L., Weaver-McClure, L., Chen, C. C., Dilsizian, V., Avila, N., Jarosinski, P., Balis, F. M., Poplack, D. G. & Horowitz, M. E. (1996). Randomized trial of the cardioprotective agent ICRF-187 in pediatric sarcoma patients treated with doxorubicin. *J Clin Oncol*. Vol. 14, No. 2, (Feb), pp. 362-372, ISSN 0732-183X

Wiseman, L. R. & Spencer, C. M. (1998). Dexrazoxane. A review of its use as a cardioprotective agent in patients receiving anthracycline-based chemotherapy. *Drugs*. Vol. 56, No. 3, (Sep), pp. 385-403, ISSN 0012-6667

Wouters, K. A., Kremer, L. C., Miller, T. L., Herman, E. H. & Lipshultz, S. E. (2005). Protecting against anthracycline-induced myocardial damage: a review of the most promising strategies. *Br J Haematol*. Vol. 131, No. 5, (Dec), pp. 561-578, ISSN 0007-1048

Xing, G., Zhang, J., Zhao, Y., Tang, J., Zhang, B., Gao, X., Yuan, H., Qu, L., Cao, W., Chai, Z., Ibrahim, K. & Su, R. (2004). Influences of Structural Properties on Stability of Fullerenols. *The Journal of Physical Chemistry B*. Vol. 108, No. 31, pp. 11473-11479, ISSN 1520-6106.

Xu, X., Persson, H. L. & Richardson, D. R. (2005). Molecular pharmacology of the interaction of anthracyclines with iron. *Mol Pharmacol*. Vol. 68, No. 2, (Aug), pp. 261-271, ISSN 0026-895X

Xu, X., Sutak, R. & Richardson, D. R. (2008). Iron chelation by clinically relevant anthracyclines: alteration in expression of iron-regulated genes and atypical changes in intracellular iron distribution and trafficking. *Mol Pharmacol*. Vol. 73, No. 3, (Mar), pp. 833-844, ISSN 1521-0111

Yen, H. C., Oberley, T. D., Vichitbandha, S., Ho, Y. S. & St Clair, D. K. (1996). The protective role of manganese superoxide dismutase against adriamycin-induced acute cardiac toxicity in transgenic mice. *J Clin Invest*. Vol. 98, No. 5, (Sep 1), pp. 1253-1260, ISSN 0021-9738

Yuhas, J. M. (1979). Differential protection of normal and malignant tissues against the cytotoxic effects of mechlorethamine. *Cancer Treat Rep*. Vol. 63, No. 6, (Jun), pp. 971-976, ISSN 0361-5960

Yuhas, J. M. (1980). A more general role for WR-2721 in cancer therapy. *Br J Cancer*. Vol. 41, No. 5, (May), pp. 832-834, ISSN 0007-0920

Yuhas, J. M., Spellman, J. M. & Culo, F. (1980). The role of WR-2721 in radiotherapy and/or chemotherapy. *Cancer Clin Trials*. Vol. 3, No. 3, (Fall), pp. 211-216, ISSN 0190-1206

Yuhas, J. M. & Storer, J. B. (1969). Differential chemoprotection of normal and malignant tissues. *J Natl Cancer Inst*. Vol. 42, No. 2, (Feb), pp. 331-335, ISSN 0027-8874

Zhang, J.-M., Yang, W., He, P. & Zhu, S.-Z. (2004). Efficient and convenient preparation of water-soluble fullerenol. *Chinese Journal of Chemistry*. Vol. 22, No. 9, pp. 1008-1011, ISSN 1614-7065.

Zhang, Y. W., Shi, J., Li, Y. J. & Wei, L. (2009). Cardiomyocyte death in doxorubicin-induced cardiotoxicity. *Arch Immunol Ther Exp (Warsz)*. Vol. 57, No. 6, (Nov-Dec), pp. 435-445, ISSN 1661-4917

Zhu, W., Zou, Y., Aikawa, R., Harada, K., Kudoh, S., Uozumi, H., Hayashi, D., Gu, Y., Yamazaki, T., Nagai, R., Yazaki, Y. & Komuro, I. (1999). MAPK superfamily plays an important role in daunomycin-induced apoptosis of cardiac myocytes. *Circulation*. Vol. 100, No. 20, (Nov 16), pp. 2100-2107, ISSN 1524-4539

6

Trastuzumab and Cardiotoxicity

M. Fiuza and A. Magalhães
Hospital de Santa Maria,
University Clinic of Cardiology, Lisbon,
Portugal

1. Introduction

In the last two decades relevant improvements have been achieved in cancer therapy with a significant increase in overall survival. However these achievements have also been accompanied by a rise in the occurrence of side effects involving several organs, in particular the cardiovascular system. Indeed, the incidence of cardiotoxicity is continuously growing which can vanish the effectiveness of cancer therapy.

Breast cancer is the second most common form of cancer in women and the leading cause of death caused by malignancy. Over the past 25 years, breast cancer incidence has risen globally, with the highest rates in industrialized countries. However, the survival rate of cancer patients has greatly increased because of early detection through screening, as well as improvement in pharmacologic treatment. Women are, therefore, now living sufficiently long for delayed consequences of treatment to become increasingly evident.

Approximately 20-25% of breast cancer overexpresses the human epidermal growth factor receptor II (HER-2). Amplification of HER-2 gene confers aggressive behavioral traits on breast cancer cells, including incresead growth and proliferation, enhanced invasiveness and metastatic capability. (Slamon, 1987)

HER-2 is a transmembrane tyrosine kinase receptor and a member of the epidermal growth factor receptor (EGFR) family,and regulate many important cell-type specific functions, particularly cell growth, proliferation and survival. (Slamon, 1987; Chien, 2006)

The use of trastuzumab (a humanized monoclonal antibody against HER-2 receptor) has changed the natural history of patients with HER-2 positive breast cancer. In the metastatic setting, the combination of trastuzumab plus chemotherapy has significantly improved survival, response rate, time to progression, and quality of life when compared with standard chemotherapy (Slamon 1987, 2001; Vogel, 2002). In the adjuvant setting, the use of trastuzumab decreased the risk of recurrence and death (Buzdar, 2005). Given these impressive results, trastuzumab has become the standard of care for treatment of patients with HER-2 positive breast cancer.

Although trastuzumab is devoid of the classical toxicities related with cancer treatment, one of major concerns noted is the occurrence of symptomatic and asymptomatic cardiac dysfunction. In fact, this treatment showed to be associated with an increased incidence of heart failure that ranged from 4.1% in the adjuvant setting to 27% in patients with metastatic disease who received concurrent anthracycline therapy (Perez E., 2004). Early identification of patients at risk for cardiotoxicity is a major challenge for both cardiologists and oncologists, for the definition of more tailored antineoplastic therapeutic interventions. The use of cardiac biomarkers such as BNP, N-terminal pro-BNP, and troponin I, has been suggested as a method for early detection of cardiotoxicity. Also, newer measurements of LV function such as strain, strain rate and speckle tracking may be sensitive tools to detect myocardial dysfunction before changes in EF are evident, possibly identifying at-risk patients at an earlier stage.

2. Diagnosis and strategies

2.1 Clinical benefits of trastuzumab

Based in substantial improvement achieved with trastuzumab in the trials performed, US Food and Drug Administration approved in 1998 this agent for the treatment of metastatic breast cancer. Indeed, in phase 2 trial was found an objective response in 12% of patients. (Baselga et al., 1996) These benefits were further confirmed in larger phase 2 and phase 3 trials (Cobleigh et al., 1999; Slamon et al., 2001). The phase 3 trial was design to compare a conventional chemotherapy regime with and without additional trastuzumab treatment. The data demonstrated that trastuzumab association to chemotherapy produced substantial response rate, improvement in time to disease progression, as well as reduction in 1-year mortality. (Slamon et al., 2001)

Since 2006 the use of trastuzumab has been extended to treat HER-2 positive early breast cancer patients. Five major randomized trials (Herceptin Adjuvant trial - HERA, National Surgical Adjuvant Breast and Bowel Project - NSABP B-31, North Central Cancer Treatment Group - NCCTG N9831, Breast Cancer International Research Group – BCIRG 006 and Finland Herceptin trial - FinHer) have proven the benefit of adjuvant trastuzumab in early breast cancer patients. More than 11 000 patients were enrolled and treatment with trastuzumab led to about 50% improvement in disease-free survival and 33% improvement in overall survival. (Romond et al., 2005; Piccart-Gebhart et al., 2005; Tan-Chiu et al., 2005; Slamon et al., 2005; Joensuu et al., 2006).

Thus, concurrent treatment with trastuzumab is actually the standard of care for patients with early HER-2 positive breast cancer.

2.2 What does cardiotoxicity mean?

A precise definition of cardiotoxicity is still lacking. The Cardiac Review and Evaluation Committee supervising trastuzumab trials created a practical and easily applicable definition, which considered chemotherapy-induced cardiotoxicity as one or more of the following: 1) cardiomyopathy characterized by a decrease in LVEF, either global or more severe in the septum; 2) heart failure (HF) symptoms; 3) signs associated with HF, such as S3 gallop, tachycardia, edema; 4) decline in initial LVEF of at least 5% to less than 55% with accompanying signs or symptoms of HF, or asymptomatic decrease in LVEF in the range of equal to or greater than 10% to less than 55% (Seidman, 2002). (Table 1)

1. Cardiomyopathy characterized by a decrease in LVEF or changes of contraction most apparent in the interventricular septum
2. Heart failure symptoms
3. Signs associated with heart failure
4. Decline in initial LVEF of at least 5% to less than 55% with signs and symptoms of heart failure or asymptomatic decrease in LVEF of at least 10% to less than 55%

Adapted from Seidman, et al. (2002). Cardiac dysfunction in the trastuzumab clinical trials experience. *Journal of Clinical Oncology,* Vol. 20, pp. 1215 - 1221

Table 1. Cardiac Review and Evaluation Committee criteria for the diagnosis of cardiac dysfunction

Cardiotoxicity can develop in a subacute, acute, or chronic manner:

a. Acute or subacute cardiotoxicity develop during the treatment period up to 2 weeks after therapy. It is characterized by electrocardiographic abnormalities such as QT-intervals changes, ventricular repolarization abnormalities, supraventricular and ventricular arrhythmias or by acute heart failure, pericarditis, myocarditis or acute coronary syndromes.
b. Chronic cardiotoxicity is the most frequent and feared form. It can be divided in 2 groups according to the timing of symptoms onset: early, when occur in the first year after treatment and late when manifests more than 1 year after chemotherapy. The most common feature of chronic cardiotoxicity is asymptomatic systolic left ventricular dysfunction that can further lead to congestive HF. The incidence of this type of cardiotoxicity depends on several factors such as, total administered dose of chemotherapy, time of follow-up, age, history of previous cardiac disease, previous mediastinal radiation, as well as on the criteria used for cardiotoxicity assessment, ranging in different studies from 5% to 65% of patients. (Dolci, 2008; Pai, 2000).

The classic example of cardiotoxicity from anticancer treatment is anthracycline-related cardiomyopathy that remains the most common cardiotoxic chemotherapy agent. However many other agents can cause cardiotoxicity, namely the monoclonal antibody trastuzumab.

The development of chemotherapy-induced cardiomyopathy has significant implications. It has not only a negative impact on the cardiac outcome of cancer patients, but also limits their therapeutic options.

2.3 Prevalence of trastuzumab induced-cardiomyopathy

Cardiotoxicity was an unexpected finding in the phase 3 trials, as early clinical trials provided little or no indication of trastuzumab-induced cardiomyopathy. Although heart failure was seen in some patients enrolled in phase 2 trials, the rate of occurrence was low and patients were at increased risk due to previous anthracycline treatment. Subsequent reports of trastuzumab-related cardiotoxicity in the phase 3 combination chemotherapy trials prompted a retrospective analysis of seven phase 2 and 3 trastuzumab trials by an independent Cardiac Review and Evaluation Committee (CREC). (Seidman, Hudis, & Pierri, 2002) An accurate assessment of cardiotoxicity in these trials has proved difficult because their design was different in what concerns the number of patients, definition of cardiotoxicity, analysis of end points and duration of follow-up. CREC used a new set of criteria to define cardiotoxicity (Table 1) and events were also classified by the New York

Heart Association (NYHA) functional classification system. Data from 1219 patients enrolled in those 7 trials were retrospectively analyzed and cardiotoxicity was detected in 112 patients (9.2%). The incidence of trastuzumab-induced cardiomyopathy ranged from 1% to 27% in different arms of trials and was higher when trastuzumab and anthracyclines were used concurrently (Seidman, Hudis, & Pierri, 2002)(Table 2)

	Incidence (%)				
Therapy	Trastuzumab monotherapy	Trastuzumab + AC	Trastuzumab + paclitaxel	AC	Paclitaxel monotherapy
CD	3-7	27	13	8	1
NYHA class III or IV	2-4	16	2	4	1

Adapted from Keefe DL (2002). Trastuzumab-associated cardiotoxicity. *Cancer,* Vol. 95, pp. 1592-1600
AC=anthracycline plus cyclophosphamide; CD=cardiac dysfunction; NYHA=New York Heart

Table 2. Retrospective analysis conducted by the Cardiac Review and Evaluation Committee of seven studies to detect trastuzumab-related cardiotoxicity.

Concerns about cardiotoxicity, together with the remarkable tumor response to this therapy, served as an impetus for several large trials collectively known as the trastuzumab adjuvant trials, which incorporate appropriate cardiac monitoring (Buzdar,2005; Perez, 2004; Cobleigh, 1999; Slamon 2001; Romond, 2005). The study protocol in these trials determined baseline assessment of LVEF using echocardiogram or myocardial scintigraphy and the exclusion of patients with impaired cardiac function, high doses of cumulative anthracycline exposure, and previous history of heart disease. Data from these trials are summarized in Table 3.

Study and reference	Treatment arm	Arm sample size	Median follow-up (months)	Baseline LVEF (%)	Grade III/IV NYHA heart failure (%)	Cardiac deaths (*n*)
NCCTG N9831 Romond *et al.* (2005)[5] Baselga *et al.* (2006)[18] Perez *et al.* (2005)[20]	AC→P	819	18	≥50[a]	0	0
	AC→P→H	981			2.2	1
	AC→PH	814			3.3	1
NSABP B-31 Romond *et al.* (2005)[5] Tan-Chiu *et al.* (2005)[6]	AC→P	1,024	28.8	≥50[a]	0.8	1
	AC→PH	1,019			4.1	0
HERA Piccart-Gebhart *et al.* (2005)[15] Smith *et al.* (2007)[16]	Protocol specified chemotherapy alone	1,698	23.5	≥55[b]	0	1
	Protocol specified chemotherapy→H	1,703			0.6	0
FinHer Joensuu *et al.* (2006)[40]	T or V→FEC	116	35	NR	3[d]	0
	HT or HV→FEC	116	37		0[d]	0
BCIRG006 Slamon *et al.* (2006)[19]	AC→T	1,073	36	≥50[c]	0.3	0
	AC→TH	1,074			1.8	0
	TCH	1,075			0.3	0
E2198 Sledge *et al.* (2006)[41]	PH→AC	115	NR	≥50[c]	2.6[d]	0
	PH→AC→H	112	NR		3.6[d]	0

Adapted form Popat & Smith. (2008). Therapy insight: anthracyclines and trastuzumab – the optimal management of cardiotoxic side effects. *Nature Clinical Practice,* Vol. 5, pp. 324-335

Table 3. Summary of trastuzumab-induced cardiotoxicity from adjuvant trials.

In the combined analysis of NCCTG N9831 and NSABP B-31 trials (administration of trastuzumab concurrent with adjuvant taxanes after anthracycline chemotherapy), was found that trastuzumab was withdrawal before 52 weeks in 31.4% of patients treated. In 14.2% of them was due to asymptomatic LVEF decline and in 4.7% due to HF symptoms (Romond et al., 2005). The 3-year cumulative incidence of NYHA class III or IV HF or death from cardiac causes reported in N9831 trial was 2.9% in the trastuzumab group, compared to 0% in the control group. In B-31 trial this endpoint was detected in 4.1% in those treated with trastuzumab and 0.8% in the control group. Twenty-seven patients from the total of 31 women who developed trastuzumab-induced cardiomyopathy, were followed for at least 6 months and only 1 patient had persistent symptoms of heart failure. (Slamon, 2001) These results were subsequently analysed by an independent group of reviewers that constituted the Adjuvant Cardiac Review and Evaluation Committee (ACREC) (Seidman, 2002). This independent review confirmed earlier risk estimates by showing that the concurrent use of trastuzumab and anthracycline based chemotherapy, increased the rate of congestive heart failure (CHF) nearly four-fold, from 0.45% to 2.0%, at a median follow-up of 1.9 and 2.0 years, respectively.

In HERA trial (Perez, 2004) was reported a smaller number of cardiac events compared with B-31 and N9831 studies. This trial is a three-group, randomized trial that compared 1 year or 2 years of trastuzumab with observation in women with HER-2 positive early breast cancer. The overall rate of trastuzumab withdrawal due to safety issues was 6.8%, with 4% stopping the treatment due to cardiac issues. The rate of symptomatic CHF was 2% in the trastuzumab group and 0.2% in the control group, with NYHA class III or IV CHF occurring in 0.6% of patients receiving trastuzumab and 0% of the control group. An asymptomatic or mildly symptomatic decline in LVEF was seen in 7.4% of women on trastuzumab and 2.3% of controls (Perez, 2004; Seidman, 2002). The overall risk of severe CHF reported in HERA was lower than that in B-31 (0.6% versus 4%) as was the proportion of patients who discontinued trastuzumab due to cardiac issues. The explanation for these differences is not clearly established, but we can speculate that it may be due to the longer interval between stopping anthracyclines and initiating trastuzumab or to the inclusion criteria that determined a LVEF≥55% in HERA trial compared to 50% for N9831/B-31 trials.

An aspect of interest in the BCIRG trial is that one arm of this study did not include concomitant or sequential therapy with anthracyclines. This fact permitted the assessment of the true effect of trastuzumab on the heart without having to adjust for previous anthracycline lesion, that otherwise interfere with interpretation of cardiotoxicity. The incidence of NYHA class III or class IV CHF was 5.1-fold greater in the anthracycline group than in the nonanthracycline arm (1.96% versus 0.38%) and the number of patients with LVEF decline of more than 10% from baseline was 19% and 9%, respectively.

2.4 Mechanism of cardiotoxicity

Cardiotoxicity came to the forefront of concerns over chemotherapy in the early 1970s, when was detected a cumulative dose-related cardiac dysfunction was detected related with anthracycline treatment.

This agent produces a cardiac dysfunction identified as type I, characterized by ultrastructural abnormalities, morphological cellular (vacuoles, myofibrillar disarray and dropout, necrosis) and heart (dilated cardiomyopathy) changes and subsequent clinical evident dysfunction. (Billingham, 1978; Lefrak, 1973; Billingham, 1978) It is dose-related and virtually irreversible. Described methods to minimize type I cardiotoxicity include prolonged infusional administration schedules (Legha, 1982) and use of the free-radical scavenger dexrazoxane (Swain, 2004). Additionally, liposomal delivery, are being studied liposomal delivery systems (Ewer, 2002) and less-toxic analogs and less toxic analogs are being study.

In contrast, type II cardiac dysfunction associated with trastuzumab therapy does not seem to cause any ultrastructural change, while a myocardial dysfunction under cardiac stress is present. (Ewer, 2005) Other specific features are: it seems not to be dose-related; it increases when trastuzumab is given concurrently with anthracyclines; it seems to be reversible; and normal cardiac function may be restored with medical management of heart failure (Seidman, 2002; Valero, 2004; Perez, 2004; Ewer, 2008). Table 4 compares type I and type II chemotherapy-related cardiac dysfunction.

	Type I (myocardial damage)	Type II (myocardial dysfunction)
Characteristic agent	Doxorubicin	Trastuzumab
Clinical course, response to CRCD therapy	May stabilize, but underlying damage appears to be permanent and irreversible; recurrence in months or years may be related to sequential cardiac stress	High likelihood of recovery (to or near baseline cardiac status) in 2-4 months (reversible)
Dose effects	Cumulative, dose related	Not dose related
Mechanism	Free radical formation, oxidative stress/damage	Blocked ErbB2 signaling
Ultrastructure	Vacuoles; myofibrillar disarray and dropout; necrosis (changes resolve over time)	No apparent ultra structural abnormalities
Noninvasive cardiac testing	Decreased ejection fraction by ultrasound or nuclear determination: global decrease in wall motion	Decreased ejection fraction by ultrasound or nuclear determination: global decrease in wall motion
Effect of rechallenge	High probability of recurrent dysfunction that is progressive, may result in intractable heart failure and death	Increasing evidence for the relative safety of rechallenge; additional data needed
Effect of late sequential stress	High likelihood of sequential stress related cardiac dysfunction	Low likelihood of sequential stress-related cardiac dysfunction

Reprinted from Ewer & Lippman (2005).Type II chemotherapy-related cardiac dysfunction: time to recognize a new entity. *Journal of Clinical Oncology*, Vol. 23, pp. 2900-2902

Table 4. Chemotherapy-related cardiac dysfunction.

The mechanisms of type I and type II cardiac dysfunction are complex and distinct. Type I cardiotoxicity is due, predominantly to iron-based oxygen free-radical that induce oxidative stress on cardiac cells. These free radicals produce peroxidation of myocyte membranes and subsequent influx of intracellular calcium, accelerated degradation of key sarcomeric protein and disruption of new sarcomere protein synthesis. (Valero, 2004; Ewer, 2002)

The molecular basis of type II chemotherapy related cardiac dysfunction is beginning to be elucidated (Speyer, 2002; Crone, 2002; Ozcelik, 2002; Sawyer, 2002; Negro, 2004). The mechanism of trastuzumab induced cardiotoxicity involves, at least in part, the ErbB2 pathway. This agent binds to the extracellular domain of the HER-2 protein and thus blocks ErbB2 signalling required for the growth, repair, and survival of cardiac cells. (Negro, 2004) ErbB2 signalling is highly complex, involving multiple ligand classes, cell systems, and pathway interactions. Of those actions, activation of the transcription factor nuclear-κB (NF-κB) seems to play an important rule. Indeed the NF-κB pathway is also involved in cardiac cells under stress, such as in myocardial infarction and hypertension and it seems to be essential in restoring the reperfusion after ischemia and also in reducing apoptosis. (Feldman, 2007).

Evidence supports a critical role for neuregulin 1 (NRG1) signalling through HER-2/HER-4 heterodimerization in cardiomyocyte survival pathways and maintenance of function. (Sawyer, 2002) NRG1 is produced by cardiac endothelial cells, binds HER-4 on cardiomyocytes and leads to heterodimerization with HER-2, with consequent activation of diverse intracellular signalling pathways, such as the PI3-kinase/AKT and MAP kinase pathways. Mouse models have given important contributes to these discovers. Mice with *HER428* and *NRG131* knockouts are both embryonically lethal.

Moreover, the essential role of HER-2 in maintenance of cardiac contractile function and structure and the possible protective effect provided by HER-2 was shown in a mouse model with a cardiac-restricted conditional HER-2 deletion mutant. Indeed, these mice stayed alive, but developed a dilated cardiomyopathy. (Negro, 2004; Crone, 2002; Ozcelik, 2002) This model provided support to the hypothesis that cardiac lesion related to trastuzumab is the result of direct targeting and inhibition of the HER-2 receptor, rather than immune-mediated or non-cardiac effects. Additionally, these mice were also sensitized to develop an anthracycline-induced cardiac dysfunction reflecting that seen clinically.

Inhibition of the previous described pathways after an insult such as anthracycline treatment could thus interfere with the heart's repair mechanisms. Indeed, de Kort et al. (2007) showed that myocardial HER-2 is upregulated in humans shortly after anthracycline exposure, providing support for the vulnerable-window hypothesis. (Fig 1.)

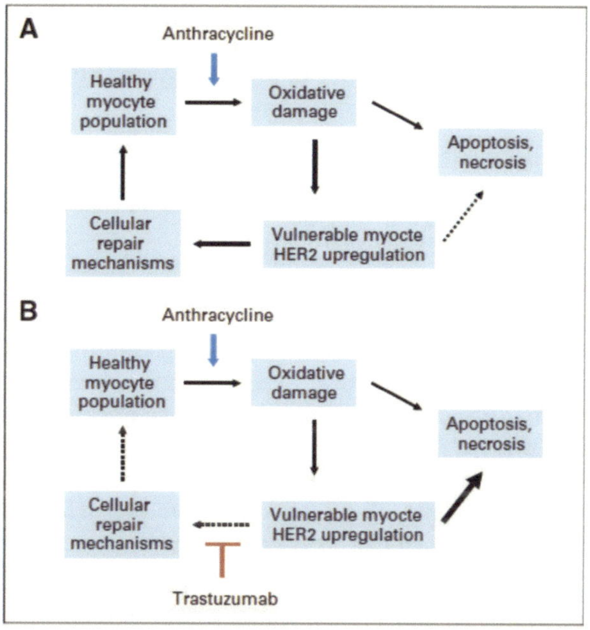

Reprinted from Ewer, M. (2010). Troponin I Provides Insight Into Cardiotoxicity and the Anthracycline-Trastuzumab Interaction. *Journal of Clinical Oncology,* Vol. 28, No. 25, pp 3901-3909

Fig. 1. (A) Simplified flow diagram of myocyte injury after anthracycline administration. Cell death is preceded by a period of vulnerability during which cell repair may take place. (B) The addition of trastuzumab inhibits cell repair compounding the loss of cardiac myocytes. HER2= human epidermal growth factor receptor 2.

Although inhibition of HER-2 signalling seems to be a central mechanism of trastuzumab-related cardiomyopathy, the pathophysiologic mechanism is likely more complex. Indeed early clinical results with lapatinib, an oral tyrosine kinase inhibitor, show minimal cardiotoxicity. (Geyer, 2006) Actually the explanation for this paradox is not sufficiently clear and remains an area of intense investigation. It is suggested that the difference between the two drugs may be explained by trastuzumab effect on adenosine triphosphate (ATP) depletion. Cardiac cells need an important quantity of ATP molecules and thus an agent that interferes with mitochondrial activity has the potential of alter normal myocyte function by decreasing the energy source. (Menendez, 2007) The binding between erbB2 and a specific antibody can unbalance $BCL\text{-}X_L/BCL\text{-}X_S$, leading to depolarization of the mitochondrial membrane potential, with reduction of ATP and subsequent alteration of contractility (Force, 2007).

2.5 Risk factors

The most established risk factors for the development of trastuzumab-induced cardiotoxicity are age > 50 years and concurrent or prior exposure to anthracycline chemotherapy (Perez, 2004; Pinder, 2007). Based on data of the NSABP B-31 trial (Tan-Chiu, et al., 2005), baseline LVEF < 55% and post-chemotherapy LVEF < 55% were also considered as significant risk factors. Current or previous treatment with antihypertensive medication and a body mass index (BMI) >25 have been shown to increase the risk of cardiotoxicity in some trials, but the results are not uniform or consistent. Prior radiotherapy to a left-sided breast cancer, race or history of smoking were not associated to a increased risk of cardiac toxicity during trastuzumab treatment.

One important aspect is that clinical trials are limited to women under 65 years old and with a good performance status (Hutchins, 1999). Thus, trastuzumab safety data only apply to a relatively young and healthy group of patients. As the incidence of cancer increases greatly with age and more than 70% of all newly diagnosed cancers are in patients >65 years, information about efficacy and safety of chemotherapy is needed in this population. This was the impetus of a recent study by C. Serrano et al (Serrano, 2011) that intended to assess the cardiac safety profile and potential cardiac risk factors associated with trastuzumab in breast cancer patients >70 years. The records of forty-five women between the ages of 70 and 92 were evaluated and was found a significantly increased incidence of cardiac events among patients with a history of cardiac disease (heart failure, arrhythmias, myocardial ischemia, or valvular heart disease) and diabetes. The overall incidence of cardiac events was 26.7%, and in 8.9% of them it was clinically evident. Thirty-three percent of women with known history of heart disease developed either asymptomatic or symptomatic cardiotoxicity compared to 9.1% with no previous cardiac disease (p=0.01). Additionally, 33.3% of diabetic women developed cardiac dysfunction compared to only 6.1% without diabetes. However, it is important to be cautious when interpreting these data given the small sample size and the very limited power to detect small differences in multivariate analysis.

In patients being simultaneous treated with anthracyclines and trastuzumab the probability of develop cardiotoxicity increases after a cumulative dose of doxorubicin superior to 300 mg/m^2 (Perez, 2004). The sequence in which chemotherapy agents are administered seem to influence the development of cardiac dysfunction. When anthracyclines and trastuzumab were administered simultaneously, the incidence of NYHA class III or IV HF was 16%. (Slamon, 2001). The interval between administration of anthracycline and trastuzumab was about 3 weeks in the NSABP B-31 and BCIRG 006 trials, and it was showed an incidence of class III or IV CHF of 4.1% and 1.9%, respectively (Romond 2005). This interval was larger in HERA trial, being approximately 3 months, and was found an incidence of cardiac dysfunction of 0.6%, similar to that obtained in the nonanthracycline arm of the BCIRG 006 trial (0.4%). (Piccart-Gebhart, 2005; Tan-Chiu, 2005; Joensuu, 2006) Thus, it seems that the greater the interval between treatment with these two drugs, the less cardiotoxicity is found. (Ewer, 2009) (Fig. 2)

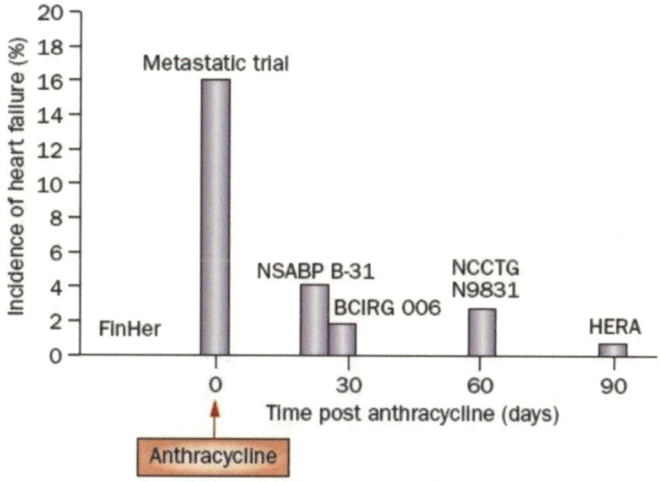

Reprinted from *Nat. Rev Cardiovasc Med* ©2010 Nature Publishing

Fig. 2. Incidence of heart failure in the different trials in what concern timing post anthracycline treatment

2.6 Clinical course

Current data on trastuzumab-induced cardiomyopathy suggest that either symptomatic or asymptomatic LVEF decline has potential to recover by stopping the agent and introducing medical therapy for HF.

In the CREC review (Seidman, 2002) of the 112 patients who developed cardiotoxicity, 79% responded to HF therapies. Further evidence of this phenomenon comes from MD Anderson series (Guarneri, 2006). In patients who developed symptomatic CHF, 79% recover after discontinuation of trastuzumab and with appropriate treatment. Of note, one patient recovered quickly with cardiac therapy during treatment with trastuzumab and one died of progressive CHF.

In those patients with asymptomatic decline of LVEF, trastuzumab was stopped in 41%. Recovery of LVEF was observed in 89% of women, independently of HF treatment. For the remainder who continued trastuzumab, LVEF recovered in 75% of patients.

Ewer et al (2005) published an observational study of 38 patients with trastuzumab-related cardiotoxicity. Thirty-one patients discontinued the agent and were treated with HF therapies. In all of them LVEF returned to baseline over a period of months (mean time: 1.5 months). In six women who stopped trastuzumab, but were not receiving HF treatment, 2 had persistent LV dysfunction during the 6 months follow-up. Trastuzumab was not withdrawal in one patient, despite evidence of cardiotoxicity, and after initiation of HF therapy was demonstrated a slight increase of LVEF. In a subgroup of patients (Ewer, 2002) treated with the maximum-tolerated doses of angiotensin converting enzyme inhibitors and beta-blockers, which had a full recovery of LVEF and had stable CHF, trastuzumab was reintroduced. The median duration of trastuzumab therapy was 8.4 months. In 88% of women (Ewer, 2005) LVEF remained stable and without recurrences of CHF; in the remainder, LVEF deteriorated and CHF reoccurred, necessitating permanent trastuzumab withdrawal. (Fig. 3) None of the patients died due to cardiac disease, and only one patient needed to be hospitalized because of CHF with volume overload.

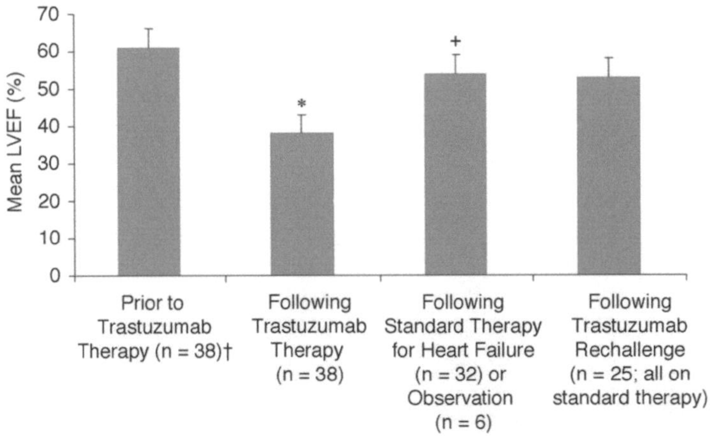

Reprinted from Ewer et al. (2005) Reversibility of trastuzumab related cardiotoxicity: new insights based on clinical course and response to medical treatment. *Journal of Clinical Oncology,* Vol. 23, pp. 7820–7826

Fig. 3. Changes in left ventricular ejection fraction from baseline to re-treatment with trastuzumab (*) P<0.05 versus before trastuzumab therapy. (+) P<0.05 versus after trastuzumab therapy.

Similar results were obtained in trastuzumab adjuvant trials. In B-31 (Tan-Chiu et al. 2005) the majority of patients who developed cardiac dysfunction recovered completely (55.5%) or partially (30.6%), as in HERA trial (Piccart-Gebhart, 2005) were there was 81% of recovery.

Although current data is limited regarding the potential long-term effects of trastuzumab on cardiac function, actual evidence of trastuzumab-induced cardiotoxicity should be evaluated in the context of the improvements in disease-free survival, response rate and quality of life attributable to trastuzumab therapy. (Table 5) Thus efforts should be placed on close cardiac function monitoring and development of strategies to early diagnosis.

2.7 Monitoring of cardiotoxicity

Outside the trials, the best cardiac monitoring strategy remains undefined. The British Society of Echocardiography (Fox, 2006) and more recently the European Society for Medical Oncology (Bovelli et al., 2010), issued a statement regarding the cardiac monitoring of patients proposed to receive trastuzumab. Clinical evaluation and assessment of cardiovascular risk factors and comorbidities should be performed to all women prior the initiation of this agent.

Study and Treatment	No. of Evaluated Patients	Absolute DFS Benefit of Tras at 3 Years (%)	DFS		Cardiac Event Rate per Study Protocol (%)	Cardiac Event Rate-Independent Review (%)	Recovery Rate from Cardiac-Independent Review (%)	Absolute OS Benefit of Tras at 3 Years (%)	OS		Cardiac Death-Independent Review (%)
			HR	95% CI					HR	95% CI	
B-31 + N9831[5,10,11,15]											
AC → Pac	1,775				0.3-0.9	0.5	43				0.11
AC → Pac + Tras	1,799	12	0.48	0.39 to 0.59	3.3-3.8	2.0	86	3	0.67	0.48 to 0.93	0.17†
HERA[12,13,13a]											
Anthracycline-based chemo*	1,698				0.6	0.7					0.1
Anthracycline-based chemo + Tras*	1,703	6	0.64	0.54 to 0.76	3.6	4.3	81	3	0.66	0.47 to 0.91	0
FinHer[3]											
Anthracycline-based chemo	116				1.7						0
Anthracycline-based chemo + Tras	116	13	0.65	0.38 to 1.12	0.9			5	0.55	0.27 to 1.11	0
BCIRG 006[6,6a]											
AC → Doc	1,073				0.7						0
AC → Doc + Tras	1,074	6	0.64	0.53 to 0.78	2.0			4	0.63	0.48 to 0.81	0
TCH (Doc, Carb, Tras)	1,075	5	0.75	0.63 to 0.90	0.4			2	0.77	0.60 to 0.99	0

Reprinted from Patrick G. et al (2010). Trastuzumab-Related Cardiotoxicity Following Anthracycline-Based Adjuvant chemotherapy: How Worried Should We Be? *Journal of Clinical Oncology*, Vol 28 , No. 21, pp 3407-3410

Table 5. Long-term cardiac risk.benefit analysis of trastuzumab-based adjuvant chemotherapy.

The statements specified that LV function must be assessed before treatment and at 3-month intervals during the administration of trastuzumab.

Echocardiography is the recommended method for evaluating LV function. (Bovelli et al., 2010) Among the imaging techniques, echocardiography has multiple advantages as it is easily accessible, with no radiation exposure and can assess LV systolic and diastolic dysfunction, heart valve disease, pericarditis and pericardial effusion.

LVEF is the most frequent parameter used for evaluation of cardiac function before initiating chemotherapy and a value less than 54% is considered a risk factor for subsequent development of HF. Extreme caution during consecutive assessment of LVEF is fundamental, in order to diminish the intra and interobserver variability. The use of 3-dimensional echocardiography or administration of contrast for left ventricle opacification can be useful strategies to achieve this proposal. However, LVEF is not a sensitive index to detect early systolic cardiac dysfunction. (Bovelli et al., 2010) Other echocardiographic techniques such as Doppler-derived parameters seem to show early changes in myocardial function in this setting. (Hare, 2009; Fallah-Rad, 2008).

Myocardial scintigraphy provides a very reliable measurement of LVEF, however does not allow evaluation of regional myocardial kinetic or diastolic function, which can be important aspects of cardiotoxicity. Additionally, it has the disadvantage of radiation exposure.

Cardiac magnetic resonance imaging (MRI) is the gold standard for accurate assessment of LV volumes and LVEF, and also allows evaluation of myocardial perfusion and tissue characterization. The common feature of trastuzumab-induced cardiotoxicity is increase of LV volumes, decrease in LVEF and delayed enhancement within the mid-myocardium portion of LV (Fallah-Rad et al., 2008). MRI has already been validated for LV function monitoring in patients treated with trastuzumab, however, due to its high cost and limited availability, it can not be used as screening test.

In this field, for an accurate monitoring oncologists and cardiologists should work as a team and prompt multidisciplinary approach to patient care, in order to detect damage caused by chemotherapy and achieve a positive resolution.

2.8 Importance of early diagnosis of trastuzumab-related cardiotoxicity

Identification of patients who will develop heart failure as a result of trastuzumab treatment remains an ongoing challenge. Currently, clinical examination and consecutive LVEF measurements have been used to determine the cardiac toxicity of chemotherapy. However, it has important limitations, namely the fact that a decline of LVEF represents a relatively late stage of cardiac dysfunction. Earlier detection of subclinical cardiac damage could lead to identifying, intervening, and possibly preventing late adverse cardiac outcomes. In the setting of trastuzumab-induced cardiotoxicity, it could allow to identify patients at higher risk that could benefit from prophylactic therapy, and also identify those who may recover from cardiac dysfunction and thus, not discontinued indiscriminately trastuzumab therapy depriving most patients from drug's effectiveness.

There is an intense research in this area, especially in what concern the role of cardiac biomarkers and new echocardiographic techniques.

2.8.1 The role of new echocardiographic techniques

Two dimensional evaluation of LVEF constitutes the most common way to assess cardiac function in chemotherapy-induced cardiomyopathy, but it has some limitations, namely low reproducibility and dependence of hemodynamic conditions.

Myocardial strain and strain rate (SR) are newer echocardiographic techniques for evaluation of LV function, offering sensitive measurement of myocardial deformation, and seem to be able to identify subclinical dysfunction in various settings, before impairment of LVEF becomes evident. (Geyer et al., 2010). These parameters can be assessed by tissue Doppler imaging (TDI) or more recently, by speckle tracking (ST).

TDI uses Doppler principles to quantify tissue-derived signals, enabling a quantitative analysis of systo-diastolic function in terms of global, regional, segmental and parietal function. Strain and SR assessed by TDI are pulsed Doppler measurements with spatial integration, obtained by determination of myocardial parietal displacement, taking into account the linear distance between the two points. (Ho & Solomon, 2006).

Speckle tracking is a distinct method to evaluate global and regional LV function. It's not Doppler based and thus, allow assessment of strain and SR independently of angle, a limitation of TDI. An important feature of this technique is the possibility of assessing longitudinal, radial and circumferential LV deformation in a single acquisition. Additionally, it is simple to perform, the processing can be done subsequently offline and has a reduced intra and interobserver variability (Geyer et al., 2010).

These echocardiographic techniques have been evaluated in murine models of chemotherapy-related cardiotoxicity and more recently, in patients with anthracycline-induced cardiomyopathy. (Neilan et al, 2006; Jassal et al, 2009)

Recently some research has been done to elucidate the role of these imaging techniques in subclinical detection of trastuzumab-induced cardiotoxicity.

Hare et al. (2009) studied 35 women treated with trastuzumab in the adjuvant and metastatic setting. LVEF measured either by 2D and 3D echocardiography, as well as myocardial E-velocity, did not demonstrate significant change in the patients evaluated. However, a reduction in longitudinal SR at 3 months after trastuzumab administration was detected in 18 patients. (Fig. 4) Three of them had a subsequent decrease in LVEF and another 2 patients showed a decline in LVEF within 20 months of follow-up. Data from this study suggest SR to be a parameter able to identify early impairment of cardiac function in trastuzumab-induced cardiomyopathy setting.

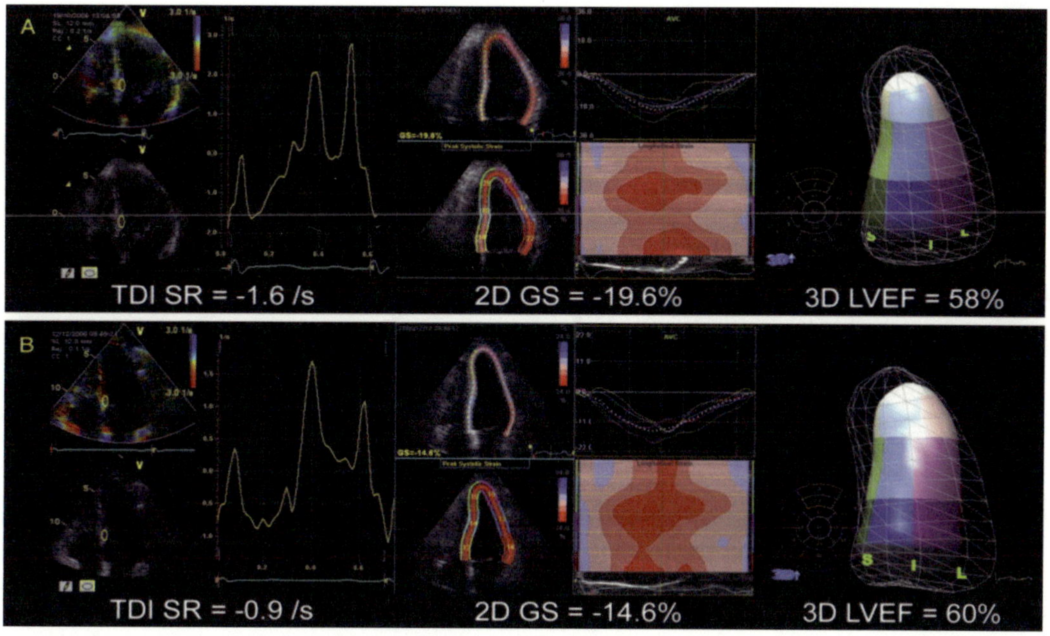

Reprinted from Hare, J. et al (2009). Natasha Woodward, Thomas H. Marwick Use of myocardial deformation imaging to detect preclinical myocardial dysfunction before conventional measures in patients undergoing breast cancer treatment with trastuzumab. *American Heart Journal*, Vol. 158, No. 2, pp. 294-301

Fig. 4. Example of preclinical reduction in myocardial deformation. Reductions in TDI SR and 2D speckle-tracking strain from initial echocardiogram (**A**) over 2 months during therapy with trastuzumab (**B**), with no concomitant reduction in 3D LVEF in a patient who ceased trastuzumab for symptoms consistent with myocardial dysfunction. *GS*, Global strain.

The study published by Fallah et al. (2011) showed similar results. Indeed it was found that an early reduction in TDI and strain values was subsequently followed by a significant decline of LVEF. Forty two patients were studied and 10 of them developed cardiac dysfunction, necessitating withdrawal of trastuzumab. There weren't significant differences in baseline TDI and strain parameters between patients who developed cardiotoxicity and those who maintain normal LVEF measurements. However, at 3 months after initiation of therapy was found a significant decrease in lateral S′ value in patients who developed cardiac dysfunction, as well as a reduction in peak global longitudinal and radial strain. Although LVEF was normal at 3 months, TDI and strain measurements were reduced in all 10 patients who demonstrated an impairment of LVEF at 6 months follow up.

A possible explanation for the increased sensitivity of strain in early detection of chemotherapy-induce cardiotoxicity can be a preferential regional pattern of damage, such that normal myocardial segments compensate the impaired function of the other, leading to a preserved LVEF.

TDI and speckle tracking imaging are thus, very promissory tools for early detection of LV systolic dysfunction in trastuzumab treated patients.

2.8.2 The role of biomarkers

Troponin I (TNI) has high sensibility and specificity to detect myocardial ischemia. Raised levels have been found after anthracycline administration and seem to predict subsequent cardiac morbidity and mortality. Indeed, Cardinale et al. 2004) showed that detectable TNI after high-dose chemotherapy is a predictor of LVEF impairment and higher rate of major cardiac events, especially in women who maintain elevation of TNI for more than a month (Fig.5).

In addition, they reported a high negative predictive value for TNI (99%), which is important to identify low-risk patients who probably don't need close monitoring after treatment.

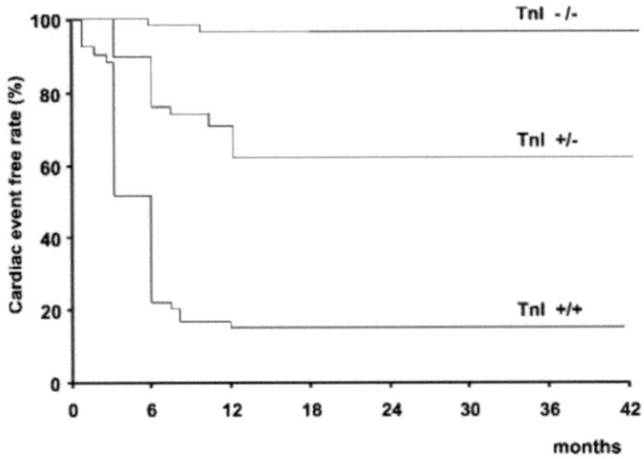

Reprinted from Cardinale, D. et al. (2004). Prognostic Value of Troponin I in Cardiac Risk Stratification of Cancer Patients Undergoing High-Dose Chemotherapy. *Circulation*, Vol. 109, pp. 2749-2754

Fig. 5. Cumulative cardiac events rate in 3 study groups. P<0.001 for TnI $^{+/+}$ vs TnI$^{-/-}$ and TnI$^{+/-}$, and for TnI $^{+/-}$ vs TnI$^{-/-}$.

The role of TNI in the clinical setting of trastuzumab-induced cardiotoxicity was recently assessed by Cardinale et al. (2010). A substantial finding of the study was that TNI assessment permits to detect patients more likely to developed LVEF impairment and to identify those who are less prone to recover. Indeed, trastuzumab-induced cardiotoxicity was detected in 72% of those who had elevation of TNI and in 7% of patients with normal TNI. From those who developed cardiac dysfunction, 60% recovered. The patients, whom LVEF did not return to baseline values had previous elevation of TNI, and additionally was found that this subgroup had a higher rate of cardiac events along the follow up (Fig.6). Interestingly, in those women with normal TNI who developed trastuzumab-related cardiotoxicity, was observed a subsequent normalization of LVEF and a lower rate of major cardiac events. These data are consistent with the hypothesis that a normal TNI value can predict LVEF recovery.

Additionally, the rate of major cardiac events, and thus increased morbidity, was higher in the patients who showed elevation of TNI.

Can be inferred that TNI permit to divide patients in two subgroups: those with good outcome, from those more prone to adverse events in whom close surveillance and prevention of further cardiotoxicity is needed.

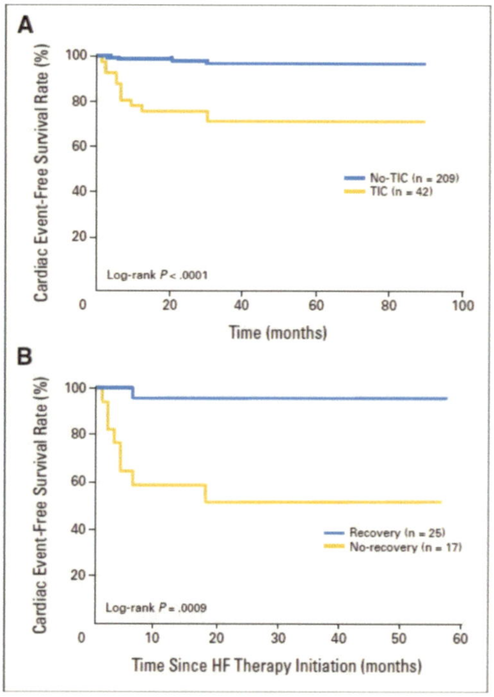

Reprinted from: Cardinale et al. (2010). Trastuzumab-Induced Cardiotoxicity: Clinical and Prognostic Implications of Troponin I Evaluation. *Journal of Clinical Oncology*, Vol. 28, No. 25, pp. 3910-3916

Fig. 6. (A) Kaplan-Meier curve of time to first cardiac event in patients developing trastuzumab-induced cardiotoxicity (TIC) and in patients who did not (No TIC). (B) Cumulative major adverse cardiac events in patients who recovered from cardiac dysfunction (Recovery) and in those who did not (No-recovery). Time zero refers to detection of cardiotoxicity and start of heart failure (HF) therapy.

Other studies such as the one published by Sawaya et al. (2011) showed similar results. Indeed an elevated TNI at three months predicted cardiac dysfunction at six months, as these patients were nine times more prone to developed cardiotoxicity than those with normal TNI values.

B-type natriuretic peptide (BNP) is a marker of increased filling pressure of LV, as it is a hormone released by myocardial cells in volume overload setting. An important feature is that it can be detectable in a subclinical stage of HF and its value reflects HF severity. (Emdin et al., 2005)

Thus it seemed reasonable to assume that BNP would be increased in patients with chemotherapy-induced cardiomyopathy. However, data currently available are heterogeneous. Some studies reported an elevation of BNP after treatment (Sandri et al., 2005; Pinchon et al., 2005), others obtained negative results (Sawaya et al., 2011). Therefore, the utility of BNP as a biomarker of cardiac damage induced by chemotherapy was not confirmed.

Larger, prospective trials are needed to elucidate BNP role in this setting.

3. Treatment and prevention strategies

Guidelines suggest HF standard therapy in patients with symptomatic or asymptomatic evidence of trastuzumab-induced cardiac dysfunction. However, as these patients have been excluded from almost all large randomized trials assessing the efficacy of HF treatment, there isn't definite evidence whether the long-term benefits of HF therapy can be directly transferred to this setting (Bovelli, 2010; Eschenhagen, 2011).

Nevertheless, data from adjuvant trials of trastuzumab and observational studies, such as the one conducted by Ewer et al (2005), support the use of HF therapy specially angiotensin converting enzyme inhibitors (ACEI) and beta-blockers.

Some other questions in this setting need to be addressed. Should we withdraw trastuzumab in patients who developed cardiotoxicity independently of the grade of LVEF impairment? Some authors proposed an evaluation scheme showed in Table 6, in which trastuzumab should be stopped in asymptomatic patients if LVEF declines more than 20 points from baseline or LVEF<30%, and in symptomatic patients if LVEF reduces more than 30 points from baseline. And should we discontinue the drug in all patients who developed cardiotoxicity or just in high-risk patients? Based on results of the study by Cardinale et al. (2010) we can speculate that patients with normal value of TNI and reduction in LVEF could be maintained in trastuzumab therapy while receiving HF therapy and close monitoring. However we don't have yet a definite answer. Another important issue is, should we treat prophylactically high-risk patients? The data from Cardinale et al. (2006) suggest that early treatment with enalapril in patients with TNI positive after high-dose chemotherapy, prevent the development of cardiac dysfunction. (Fig. 7) Indeed, in those patients treated with ACEI, LVEF remained normal and compared with the untreated patients, a lower rate of adverse cardiac events was seen. (Table 6)

	Total (n=114), n (%)	ACEI Group (n=56), n (%)	Control Subjects (n=58), n (%)	*P*
Sudden death	0 (0)	0 (0)	0 (0)	1.0*
Cardiac death	2 (2)	0 (0)	2 (3)	0.49*
Acute pulmonary edema	4 (3)	0 (0)	4 (7)	0.07*
Heart failure	14 (12)	0 (0)	14 (24)	<0.001
Arrhythmias requiring treatment	11 (10)	1 (2)	10 (17)	0.01
Cumulative events	31	1	30	<0.001

Reprinted from Cardinale, D. et al. (2006). Prevention of high-dose chemotherapy-induced cardiotoxicity in high-risk patients by angiotensin-converting enzyme inhibition. *Circulation*, Vol. 114, pp. 2474-2481

Table 6. Cardiac events in the study groups

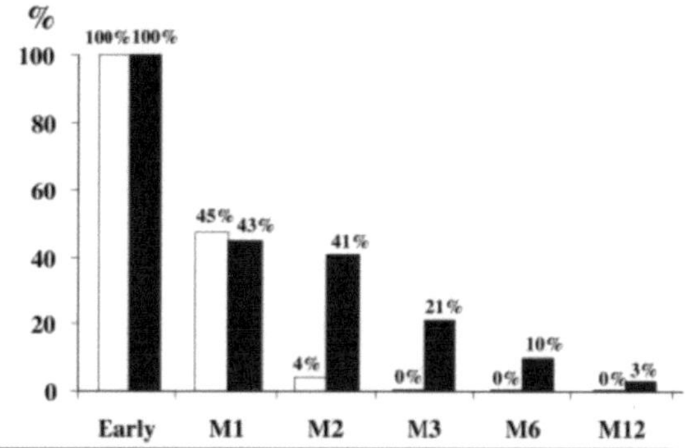

		Early	M1	M2	M3	M6	M12
ACEI-group	n.	56	56	56	56	56	55
	TnI (ng/ml)	0.18±0.38	0.15±0.34	0.02±0.02	0.01±0.01	0.01±0.01	0.00±0.01
Controls	n.	58	58	58	58	57	55
	TnI (ng/ml)	0.23±0.44	0.14±0.31	0.10±0.17*	0.09±0.29*	0.03±0.06	0.01±0.02

Reprinted from Cardinale, D. et al. (2006). Prevention of high-dose chemotherapy-induced cardiotoxicity in high-risk patients by angiotensin-converting enzyme inhibition. *Circulation*, Vol. 114, pp. 2474-2481

Fig. 7. Patients showing increased TNI value during follow-up in the ACEI group (open bars) and control subjects (solid bars). P<0.001 (log-rank test). Mean ± SD TNI values at each considered step are given at the bottom. *P<0.05 vs ACEI group.

Kalay et al. (2006) studied the impact of prophylactic carvedilol use in patients receiving anthracycline chemotherapy and showed that LVEF maintained stable in those treated with beta-blocker, contrary to what occurred in the untreated group.

Probably the MANTICORE - Multidisciplinary Approach to Novel Therapies In Cardiology Oncology Research - trial, will add some light to this issue. This is a randomized, placebo-controlled trial that aims to determine if standard HF therapies can prevent trastuzumab-induced cardiotoxicity. (Pituskin, 2011)

Physical status	LVEF	Trastuzumab	Monitor LVEF	Therapeutic guidelines
Asymptomatic	>50%	Continue	Repeat in 4 weeks	
	↓ >10 points but normal	Continue	Repeat in 4 weeks	Consider βB
	↓ 10-20 points and LVEF >40%	Continue	Repeat in 2-4 weeks	Treat CF
	↓>20 points or LVEF <30%	Suspend	If improved: surveillance	Treat CF
			If not improved/no change: stop	
			Repeat in 2 weeks	
			If improved (>45%): restart	
			If not improved/no change: stop	
Symptomatic	↓ <10 points	Continue		NC?
	↓ <10 points and LVEF >50%	Continue	Repeat in 2-4 weeks.	Anemia?
	↓ <30 points	Stop	If improved/no change:	Treat CF
			surveillance	Treat CF
			If not improved: stop	

Adapted from Keefe DL. (2002). Trastuzumab-associated cardiotoxicity. *Cancer*, Vol. 95, pp. 1592-1600
↓=decrease; βB=beta-blockers; CF=cardiac failure; LVEF=left ventricular ejection fraction; NC=noncardiac pathology. trastuzumab

Table 7. Proposal for the evaluation and treatment of heart failure in patients undergoin treatment with trastuzuma

Some authors suggest other strategies to minimize cardiotoxicity (Sengupta, 2008), such as the adoption of non-anthracyclines regimes, to prefer larger intervals between the administration of anthracyclines and trastuzumab or to diminish the duration of trastuzumab adjuvant therapy. However, our conviction is that we should prompt effort in early diagnosis of cardiac dysfunction and appropriate treatment, in order to not deprive patients to a treatment with such substantial therapeutic benefits and propose the algorithm presented in Figure 8, for the management of patients receiving trastuzumab.

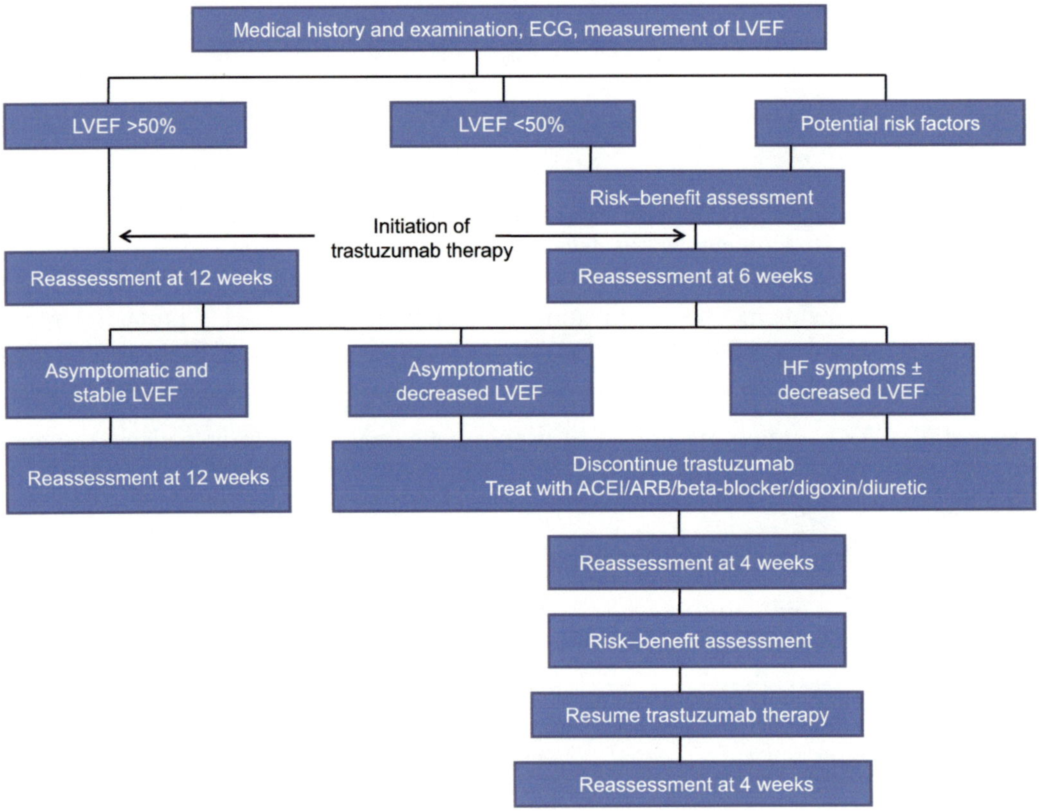

Abbreviations: ACEI, angiotensin-converting enzyme inhibitor; ARB, angiotensin II receptor blocker; ECG, electrocardiography; HF, heart failure; LVEF, left ventricular ejection fraction (adapted from Martin M et al (2009);

Fig. 8. Proposed algorithm for the management of patients receiving treatment with trastuzumab.

4. Conclusion

Trastuzumab is the standard of care for treatment of patients with ERB2-positive breast cancer. When used in combination with chemotherapy, trastuzumab can improve overall survival in patients with ERB2-positive metastatic breast cancer and disease free survival and overall survival in patients with early ERB2-positive breast cancer. Because of the risk of cardiac dysfunction associated with trastuzumab therapy, cardiac function should be monitored closely (Carver, 2010).

Cardiotoxicity has a strong impact on patients with cancer. This paradigm suggests that a multidisciplinar team of cardiologists and oncologists may provide a more comprehensive care to this complex patient population.

The main strategy is early detection of high risk patients and prompt prophylatic treatment. New echocardiographic methods to detect subclinical myocardial changes, measurement of cardiospecific biomarkers may become useful routine methods for identifying patients more prone to developing cardiotoxicity and in whom a preventive pharmacologic approach together with a closer cardiac monitoring could reduce a major cause of mortality in women with breast cancer.

5. References

Baselga, J.; Tripathy, D.; Mendelsohn, J. et al. (1996). Phase II study of weekly intravenous recombinant humanized anti-p185HER2 monoclonal antibody in patients with HER2/neu-overexpressing metastatic breast cancer. *Journal of Clinical Oncology,* Vol. 14, No.3, pp. 737-744

Billingham, M (1978). Use of the myocardial biopsy to monitor cardiotoxicity. *Cancer Treatment Reports,* Vol. 62, pp. 1607

Billingham, M.; Mason, J.; Bristow, M. & Daniels JR. (1978). Anthracycline cardiomyopathy monitored by morphological changes. *Cancer Treatment Reports,* Vol. 62, pp. 865-72

Bovelli, D.; Plataniotis, G. & Roila, F. (2010). Cardiotoxicity of chemotherapeutic agents and radiotherapy-related heart disease: ESMO Clinical Practice Guidelines. *Annals of Oncology,* Vol.21 (Supplement 5), pp. 277–282

Buzdar, I. (2005). Significantly higher pathological complete remission rate after neoadjuvant therapy with trastuzumab, paclitaxel, and epirubicin chemotherapy: results of a randomized trial in human epidermal growth factor receptor2-positive operable breast cancer. *Journal of Clinical Oncology,* Vol. 23, pp. 3676-85

Cardinale, D.; Sandri, M.; Colombo, A. et al. (2004). Prognostic Value of Troponin I in Cardiac Risk Stratification of Cancer Patients Undergoing High-Dose Chemotherapy. *Circulation,* Vol. 109, pp. 2749-2754

Cardinale, D.; Colombo, A.; Sandri, T. et al. (2006). Prevention of high-dose chemotherapy-induced cardiotoxicity in high-risk patients by angiotensin-converting enzyme inhibition. *Circulation,* Vol. 114, pp. 2474-2481

Cardinale, D.; Colombo, A.; Torrisi, R.; Sandri, M. et al. (2010). Trastuzumab-Induced Cardiotoxicity: Clinical and Prognostic Implications of Troponin I Evaluation. *Journal of Clinical Oncology,* Vol.28, No.25, pp. 3910-3916

Carver, J. (2010). Management of trastuzumab-related cardiac dysfunction. *Progr Cardiovascular Disease,* Vol. 53, pp. 130-139.

Chien, K. (2006). Herceptin and the heart—a molecular modifier of cardiac failure. *New England Journal of Medicine,* Vol. 8, pp. 789-790.

Cobleigh, M; Vogel, C.; Tripathy, D. et al. (1999). Multinational study of the efficacy and safety of humanized anti-HER2 monoclonal antibody in women who have HER2-overexpressing metastatic breast cancer that has progressed after chemotherapy for metastatic disease. *Journal of Clinical Oncology,* Vol.17, No.9, pp. 2639-2648

Crone, S.; Zhao, Y.; Fan, L. et al. (2002). ErbB2 is essential in the prevention of dilated cardiomyopathy. *Nature Medicine,* Vol. 8, pp. 459-465

Dolci, A.; Dominici, R.; Cardinale, D.; Sandri, M. & Panteghini, M. (2008). Biochemical markers for prediction of chemotherapy-induced cardiomyopathy: systematic review of the literature and recommendations for use. *American Journal of Clinical Pathology*, Vol. 130, pp. 688-695

Emdin, M.; Clerico, A.; Clemenza, F. et al. (2005). Recommendations for the clinical use of cardiac natriuretic peptides. *Italian Heart Journal*, Vol.6, pp. 430-446.

Eschenhagen, T.; Force, T.; Ewer, M. et al. (2011). Cardiovascular side effects of cancer therapies: a position statement from the Heart Failure Association of the European Society of Cardiology. European *Journal of Heart Failure*, Vol. 13, pp. 1–10

Ewer, M.; Martin, F.; Henderson, I. et al. (2002). Cardiac safety of liposomal anthracyclines. *Seminary Oncology*, Vol. 31 (suppl 13), pp. 161-181.

Ewer, M.; Vooletich, M.; Valero, V. et al. (2002). Trastuzumab (Herceptin) cardiotoxicity: Clinical course and cardiac biopsy correlations. *Proceedings American Society of Clinical Oncology*. Vol.21, pp. 123

Ewer, M. & Lippman, S. (2005). Type II chemotherapy-related cardiac dysfunction: time to recognize a new entity. *Journal of Clinical Oncoloy*, Vol. 23, No.13, pp. 2900-2902.

Ewer, M., Vooletich, M. et al. (2005). Reversibility of trastuzumab related cardiotoxicity: new insights based on clinical course and response to medical treatment. *Journal of Clinical Oncology*, Vol.23, No.31, pp. 7820–7826

Ewer, M. & Ewer, S. (2010). Troponin I Provides Insight Into Cardiotoxicity and the Anthracycline-Trastuzumab Interaction. *Journal of Clinical Oncology*, Vol. 28, No. 25, pp 3901-3909

Ewer, S. & Ewer, M. (2009). Anthracycline cardiotoxicity: why are we still interested? *Oncology*, Vol. 23, pp. 134-234

Ewer, S. & Ewer, M. (2008). Cardiotoxicity profile of trastuzumab. *Drug Safety*, Vol.22, pp. 322-329

Fallah-Rad, N.; Lytwyn, M.; Fang, T.; Kirkpatrick, I. et al. (2008). Delayed contrast enhancement cardiac magnetic resonance imaging in trastuzumab induced cardiomyopathy. *Journal of Cardiovascular Magnetic Resonance*, Vol. 10, pp 5.

Feldman, A.; Koch, W. & Force, T. (2007). Developing strategies to link basic cardiovascular sciences with clinical drug development: another opportunity for translational sciences. *Clinical Pharmacology Therapy*, Vol.81, pp. 887-92

Force, T.; Krause, D. & Van, E. (2007). Molecular mechanisms of cardiotoxicity of tyrosine kinase inhibition. *Nature Reviews Cancer*, Vol. 7, pp. 332-344

Geyer, C.; Forster, J.; Lindquist, D. et al. (2006). Lapatinib plus capecitabine for HER2-positive advanced breast cancer. *New England Journal of Medicine*, Vol. 355, pp. 2733-2743

Geyer, H.; Caracciolo, G.; Abe, H.; Wilansky, S.; Carerj, S.; Gentile, F. et al. (2010). Assessment of Myocardial Mechanics Using SpeckleTracking Echocardiography: Fundamentals and Clinical Applications. *Journal of American Society of Echocardiography*, Vol. 23, No.4, pp. 351-69

Guarneri, V. e. (2006). Long-term cardiac tolerability of trastuzumab in metastatic breast cancer: the MD Anderson Cancer Center experience. *Journal of Clinical Oncology*,Vol. 24, pp. 4107–4115

Hare, J.; Brown, J.; Leano, R. & Jenkins, C. (2009). Use of myocardial deformation imaging to detect preclinical myocardial dysfunction before conventional measures in patients undergoing breast cancer treatment with trastuzumab. *American Heart Journal*, Vol. 158, No. 2, pp. 294-301

Ho, C. & Solomon, S. (2006). A Clinician's Guide to Tissue Doppler Imaging. *Circulation*, Vol.113, pp. 396-398

Hutchins, L.; Unger, J.; Crowley, J. et al. (1999). Underrepresentation of patients 65 years of age or older in cancer-treatment trials. *New England Journal of Medicine*, Vol.341, pp. 2061–2067

Jassal, D.; Han, S.; Hans, C. et al. (2009). Utility of tissue Doppler and strain rate imaging in the early detection of trastuzumab and anthracycline mediated cardiomyopathy. *Journal of American Society of Echocardiography*, Vol. 22, pp. 418-24

Joensuu, H.; Kellokumpu-Lehtinen, P.; Bono, P. et al. (2006). Adjuvant docetaxel or vinorelbine with or without trastuzumab for breast cancer. *New England Journal of Medicine*, Vol. 354, pp. 809–820

Kalay, N.; Basar, E.; Ozdogru, I. et al. (2006). Protective effects of carvedilol against anthracycline-induced cardiomyopathy. *Journal of American College of Cardiology*, Vol. 48, No. 11, pp.2258-2262

Keefe, D. (2002). Trastuzumab-associated cardiotoxicity. *Cancer*, Vol. 95, pp. 1592-1600

Korte, M. ; Vries, E.; Lub-de Hooge, M. et al. (2007). 111Indiumtrastuzumab visualises myocardial human epidermal growth factor receptor 2 expression shortly after anthracycline treatment but not during heart failure: A clue to uncover the mechanisms of trastuzumab-related cardiotoxicity. *European Journal of Cancer*, Vol. 43, pp. 2046-2051

Lefrak, E.; Pitha, J.; Rosenheim, S. et al. (1973). A clinicopathologic analysis of adriamycin cardiotoxicity. *Cancer*, Vol. 32, pp. 302-314

Legha, S.; Benjamin, R.; Mackay, B. et al. (1982). Reduction of doxorubicin cardiotoxicity by prolonged continuous intravenous infusion. Annals of Internal Medicine, Vol. 96, pp. 133-139

Martin, M. (2009). Minimizing cardiotoxicity while optimizing treatment efficacy with trastuzumab: review and expert recommendations. *The Oncologist*, Vol. 14, pp. 1-11

Menendez, J. & Lupu, R. (2007). Targeting human epidermal growth factor receptor 2: it is time to kill kinase death human epidermal growth factor receptor 3. *Journal of Clinical Oncology*, Vol.25, pp. 2496-2498

Negro, A.; Brar, B. & Lee, K. (2004). Essential roles of Her2/erbB2 in cardiac development and function. *Recent Progress in Hormone Research*, Vol. 59, pp. 1-12

Neilan, T.; Jassal, D.; Perez-Sanz, T. et al. (2006). Tissue Doppler imaging predicts left ventricualr dysfunction in a murine model of cardiac injury. *European Heart Journal*, Vol. 27, pp. 1868-75

Ozcelik, C.; Erdmann, B.; Pilz, B. et al. (2002). Conditional mutation of the ErbB2(HER2) receptor in cardiomyocytes leads to dilated cardiomyopathy. *Proceedings of the National Academy of Sciences*, Vol. 99, pp. 8880-8885

Pai, V. & Nahata, M. (2000). Cardiotoxicity of chemotherapeutic agents: incidence, treatment and prevention . *Drug Safety*, Vol. 22, No. 4, pp. 263 - 302

Perez, E. & Rodeheffer, R. (2004). Clinical cardiac tolerability of trastuzumab. *Journal of Clinical Oncology*, Vol. 22, No.2, pp. 322-329

Piccart-Gebhart, M.; Procter, M.; Leyland-Jones, B. et al. (2005). Trastuzumab after adjuvant chemotherapy in HER2-positive breast cancer. *New England Journal of Medicine*, Vol.353, pp.1659–1672

Pichon, M.; Cvitkovic, F.; Hacene, K. et al. (2005). Drug-induced cardiotoxicity studied by longitudinal B-type natriuretic peptide assays and radionuclide ventriculography. *In Vivo*, Vol. 19, pp. 567-576

Pinder, M.; Duan, Z.; Goodwin, J.; Hortobagyi, G. & Giordano, S. (2007). Congestive heart failure in older women treated with adjuvant anthracycline chemotherapy for breast cancer. *Journal of Clinical Oncology*, Vol. 25, pp. 3808-3815

Pituskin, E. et al. (2011). Rationale and design of the Multidisciplinary Approach to Novel Therapies in Cardiology Oncology Research Trial (MANTICORE 101 - Breast): a randomized, placebo-controlled trial to determine if conventional heart failure pharmacotherapy can prevent trastuzumab-mediated left ventricular remodeling among patients with HER2+ early breast cancer using cardiac MRI. *BMC Cancer*, Vol. 11, pp. 318

Romond, E.; Perez, E.; Bryant, J. et al. (2005). Trastuzumab plus adjuvant chemotherapy for operable HER2-positive breast cancer. *New England Journal of Medicine*, Vol. 353, pp. 1673–1684

Sandri, M. ; Salvatici, M. ; Cardinale, D. et al. (2005). N-terminal pro-B-type natriuretic peptide after high-dose chemotherapy: a marker predictive of cardiac dysfunction? *Clinical Chemistry*, Vol. 51, pp. 1405-1410

Sawaya et al. (2011). Early detection and Prediction of Cardiotoxicity in Chemotherapy-treated patients, *American Journal of Cardiology*, Vol. 107, No.9, pp. 1375-1380

Sawyer, D.; Zuppinger, C.; Miller, T. et al. (2002). Modulation of anthracycline induced myofibrillar disarray in rat ventricular myocytes by neuregulin-1_and anti-erbB2–potential mechanism for trastuzumab-induced cardiotoxicity. *Circulation*, Vol. 105, pp. 1551-1554

Seidman, A.; Hudis, C.; Pierri, M. et al. (2002). Cardiac dysfunction in the trastuzumab clinical trials experience. *Journal of Clinical Oncoloyg*, Vol. 20, No. 5, pp. 1215 – 1221

Sengupta, P.; Northfelt, D.; Gentile, F. et al. (2008). Trastuzumab-induced cardiotoxicity: heart failure and crossroads. *Mayo Clinic Proceedings*, Vol. 83, No.2, pp. 197-203

Serrano, C.; Corte, J.; De Mattos-Arruda, L. et al. (2011). Trastuzumab-related cardiotoxicity in the elderly: a role for cardiovascular risk factors. *Annals of Oncology*

Slamon, D.; Clark, G.; Wong, S.; Levin, W.; Ulrich, A. & McGuire, W. (1987). Human breast cancer: correlation of relapse and survival with amplification of the HER-2/neu oncogene. *Science*, Vol.235, pp. 177-82

Slamon, D.; Leyland-Jones, B.; Shak, S. et al. (2001). Use of chemotherapy plus a monoclonal antibody against HER2 for metastatic breast cancer that overexpresses HER2. *New England Journal of Medicine*, Vol. 344, No.11, pp. 783-792

Speyer, J. (2002). Cardiac dysfunction in the trastuzumab clinical experience. *Journal of Clinical Oncology*, Vol. 20, pp.1156-1157

Swain, S. & Vici P. (2004). The current and future role of dexrazoxane as a cardioprotectant in anthracycline treatment: Expert panel review. *Journal of Cancer Research and Clinical Oncology*, Vol.130, pp. 1-7

Tan-Chiu, E. ; Yothers, G. ; Romond, E. et al. (2005). Assessment of cardiac dysfunction in a randomized trial comparing doxorubicin and cyclophosphamide followed by paclitaxel, with or without trastuzumab as adjuvant therapy in node-positive, human epidermal growth factor receptor 2-overexpressing breast cancer: NSABP B-31. *Journal of Clinical Oncology*, Vol.23, No.9, pp. 7811–7819.

Valero, V.; Gill, E.; Paton, V. et al. (2004). Normal cardiac biopsy results following co-administration of doxorubicin, cyclophosphamide and trastuzumab to women with HER2 positive metastatic breast cancer. *Journal of Clinical Oncoloy*, Vol.22, pp. 572

Vogel, C. (2002). Efficacy and safety of trastuzumab as single agent in first-line treatment HER2- overexpressing metastatic breast cancer. *Journal of Clinical Oncology*,Vol. 20, pp. 719-26.

7

Early Detection and Prediction of Cardiotoxicity – Biomarker and Echocardiographic Evaluation

Elena Kinova and Assen Goudev
UMHAT "Tsaritsa Yoanna - ISUL",
Cardiology Department,
Bulgaria

1. Intoduction

In recent years with new anticancer therapies, many patients can have a long life expectancy. According to recently published data there are at present more than 12 million cancer survivors in the United States and in Europe (CDC, 2011; Coleman et al., 2003). These patients are prone to higher risk of cardiovascular death than the risk of tumor recurrence, particularly in childhood cancer survivors in which the cardiac mortality rate is sevenfold higher (Scully et al., 2007). However, cardiac toxicity remains an important side effect of anticancer therapies, leading to increased mortality due to mainly heart failure, but also myocardial ischemia, arrhythmias, hypertension, thromboembolism. The time from early development of cardiac dysfunction to the modification or end of chemotherapy and beginning of heart failure therapy, is an important determinant of the extent of recovery. Using conventional strategies with serial measurement of left ventricular ejection fraction, the time from first asymptomatic cardiac changes to clinical onset of cardiac dysfunction with heart failure may be lost for preventive therapy. This underlines the need for a real-time diagnosis of cardiac injury which represents the main goal for cardiologists and oncologists.

According to the general consensus the definition of chemotherapy-related cardiotoxicity include decrease in left ventricular ejection fraction by more than 20% to a value >50%, a decrease of ejection fraction by more than 10% to a value <50%, or clinical manifestations with signs and symptoms of congestive heart failure. Some of the most accurate clinical criteria of preliminary diagnosis of cardiotoxicity are established by cardiac review and evaluation committee for trastuzumab clinical trials: (1) cardiomyopathy characterized by a decrease in cardiac left ventricular ejection fraction that was either global or more severe in the septum; (2) symptoms of congestive heart failure; (3) associated signs of congestive heart failure, including but not limited to S3 gallop, tachycardia, or both; (4) decline in left ventricular ejection fraction of at least 5% to less than 55% with accompanying signs or symptoms of congestive heart failure, or a decline in left ventricular ejection fraction of at least 10% to below 55% without accompanying signs or symptoms (Seidman et al., 2002). Any of the four criteria was sufficient to confirm a diagnosis of cardiac dysfunction.

The incidence of cardiotoxicity depends on treatment-related factors (type of drug, cumulative dose and schedule of administration, combination of potentially cardiotoxic drugs, or association with radiotherapy) or patient related factors (age, presence of cardiovascular risk factors or coexisting cardiac disease, and previous mediastinal irradiation) (Jurcut et al., 2008b). Heart injury usually is subclinical and may present as acute or early onset during therapy, chronic onset - within the first year, or late onset - 1 year or more after completion of treatment. The later form is usually irreversible, and its prediction is the most important challenge.

The chemotherapeutic class of antracyclines is the most frequently implicated group and can cause an irreversible and sometimes fatal cardiomyopathy. The reported incidence of doxorubicin-induced cardiac dysfunction varies from 4%, at a cumulative dose of 500–550 mg/m^2, to >36% in patients receiving 600 mg/m^2 or more (Singal et al., 1998). Moreover, in children, the estimated risk of antracycline-induced clinical heart failure increased with time to 5.5% at 20 years after the start of therapy (van Dalen et al., 2006), and in patients treated with a cumulative antracycline dose of 300 mg/m^2 or more, the risk was even higher, almost 10%.

For treatment of breast cancers with Her-2 amplification, doxorubicin is administered in combination with trastuzumab - a monoclonal antibody against the Her-2/neu receptor (also known as ErbB2 – epidermal growth factor receptor 2). The results from trials using combination of trastuzumab with anthracycline plus taxane-based adjuvant chemotherapy, suggest that approximately 5% of patients will develop objective evidence of cardiac dysfunction, 2% will develop symptomatic congestive heart failure, and 1% will develop severe heart failure (New York Heart Association class III or IV), (Slamon et al., 2001). Her-2/neu receptors are superexpressed over the carcinoma cells in some kind of breast cancer but they are present at regulation of sarcomeric proteins which define the myocardial changes. However, in contrast to anthracyclines, cardiac failure due to trastuzumab administration appears, to a large extent, reversible.

The therapeutic management of oncologic patients includes combinations of drugs, radiation therapy and surgery. Irradiation with a thoracic field (as used in lymphomas and breast or lung cancer) can damage the myocardium by injuring capillary endothelial cells, which leads to ischemia and then to myocardial cell death and fibrosis. These effects can be amplified by the use of other cardiotoxic chemotherapeutic agents.

Although multiple mechanisms involved in doxorubicin cardiotoxicity have been studied there is no clinically proven treatment established for cardiotoxicity. Several approaches have been studied in order to reduce anticancer therapy-induced cardiotoxicity, from developing newer molecules (e.g., pegylated liposomal anthracyclines) (Batist et al., 2001), to the use of cardioprotective agents (dexrazoxane), and angiotensin converting enzyme inhibitors and β-blockers (Shi et al., 2011). Vascular progenitor cells have been the focus of much attention in recent years, both from the point of view of their pathophysiological roles and their potential as therapeutic agents (Jevon et al., 2008) with the ability to differentiate into mature endothelial and vascular smooth muscle reportedly reside within a number of different tissues - bone marrow, spleen, cardiac muscle, skeletal muscle and adipose tissue. Progenitor cells remain quiescent, until mobilized in response to injury or disease. Mobilized, these progenitor cells enter the circulation and migrate to sites of damage, where they contribute to the remodeling process. The number of circulating endothelial progenitor cells inversely correlates with exposure to cardiovascular risk factors and numbers of animal models and human studies have demonstrated therapeutic roles for endothelial progenitor cells, which can be enhanced by manipulating them to overexpress vasculo-protective genes (Jevon et al., 2008; Rodriquez-Losada et al., 2008).

Until prophylaxis and therapeutic strategies for chemotherapy-related cardiotoxicity are established, close and accurate monitoring of cardiac function is recommended. Using a robust technique is important for early detection of cardiac dysfunction during anticancer therapy. Most international consensus guidelines for chemotherapy recommend serial measurement of left ventricular ejection fraction at the beginning of anticancer therapy, after administration of the half total cumulative dose and before every subsequent dose, as well as assessment at 3, 6 and 12 months after the end of treatment (Bovelli et al., 2010). Using this monitoring strategy the heart failure risk has been reduced to less than 3% in patients examined with equilibrium radionuclide angiocardiography (Mitani et al, 2003). However, subsequent reduction of ejection fraction by more than 10% or less than 50% as absolute value that was proposed as a criterion for suspending treatment (Schwartz et al., 1987, as cited by Dolci et al., 2008), is a relatively insensitively parameter for early cardiotoxicity detection. The possible explanation is that systolic dysfunction appears after a critical amount of myocardium has become damaged. Furthermore, the lack of reduction of ejection fraction does not exclude development of late cardiotoxicity (Aleman et al., 2007). Regardless of these limitations evaluation of ejection fraction has been used for monitoring left ventricular function in both clinical practice and clinical trials. Currently, there is no consensus statement on the method for efficient identification of patients at high risk for development of chemotherapy related cardiotoxicity.

2. Biomarkers

In recent years the biomarkers - enzymes, hormones, markers of cardiac stress and malfunction, as well as myocyte injury of inflammation, appear to have growing clinical importance and have become the subject of intense inquiry. A biomarker should fulfill three criteria to be useful clinically. First, accurate, repeated measurements must be available at a reasonable cost and with short times; second, the biomarker must provide additional information; and third, knowing the measured level should aid in medical decision making. The biomarkers that were proved to predict heart failure could be divided into six categories according to their origin or effects (inflammation, oxidative stress, extracellular matrix remodeling, neurohormones, myocyte injury, myocyte stress), and a seventh category of new biomarkers that have not yet been fully characterized (Braunwald et al., 2008). Heart failure, including in cardiotoxicity, appears to result from a complex interplay among genetic, neurohormonal, inflammatory, and biochemical changes acting on cardiac myocytes, the cardiac interstitium, or both.

2.1 C-reactive protein

C-reactive protein is an acute-phase reactant synthesized by hepatocytes in response to the proinflammatory cytokine interleukin-6. Increased levels of C-reactive protein correlate with the severity of heart failure and is an independent predictor of adverse outcomes in patients with acute or chronic heart failure (Anand et al., 2008). C-reactive protein has direct effects on the vascular endothelium by reducing nitric-oxide release and increasing endothelin-1 production, as well as by inducing expression of endothelial adhesion molecules (Venugopal et al., 2005). This marker may be useable in wide population because of the low-cost and high-sensitivity test was developed. In most studies C-reactive protein has been investigated as risk factor and prognostic variable in patients with various malignances. In patients with small cell lung cancer the baseline serum concentrations of the C-reactive protein were raised in most of patients and doubled during induction chemotherapy in chemosensitive patients but it did not in non-responders (Milroy et al., 1989). In prospective study including ninety-five patients with breast cancer treated with dose-dense doxorubicin and cyclophosphamide, than weekly paclitaxel with trastuzumab and lapatinib, the levels of C-reactive protein were measured every 2 weeks during chemotherapy then at months 6, 9 and 18. During chemotherapy a detectable C-reactive protein was seen in 78% but did not correlate with ejection fraction declines (Morris et al., 2010).

2.2 Tumor Necrosis Factor α (TNF-α)

Tumor necrosis factor α (TNF-α) and three interleukins (interleukins 1, 6, and 18) are considered to be proinflammatory cytokines and are produced by nucleated cells in the heart (Anker et al., 2004). According to the cytokine hypothesis of heart failure, proinflammatory cytokines are produced by the damaged myocardium, which is enhanced by stimulation of the sympathetic nervous system. Injured myocardium, as well as skeletal muscle, which is hypoperfused because of reduced cardiac output, activate monocytes to produce the same cytokines, which act on and further impair myocardial function as a result of apoptosis and necrosis. Interleukin-6 induces a hypertrophic response in myocytes, whereas TNF-α causes left ventricular dilatation through activation of matrix metalloproteinases. Interleukin-6 and TNF-α levels could be used to predict the future development of heart failure in asymptomatic elderly subjects (Lee et al., 2005) though blockade of TNF-α has not resulted in clinical benefit in patients with heart failure (Anker et al., 2004). The increased levels of soluble members of the TNF-superfamily of apoptosis-related protein have been reported after a median follow-up of more than 6 years in patients after epirubicin-containing chemotherapy and chest wall irradiation for breast cancer especially after high-dose chemotherapy (Perik et al., 2006). To investigate if high TNF-protein levels are related to cardiac function, 40 breast cancer patients were examined following surgery, one month and one year after epirubicin-based chemotherapy. Significant but transient changes in soluble apoptotic protein levels were obsereved, particularly after high-dose chemotherapy but no relation was found between TNF-proteins and carditoxicity, assessed by electrocardiogram, conventional echocardiography and plasma natriuretic peptid.

2.3 Markers of the oxidative stress

Increased oxidative stress results from an imbalance between reactive oxygen species and endogenous antioxidant defense mechanisms. Since it is difficult to measure reactive oxygen species directly in humans, indirect markers of oxidative stress - plasma-oxidized low-density lipoproteins, malondialdehyde and myeloperoxidase have been sought. In animal models administration of doxorubicin resulted in higher myeloperoxidase activity and lipid peroxidation (Fadillioglu et al., 2004). In twenty-two patients with non-Hodgkin's lymphoma or Hodgkin's disease, treated with doxorubicin-containing regimen the flow-mediated dilation was monitored (Nagi et al., 2001). During the same time biochemical markers were measured - the marker of lipid peroxidation (malondialdehyde), the amounts of the ratio of reduced to oxidized glutathione and the marker of free radical generating capacity of neutrophils (myeloperoxidase). No significant alterations were found in these biomarkers concentrations after doxorubicin bolus.

2.4 Sympathetic nervous system and renin–angiotensin–aldosterone system

The sympathetic nervous system is activated in patients with heart failure and this lead to higher plasma levels of norepinephrine which was proved as an independent predictor of mortality (Cohn et al., 1984). Attention focused on big endothelin-1, secreted by vascular endothelial cells and then undergoes conversion into the active neurohormone endothelin-1, which is a powerful stimulant of vascular smooth-muscle contraction and proliferation and ventricular and vessel fibrosis. Besides the activation of sympathetic nervous system, the renin–angiotensin–aldosterone system becomes activated in patients with heart failure as well. In the Randomized Aldactone Evaluation Study (RALES) of patients with severe heart failure administration of the aldosterone blocker spironolactone was associated with a reduction of plasma procollagen type III and clinical benefit, but only in patients whose baseline levels of the procollagen were above the median (Zannad et al., 2000). Moreover, in Troponin I positive patients after high-dose chemotherapy, early starting of treatment with enalapril prevent the development of late cardiotoxicity (Cardinale et al., 2006b). Obviously, blockers of rennin-angiotensin-aldosterone system slow the progression of left ventricular dysfunction.

2.5 Natriuretic peptides

Natriuretic peptides - brain natriuretic peptide (BNP) and N-terminal probrain natriuretic peptide (NT-proBNP), are synthesized in the myocytes in response to high wall stress and pressure overload (Yasue et al., 1994). Brain natriuretic peptide causes arterial vasodilatation, diuresis, and natriuresis, and reduces the activities of the renin-angiotensin–aldosterone system and the sympathetic nervous system. Measuring the BNP levels not only increases the accuracy of the diagnosis of heart failure in patients presenting with dyspnea, when a level of more than 400 pg/ml makes the diagnosis likely, but appears to be useful in risk stratification of patients with chronic heart failure (Sugiura et al., 2005) and in screening for acute or late cardiotoxic effects associated with cancer chemotherapy (Suzuki et al., 1998). Normal plasma concentrations exclude heart failure with high negative predictive value of the test. Two studies which have directly compared BNP and NT-proBNP, found that the N-terminal prohormone was slightly superior to BNP for predicting death or rehospitalization for heart failure because of the longer half-life of NT-pro-BNP (Masson et al., 2006).

The predictive role of NT-proBNP in patients treated with high dose chemotherapy was evaluated. In 52 patients after 62 chemotherapy treatments for aggressive malignancies the levels of NT-proBNP were measured before the start of high-dose chemotherapy, at the end of administration, and 12, 24, 36, and 72 h thereafter (Sandri et al, 2005). Thirty three percent of patients had persistently increased NT-proBNP, 36% - only transient increases and 31% had no increased values at 72 h. Only patients with persistently increased NT-proBNP developed significant worsening of the left ventricular diastolic indexes from baseline to 12 months and of the ejection fraction from 62% to 45.6%. In 44 patients BNP-levels at 6-th month were significantly increased and in 4 patients they exceeded the upper normal limit 100 pg/ml, although the patients were asymptomatic (Krastev et al., 2010a).

2.6 Markers of myocyte injury

Myocyte injury results from severe ischemia usually, but in heart failure it is also a consequence of stresses on the myocardium such as inflammation, oxidative stress, and neurohormonal activation. During the past two decades, the myofibrillar proteins – the cardiac troponins T and I – have emerged as sensitive and specific markers of myocyte injury. Cardiac troponin I was detectable (≥0.04 ng/ml) in approximately half of patients with advanced, chronic heart failure without ischemia and after adjustment it remained an independent predictor of death (Horwich et al., 2003). Cardiac troponin T levels greater than 0.02 ng/ml in patients with chronic heart failure were associated with a hazard ratio for death of more than 4 (Hudson et al., 2004). The serum levels of troponin T have been shown to increase in the early stages of antracyclin therapy and it was associated with diastolic dysfunction of the left ventricle (Kilickap et al., 2005). The ability of troponin I to predict cardiotoxicity has been tested in 251 women with breast cancer treated with trastuzumab (Cardinale et al., 2010c). Positive troponin I was found in 14% of patients and in some of them troponin was already positive at baseline, possibly due to myocardial injury caused by previous chemotherapy. In the rest of patients the levels of troponin increased during therapy with first positive troponin soon after the first trastuzumab cycle. Most patients showed only transient positive troponin that normalized within 3 months. In patients with positive troponins cardiotoxicity occurrence was observed in period from 1 to 8 months after the first detection of positive marker. At multivariate analysis positive troponin was the strongest independent predictor of cardiotoxicity with hazard ratio 17.6. In addition to predict cardiotoxicity, troponin I predicts lack of cardiac function recovery with positive predictive value 65% (lack of ejection fraction recovery in troponin positive patients) and negative predicting value 100% (ejection fraction recovery in patients with normal troponin I level). Therefore, the authors propose troponin as a criterion standard marker for the assessment of cardiac risk of both old and new antineoplastic treatments (Cardinale et al., 2010a).

Other marker is creatine kinase MB fraction (CK-MB) which also circulates in stable patients with severe heart failure and is an accurate predictor of death or hospitalization for heart failure (Sugiura et al., 2005). During preparative regimen and hematopoietic cell transplantation in nineteen patients with acute leukemia, CK-MB mass and troponin T concentrations stayed negative, which mean that there was no detectable damage of cardiomyocyte structure. At the same time persistent N-terminal pro-brain natriuretic peptide elevations were registered, indicated significant cardiotoxicity with risk for development of heart failure (Horacek et al., 2007). In 47 adult acute leukemia patients after first chemotherapy the levels of Troponin I became elevated (above 0.40 µg/L) in 2 (8.3%) patients after first and last chemotherapy with anthracyclines. Both patients with Troponon I positivity had elevated glycoprotein phosphorylase. The CK-MB mass stayed in normal limits (Horacek et al., 2010).

2.7 Heat shock proteins

Heat shock proteins (HSP) are present in cells in normal conditions but are expressed at high levels in high temperature exposition or other stress. HSP27, 70, 90 and 110 increase to become the dominantly expressed proteins after stress (Hickey & Weber, 1982, as cited by Ciocca & Calderwood, 2005). Heat shock proteins become overexpressed in cancer by multiple mechanisms and they are effective biomarkers for carcinogenesis in some tissues and signal the degree of differentiation and aggressiveness of certain cancers. The levels of HSP and anti-HSP antibodies in the serum of cancer patients are useful in tumor diagnosis. Moreover, some HSP are implicated with the prognosis of specific cancers and may also predict the response to some anticancer treatments which was summarized in review by Ciocca et al. (Ciocca & Calderwood, 2005).

Implication of HSP in tumor progression and response to therapy has led to its targeting in therapy by two main strategies: pharmacological modification of HSP expression or molecular chaperon activity, and use of HSPs as adjuvants to present tumor antigens to the immune system. Furthermore, it was established that some heat shock proteins have been increased by doxorubicin treatment. In vivo rat model the levels of HSP90, known ErbB2 (epidermal growth factor receptor-2) protein stabilizer and chaperon, are increased by treatment with doxorubicin, with revealed binding of HSP90 to ErbB2. Registered in vivo increases in HSP90 and ErbB2 cardiac proteins occur even before cardiac dysfunction is detected by echocardiography. If a similar relationships occurs in humans this change could potentially be used to predict which patients receiving anti-ErbB2 treatment are at risk for developing cardiac symptoms. After treatment with HSP90 inhibitor, isolated cardiomyocites are more susceptible to doxorubicin, suggesting the protective role of HSP90 during doxorubicin treatment (Gabrielson et al., 2007). Chronic cyclosporine A treatment also induces in vivo HSP90 expression in the heart and is associated with modulation of protective endothelial nitric oxide synthase signaling (Rezzani et al., 2003). HSP 70 protects the heart from hypoxia or reoxygenation and postinfarction stresses in the heart (Iwaki et al., 1993; Marber et al., 1995). The results about HSP70 dynamic during chemotherapy are contradictive possibly due to the multitude of roles of HSP70s (Kampinga et al., 2010). In animal models the short term cardiotoxicity of dideoxycytidine causes multiple complex reactions and depression of HSP 70 levels (Skuta et al., 1999; Šimončiková et al., 2008).

The new biomarkers which are under investigation are chromogranin A (polypeptide hormone produced by the myocardium), galectin-3 (a protein produced by activated macrophages) and osteoprotegerin (a member of the tumor necrosis factor receptor superfamily) (Braunwald, 2008).

A multimarker approach is proved to be useful in improving the prognostic significance and early detection of development of heart failure. The combination of four biomarkers troponin I, NT-pro-BNP, C-reactive protein, and cystatin C, improved risk stratification for death from cardiovascular causes among elderly men beyond that of the model based on established risk factors (Zethelius et al., 2008).

The new methods, as the evaluation of proteins using mass spectrometric analysis coupled with high-pressure liquid chromatography, is likely to yield totally new classes of biomarkers for development of heart failure (Arab et al., 2006). Large platforms that would facilitate the study of hundreds of proteins are likely to become available, which may provide a greatly expanded approach to the early detection of ventricular dysfunction, elucidating its pathogenesis and making it possible to monitor the therapy.

3. Echocardiography

Imaging techniques are conventionally applied in monitoring of chemotherapy-related cardiotoxicity to determine left ventricular ejection fraction, on whose drops the definition of cardiotoxicity is based. Endomyocardial biopsy has been accepted as the "gold standart" test for the evaluation of antracycline-induced cardiomyopathy (Friedman et al., 1978). However, the biopsy is an invasive technique with associated risk, which makes it a less acceptable method for monitoring the occurrence of cardiotoxicity.

3.1 Conventional echocardiography

3.1.1 Current recommendations for monitoring cardiac function by ejection fraction and pulsed-wave Doppler echocardiography

Echocardiography has become the dominant cardiac imaging technique due to its portability and versatility. Two-dimensional (2D) echocardiography is currently the first-line imaging modality for assessing global and regional function. 2D echocardiography offers the opportunity to measure end-diastolic and end-systolic volumes (EDV, ESV), and thereby to calculate left ventricular (LV) ejection fraction [1].

$$\text{Ejection fraction} = (\text{EDV} - \text{ESV})/\text{EDV} \quad (1)$$

According to European Society for Medical Oncology (ESMO) clinical practice guidelines, baseline assessment and periodic monitoring of cardiac function with Doppler echocardiography is suggested (Bovelli et al., 2010):

Baseline assessment of left ventricular systolic and diastolic function is recommended before treatment with monoclonal antibodies [III, A] or antracyclines and their derivates in patients aged above 60 years, or with cardiovascular risk factors, or previous treatment with 5-hydroxytryptamine-2B agonists, or documented cardiopathy or previous thoracic radiotherapy [III, A].

In all patients evaluation of ejection fraction is recommended after administration of half the planned dose of anthracycline, or after administration of cumulative dose of doxorubicin 300 mg/m^2, epirubicin 450 mg/m^2 or mitoxantrone 60 mg/m^2 [III, A] or after administration of a cumulative dose of doxorubicin of 240 mg/m^2 or epirubicin 360 mg/m^2 in patients aging under 15 years or above 60 years [III, B].

Echocardiography should be repeated before every next administration of anthracycline [III, A], after 3, 6, and 12 months from the end of therapy with anthracycline [III, B].

During echocardiography patterns of PW-Doppler of left ventricular in-flow tract and pulsed Tissue Doppler Imaging (TDI) of mitral annulus should be evaluated to detect initial signs of left ventricular dysfunction that may occur before reduction of ejection fraction. For patients receiving monoclonal antibodies, especially if previously treated with anthracycline, periodic monitoring every 12 weeks is also suggested [III, A].

Assessment of cardiac function is recommended 4 and 10 years after anthracycline therapy in patients who were treated at <15 years of age [III, B], or at age >15 years but with cumulative dose of doxorubicin of >240 mg/m² or epirubicin >360 mg/m² [III, B].

Reassessment or discontinuation of therapy with further frequent clinical and echocardiographic checks are needed in cases with ejection fraction reduction of ≥20% from baseline despite normal function or ejection fraction decline <50%. Mandatory these patients, even asymptomatic, should be aggressively medically treated with ACE inhibitors and β-blockers.

According to the guidelines, biomarkers are not included as routine screening measurements because their predictive role for cardiotoxicity is not well defined yet. Despite all, a persistent increases in cardiac troponin I and BNP levels seem to identify high risk patients for cardiotoxicity but this approach is costly and controversial. Using these methods patients who need further cardiac assessment may be identified [III, C]. Baseline assessment of biomarker concentrations is required and periodic measurements during therapy - at the end of therapy administration, after 12, 24, 36, 72 h and 1 month later for troponin I, and at the end of medical infusion and after 72 h for BNP.

The American Society of Echocardiography together with the European Association of Echocardiography has updated the recommendations for quantifying cardiac chambers. To perform adequate chamber quantification several main requirements should be fulfilled: to achieve minimal translational motion of the image, to maximize image resolution, to avoid apical foreshortening and maximize endocardial border (Lang et al., 2006). The most commonly used for volume measurements is the biplane method of discs (modified Simpson's rule,) and is the currently recommended method of choice. The principle of this method is that the total left ventricular volume is calculated from the summation of a stack of elliptical discs. The height of each disc is calculated as a fraction of the left ventricular long axis based on the longer of the two lengths from the two- and four-chamber views. Normal values of left ventricular ejection fraction are ≥55% for both genders (Lang et al., 2006). The alternative method to calculate volumes when apical endocardial definition is not possible is the area-length method where the left ventricle is assumed to be bullet-shaped. However, the accuracy of measured left ventricular volumes and ejection fraction depends on the expertise of the reader, resulting in large intra- and interobserver variability, and are preload-dependent parameters. If a transthoracic window yield unacceptable cardiac images because of local surgery or radiation-related changes, an alternative imaging modality like radionuclide scanning should be considered (Sengupta et al., 2008). Moreover, ejection fraction is not a very sensitive parameter in detecting early alterations in myocardial function as they occur in early cardiotoxicity (Schmitt et al., 1995).

It was established that cardiotoxocity lead to diastolic dysfunction of the left ventricle which can be registered with Doppler echocardiography before systolic function occurs (Schmitt et al., 1995). The impairement was not lineary related to the cumulative dose of antracyclines, but may persist years after treatment with antracyclines (Bu'lock et al., 1995; Hausdorf et al., 1988). Conventional Doppler echocardiography with measurements of the velocities of mitral inflow (early peak E wave and late peak A wave), deceleration time of early filling and isovolumic relaxation time, characterizes the pattern of left ventricular filling (fig. 1 and fig. 2) but is not sufficient to differentiate pseudonormal from normal filling because of preload dependence.

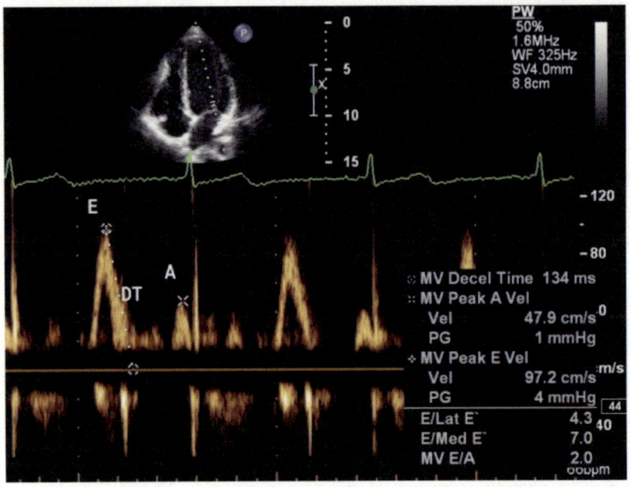

Fig. 1. Pulsed-wave Doppler of mitral filling. E-wave – early diastolic filling, A-wave – late diastolic filling, DT – deceleration time of early mitral filling.

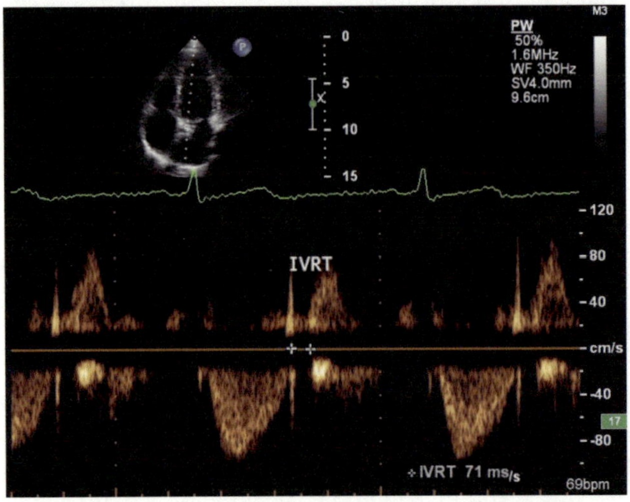

Fig. 2. Isovolumic relaxation time, measured from aortic valve closure to onset of mitral filling.

An algorithm for monitoring cardiac function during trastuzumab therapy is proposed (Sengupta et al., 2008). During chemotherapy, if new diastolic dysfunction, independently of ejection fraction and clinical symptoms manifestation, is detected, patients should be reassessed for risk-benefit of cancer treatment. Heart failure therapy should be started and echocardiography performed every 1 week. If heart failure is presented and worsens, chemotherapy discontinuation should be considered. If symptoms reverse and left ventricular function stabilizes, chemotherapy may be reinstituted. Echocardiographic evaluation of ejection fraction and diastolic function continues once every 8 week.

3.1.2 Additional echocardiographic methods for early detection of cardiac dysfunction

3.1.2.1 Tei-index

Tei-index is a combined index for estimation of systolic and diastolic left venrtricular function, calculated from the ratio of the difference between time interval from the end to the start of transmitral flow (a), and the left ventricular ejection time (b) to the duration of ejection time b [2] (Tei et al., 1995).

$$\text{Tei-index} = (a - b)/b \qquad (2)$$

The interval (a) includes the isovolumic contraction time, ejection time and the isovolumic relaxation time, and is derived by pulsed-wave Doppler echocardiography with sample volume at the tips of the mitral valve leaflets in the 4-apical chamber view (fig. 3). The time interval (b) are derived with sample volume in the left ventricular outflow tract from 5-chamber view (fig. 4). Tei-index may also be expressed as [3]:

$$\text{Tei-index} = (IVCT + IVRT)/ET \qquad (3)$$

IVCT - isovolumic contraction time, IVRT - isovelocity relaxation time, ET - ejection time

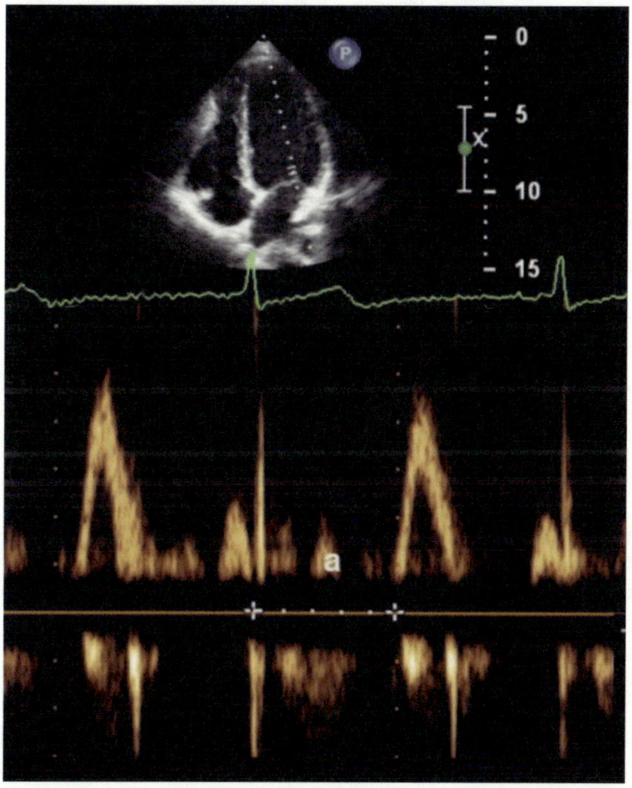

Fig. 3. Measurement of interval (a) which includes the isovolumic contraction time, ejection time and the isovolumic relaxation time. The spectrogram is registered with PW-Doppler at the tips of mitral valve leaflets from apical 4-chamber view.

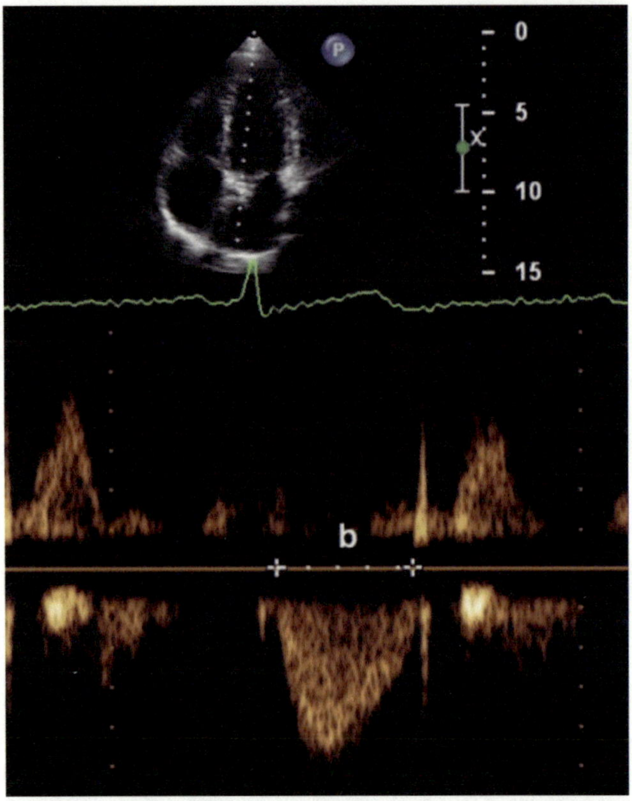

Fig. 4. Measurement of interval (b) which represents the ejection time. The spectrogram is registered with PW-Doppler in the left ventricular outflow tract from apical 5-chamber view.

Calculation of Tei-index is easily obtained and has been proven to be a reliable method for evaluation of left ventricular systolic and diastolic performance, because of its load, heart rate and age independence, although it is not applicable in patients with rhythm and conduction disorders. It appears to be promising parameter for evaluation of myocardial dysfunction in large number of diseases but future studies are needed to confirm its prognostic power (Lakoumentas et al., 2005).

According to the results from serial echocardiographic examination of 23 patients on anthracycline treatment, the Tei-index is a more sensitive indicator of early cardiotoxicity than left ventricular ejection fraction regardless of its value before treatment (Senju et al., 2007). An additional anthracycline dose significantly correlated with a change in Tei-index, in contrast to ejection fraction.

In 61 cancer patients on chemotherapy, the left ventricular Tie index was significantly increased from 0.33 at baseline to 0.44 at 6-th month from chemotherapy, which confirm early changes in cardiac function, undetectable by traditional echocardiography (Krastev et al., 2010c). Moreover, Tei-index calculated for right ventricle was increased also.

In 67 consecutive patients on doxorubicin-containing chemotherapy, 26% of patients developed cardiotoxicity (Belham et al., 2007). The Tei-index detected declines in left ventricular function earlier in the course of anthracycline treatment and to a greater significance than others standard echocardiographic measurements but did not predict functional cardiotoxicity.

Other authors did not find Tei-index to detect early adriamycin cardiotoxicity in adults in echocardiographic examination performed at baseline, at an-intermediary cycle and at the end of chemotherapy (Rohde et al., 2007). The comparison of its predictive value has been done with left ventricular ejection fraction measured by radionuclide ventriculography.

3.1.2.2 Color-M-mode flow propagation velocity

Flow propagation velocity Vp, measured with color M-mode Doppler echocardiography as a slope of the first color-aliasing from mitral annulus to 4 cm into left ventricular cavity (fig. 5), is a relatively preload and heart rate independent parameter. It has been shown that Vp <45 cm/s to be robust predictor of high left ventricular pressures and cardiovascular mortality (Garcia et al., 2000). Moreover, the ratio of E-wave mitral velocity/propagation velocity (E/Vp) ≥ 1.5 predicts a left ventricular end-diastolic pressure >15 mmHg and differentiates sufficiently pseudonormal from normal left ventricular filling (Garcia et al., 1997). It has been shown that E/Vp ratio to have prognostic value in postmyocardial infarction patients (Moller et al, 2000; Kinova et al, 2004). This method has been validated in a heterogeneous group of pediatric patients by comparing the flow propagation velocity Vp and septal mitral annular myocardial velocity with simultaneously obtained invasive indices of diastolic function (Border et al., 2003). Propagation velocity correlated significantly with the time constant of isovolumic relaxation τ (r= -0.56, p=0.01) and with peak negative dp/dt (r=0.5, p<0.03), and septal mitral annular myocardial velocity - with the time constant of isovolumic relaxation τ (r= -0.58, p=0.01). The E/Vp ratio correlated significantly with left ventricular end-diastolic pressure (r=0.71, p <0.001).

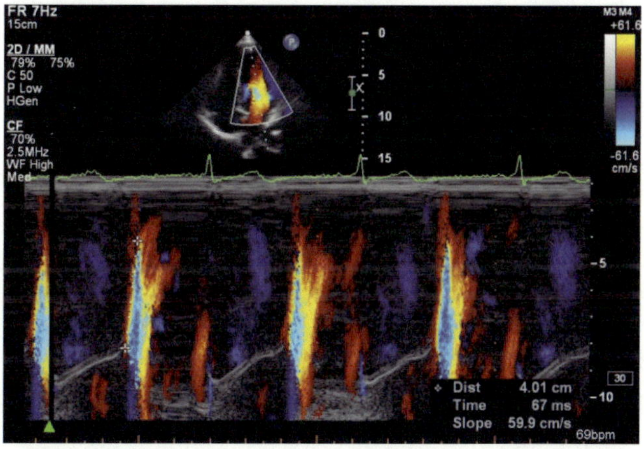

Fig. 5. Color M-mode Doppler flow velocity propagation Vp, measured as the first color aliasing from mitral annulus to 4 cm into left ventricular cavity from 4-chamber apical view.

3.2 Tissue Doppler echocardiography

Tissue Doppler imaging (TDI) uses Doppler principles to measure the velocities of myocardial motion which are lower and have higher amplitude than the velocities of blood flow. Myocardial velocities are measured only in direction of the ultrasound beam and reflected the absolute tissue motion but with impossibility to discriminate passive from active motion. This is the reason for inability of TDI-velocities to differentiate translation or tethering motion from myofiber shortening and lengthening. Tissue Doppler Imaging can be performed in pulsed-wave and color modes.

3.2.1 Pulsed-wave tissue Doppler imaging

In pulsed-wave (PW) Tissue Doppler Imaging (TDI) the Doppler signal from one sample region is collected. The spectrogram is represented with Doppler frequency on the vertical axis and time on the horizontal axis and it consists of peak systolic myocardial velocity (S-velocity) and early and late diastolic velocities (E′ and A′ respectively), fig. 6. In apical views PW-TDI measures the long-axis ventricular motion well because the longitudinally oriented endocardial fibers are parallel to the ultrasound beam. The sample volume is placed in the basal myocardial segments adjacent to the annulus and thus PW-TDI has high temporal resolution but does not allow simultaneous analysis of multiple myocardial segments.

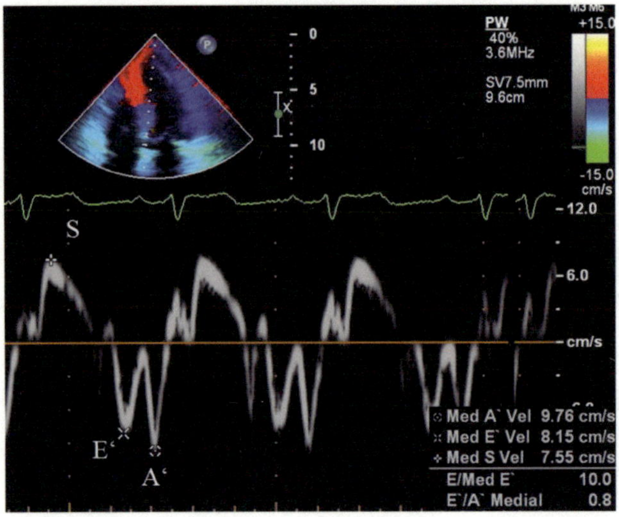

Fig. 6. Pulsed Tissue Doppler of the medial mitral annulus. S – systolic velocity above the baseline as a result of annular movement toward the apex, E′m – early diastolic velocity below the baseline due to annular movement away from the apex, A′m – late diastolic velocity, at the time of atrial contraction.

A heterogeneous pattern of systolic and diastolic myocardial velocities was observed between individual wall segments and between basal and mid segments of each myocardial wall (Galiuto et al., 1998). The velocities are lower in the septum, with higher basal to midwall difference. This heterogeneity should be taken into account in clinical application.

Systolic velocity correlates with peak dp/dt of the left ventricular pressure curve and may be useful for noninvasive evaluation of global left ventricular systolic function (Yamada et al., 1998). Moreover, TDI of the mitral annulus is an established method for assessment of the global diastolic function due to the moving mitral annulus and relatively stationary apex throughout the cardiac cycle. The ratio of early mitral velocity E/early mitral annular diastolic velocity E′ (E/E′) correlates closely with LV filling pressures (Nagueh et al., 1997; Sohn et al., 1997). Mitral E-wave depends on left atrial driving pressure, left ventricular relaxation and age, and E′ depends mostly on left ventricular relaxation and age. Hence, in the ratio E/E′, effects of left ventricular relaxation and age are eliminated and the ratio becomes a measure of left atrial driving pressure or LV filling pressure. Early diastolic E′-velocity can be conceptualized as the amount of blood entering the LV during early filling, whereas mitral E-wave represents the gradient necessary to make this blood enter the left ventricle. When the ratio E/E′ exceeds 15, left ventricular filling pressures are elevated, and when the ratio is lower than 8, left ventricular filling pressures are low(Paulus et al., 2007).

The early and late anthracycline effects in 20 adults were evaluated with conventional echocardiography and tissue Doppler imaging. Early after chemotherapy (1-3 months) changes in left ventricular diastolic function were observed (Tassan-Mangina et al., 2006). The mitral E peak velocity and early diastolic myocardial velocity Em of the basal segments of lateral and posterior wall decreased significantly. Changes in systolic function with lower ejection fraction and systolic myocardial velocities occurred later (3.5 ± 0.6 years) together with even more pronounced diastolic changes with decline in late diastolic velocities Am of the lateral and posterior wall and early and late diastolic mitral annular velocities. Moreover, a short isovolumic relaxation time <80 ms, measured at the mitral annulus level early after chemotherapy, predicted with accuracy a late decline of LV ejection fraction below 50%.

In patients with breast cancer cardiac function has been monitored using Tissue Doppler imaging which is found to be more sensitive than standard Doppler for assessment of left ventricular diastolic function and 2-dimensional echocardiography for systolic function (Di Lisi et al., 2011). These results show that TDI should be integrate in echocardiographic examination in monitoring chemotherapy-related cardiotoxicity.

The applicability of the conventional and tissue Doppler echocardiography for detection of late or subclinical cardiotoxicity, following anthracycline chemotherapy was compared in forty women (Nagi et al., 2008). After one year diastolic left ventricular function was impaired in 97.5% of patients, and in 25% of them diastolic dysfunction could only be detected with TDI. At the end of the study the rate of undetectable diastolic dysfunction, registered with conventional E/A ratio, rose to 32.5% and TDI was the method for identifying these patients.

In 61 cancer patients treated with cytostatics with known cardiotoxic effects no changes in conventional echocardiographic parameters of systolic and diastolic function were observed. However, at 6-th month systolic velocity of lateral mitral annulus Sl and all medial and lateral annular diastolic velocities (E′m, A′m, E′l, A′l) were significantly reduced (Krastev et al., 2010c). Asymptomatic diastolic dysfunction was developed despite of normal ejection fraction during and after chemotherapy (Krastev et al., 2010b).

Serial evaluation of cardiac function in 37 breast cancer patients revealed progressive decrease in systolic velocity and early diastolic velocity of medial mitral annulus, and early diastolic velocities of inferior and anterior mitral annulus (Tanindi et al., 2011). Pulsed-wave TDI is able to detect even subtle changes in right ventricular function during cancer therapy. Systolic and early diastolic velocity of lateral tricuspid annulus showed significant reduction from baseline to the day after the completion of the first cure, and then to the day after the completion of two cures. Late diastolic velocity decreased later after the second cure of chemotherapy.

Based on the results for possibility of TDI to identify early diastolic changes in left ventricular function in patients on chemotherapy, a randomized clinical trial the Liposomal doxorubicin-investigational chemotherapy-Tissue Doppler imaging Evaluation (LITE) to compare the safety of lisosomal doxorubicin vs. standard epirubicin in terms of clinical and subclinical cardiotoxicity, has been started (Lorionte et al., 2009). The primary end-point will be the comparison of changes from baseline to 12-month follow-up of left ventricular systolic function TDI-parameters and the co-primary end-point will be based on changes in TDI-diastolic parameters.

3.2.2 Color tissue Doppler imaging

Color TDI overcomes the limitations of PW-TDI for performing simultaneous analysis of different myocardial segments. It represents color-coded myocardial velocities of multiple segments at the same time during the cardiac cycle, superimposed on gray-scale 2-dimensional or M-mode images, in a single view. This improves the spatial resolution. Off-line analysis allows derivation of time-velocity plots (fig. 7). Velocities measured off-line represent regional mean velocity and are lower than peak velocity obtained with PW-TDI. The reason is that Doppler signal is collected for each depth and each ultrasound beam which limits the ability to calculate full-signal spectra for each position of the image.

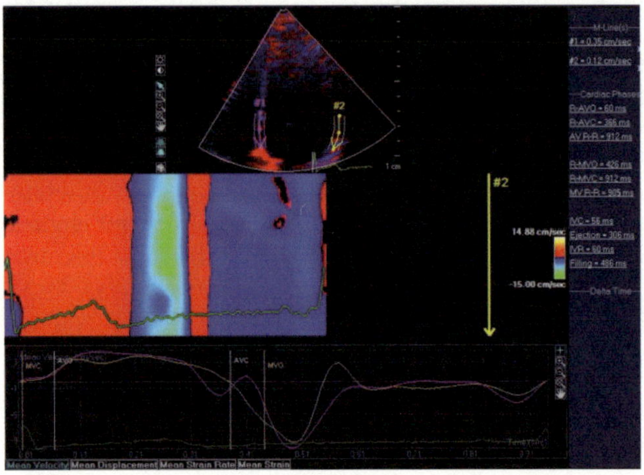

Fig. 7. Tissue Doppler Imaging for assessment of regional myocardial velocities. Apical 4-chamber view with regional analysis of the septal and lateral walls. Region of interest include the basal segments and systolic and diastolic velocities in the averaged cardiac cycle are presented as color M-mode imaging and curves over time.

3.2.3 Strain rate imaging by tissue Doppler

Recently, strain rate imaging, using color-coded tissue Doppler imaging, have emerged as a quantitative technique to estimate myocardial function and contractility (Hashimoto et al., 2003). This method uses Doppler measurements of the myocardium to extract parameters such as deformation, strain rate (fig. 8) and strain (fig. 9).

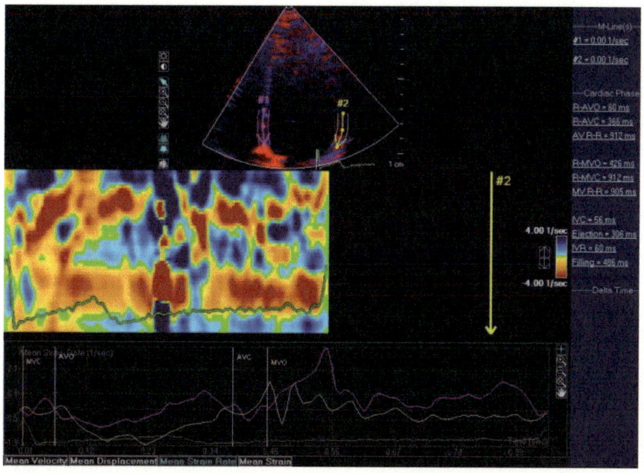

Fig. 8. Color M-mode longitudinal strain rate image and strain rate waveforms obtained from the same region of interest as the velocity curves - basal septal and lateral walls from 4-chamber apical view.

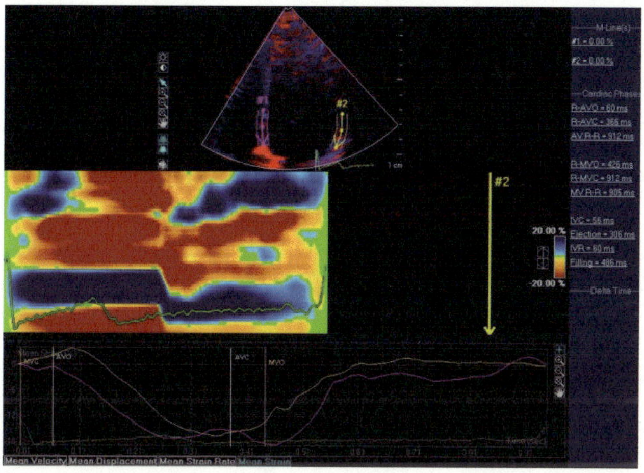

Fig. 9. Color M-mode longitudinal strain image and strain waveforms obtained from the same region of interest as the velocity curves - basal septal and lateral walls from 4-chamber apical view.

TDI-Strain rate provides differentiation of true contractility from passive myocardial motion by accounting relative changes in tissue velocity. Left ventricular function can be assessed in one dimension by the analysis of myocardial wall velocity, or by the analysis of wall deformation of a myocardial segment (strain rate) and deformation over time (strain). These parameters can be measured with sufficient spatial and very good temporal resolution. Using TDI-based Strain rate imaging, derivation of longitudinal strain rate and strain in apical views, and radial strain rate and strain in short axis views is possible. So far, several diseases with subtle impairment of left ventricular function have already been evaluated by Strain rate Imaging (SRI), including cardiomyopaties, hypertensive heart disease, ischemic heart disease and proved to be more sensitive than conventional measurements (Abraham et al., 2007).

In a population of children treated with anthracyclines myocardial deformation parameters had already changed, while conventional echocardiography did not show any decline in left ventricular ejection fraction or fractional shortening after the first two cycles of treatment (Ganame et al., 2007a). Regional left ventricular longitudinal and radial systolic strain and strain rate were reduced within 2 h after the first dose of anthracyclines.

In 56 late survivors of childhood cancer, previously treated with anthracyclines at supposedly safe doses lower than 300 mg/m^2, both radial and longitudinal myocardial strain was reduced by 15% in patients compared to controls, while ejection fraction remained within normal limits at a median of 5.2 years after the completion of therapy (Ganame et al., 2007b).

The feasibility and sensitivity of Doppler-based strain rate imaging in detection of cardiac effects of pegylated liposomal doxorubicin have been tested in 16 women with breast cancer at baseline and 6 cycles of treatment (Jurcut et al., 2008a). Longitudinal and radial strain and strain rate were significantly reduced after 6 cycles. Changes in radial function appeared earlier and were more pronounced then longitudinal function.

The angle-dependence of tissue Doppler-based velocities and strain is the main limitation of the method and this makes the measurements of apical segmental velocities and strain difficult. The angle dependency is the reason for inability to analyse anything than movement in longitudinal direction. The inability of TDI-velocities to reflect the motion caused by tethering to adjacent segments is overcome through derivation of strain rate and strain, but spatial resolution is impaired by imaging at high temporal resolution. Higher spatial resolution is achieved by using of a narrow imaging sector and lower depth but decreases the lateral resolution (Marwick et al., 2006). These limitations on lateral resolution significantly limit the ability of this technique to assess longitudinal subendocardial and subepicardial deformation.

3.3 Two-dimensional speckle tracking echocardiography

The real power of speckle analysis is the ability to examine several components or planes (i.e. radial, longitudinal and circumferential) in a single data set (Goffinet et al., 2007; Gorcsan et al., 2011). By analyzing speckle motion each speckle can be identified and tracked by calculating frame to frame changes throughout the cardiac cycle. Speckle tracking echocardiography (STE) offers the opportunity to assess myocardial tissue velocity, strain and strain rate independently of cardiac translation and beam angle. It requires acquiring at least two cardiac cycles for further offline processing and interpretation. Deformation parameters are derived for each left ventricular segment and thus allow regional function assessment. Global circumferential, radial and longitudinal strain is calculated from the mean of all cardiac segments (fig. 10, 11, 12).

Myocardial strain quantification by speckle tracking echocardiography has been well validated, using sonomicrometry and tagged cardiac magnetic resonance as reference methods (Amundsen et al., 2006).

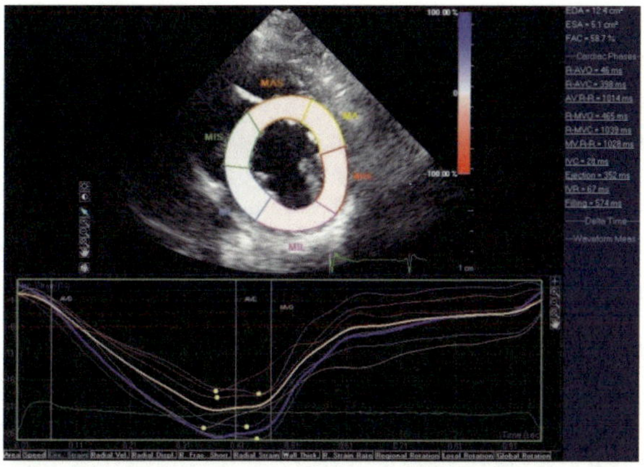

Fig. 10. 2D-speckle tracking analysis of circumferential strain from parasternal short axis view at the level of papillary muscles.

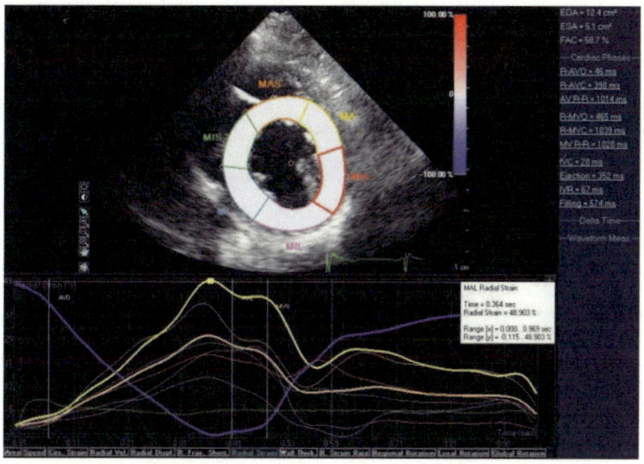

Fig. 11. 2D-speckle tracking analysis of regional and global radial strain from parasternal short axis view at the level of papillary muscles.

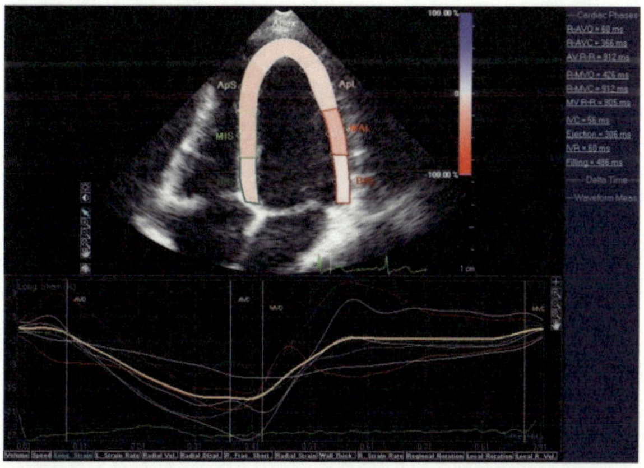

Fig. 12. 2D-speckle tracking analysis of regional and global longitudinal strain from apical 4-chamber view.

Due to the orientation of left ventricular muscle fibers, varying across the left ventricular wall, the shortening of obliquely oriented fibers generates a wringing motion responsible for left ventricular torsion. During the cardiac cycle, a systolic twist and an early diastolic untwist are generated by opposite basal and apical rotations. Twist or torsion (twist/left ventricular length) plays an important role in ejection and in the storage of potential energy at end-systole, the release of this energy as elastic recoil during early diastole assists ventricular suction. Since left ventricular rotation is sensitive to changes in function it is, therefore, of obvious clinical interest to assess left ventricular torsion non-invasively.

Until recently, tagged cardiac magnetic resonance was the only method capable of assessing left venricular torsion non-invasively. Speckle tracking echocardiography has the opportunity to assess torsional deformation of the left ventricle (Notomi et al., 2005).With the advent of speckle tracking echocardiography, left ventricular torsional deformation can be assessed, thus permitting a broader use of this new functional approach. The tissue motion quantification software allows the assessment of rotation in subendocardial, midwall and subepicardial layers at basal and apical levels (fig. 13 and fig. 14) and thus calculating torsion and untwisting.

Myocardial deformation parameters are superior to conventional measures for detection of early subtle alterations in left ventricular function. In 35 female patients treated with trastuzumab, ejection fraction with 2D- and 3D-echocardiography and strain and strain rate with TDI and 2D speckle tracking echocardiography, were measured every 3 months between baseline and 12 months. During the period no overall changes in 2D and 3D ejection fraction, myocardial E-velocity and strain were observed. However, significant reduction in TDI strain rate, 2D longitudinal strain rate and 2D radial strain rate were registered. Three out of 18 patients with reduced longitudinal strain rate had a reduction in ejection fraction ≥10% and another 2 developed a reduction over 20 months follow-up (Hare et al., 2009).

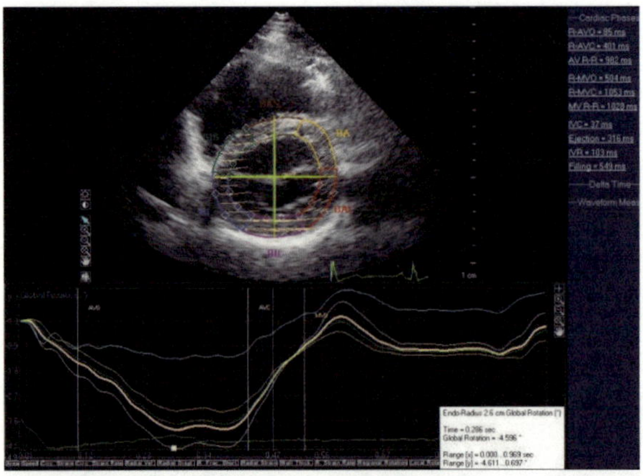

Fig. 13. Rotation by speckle tracking echocardiography.The curves represents rotation in subendocardial, mural and subepicardial layers at the basal left ventricular level from parasternal short axis view.

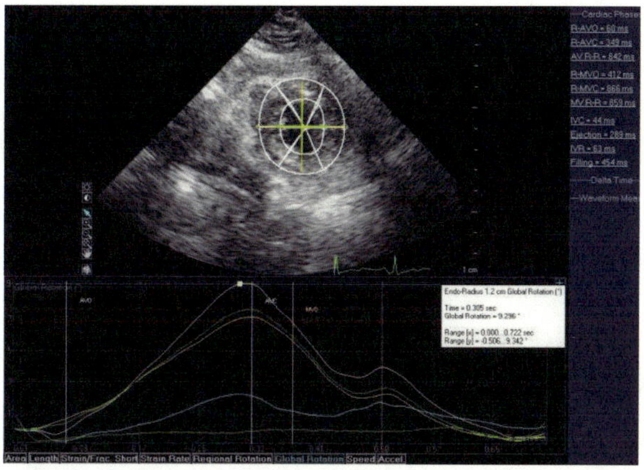

Fig. 14. Rotation by speckle tracking echocardiography. The curves represents rotation in subendocardial, mural and subepicardial layers at the apical left ventricular level from parasternal short axis view.

The data about the possibility of 2D speckle tracking echocardiography to detect early changes in cardiac function during chemotherapy is limited nowadays. However, the results of the currently recruiting participants study "Early detection of anthracycline cardiotoxicity by echocardiographic analysis of myocardial deformation in 2D strain - CA2D" for analysis of myocardial deformation in patients with leukemia, is expected to determine the reliability and reproducibility of this method for diagnosis of cardiotoxicty (University Hospital, Bordeaux, 2011).

3.4 Three-dimensional echocardiography

The interpretation of echocardiographic images requires a complex mental integration of multiple image planes for a true understanding of anatomic and pathologic structures. The representation of images in a 3-dimensional format more closely resembles reality and could therefore enhance image interpretation (Hung et al., 2007). Newer developments use a transthoracic probe technology with volumetric scanning capabilities, which allows simultaneous acquisition of an entire 3D-data set.

3D-reconstructions have also been applied to the color Doppler information allowing a three dimensional representation of jets superimposed on the 3D-grayscale image. Three-dimensional transthoracic imaging can be performed with mechanical steering devices, which are attached to standard transducers. These devices steer the transducer motion causing incremental changes in the scan plane either by rotating, shifting or fanning the probe. The advantage of this technique is that freely definable image planes can be chosen allowing for more flexibility. This method is capable to increase the reproducibility of measured left ventricular ejection fraction as well as is suitable for valve pathology assessment.

Volumetric real-time echocardiography is a recently developed technique based on the design of an ultrasound transducer with a matrix array that instantaneously acquires the image and allows instant (real-time) acquisition of a complete 3-dimensional data set without complex post-processing (Kisslo et al., as cited by Binder, 2002). 3D-echocardiography is reliable, although image quality can be a problem in some patients. Magnetic resonance imaging is suitable in these patients.

The use of new echocardiographic methods requires additional time to the conventional echo study and further studies are needed to determine the most feasible parameters and their cut-off values, which can be used for prediction of deterioration of global ventricular function with heart failure.

4. Disadvantages of using biomarkers and echocardiography for early cardiotoxicity detection

Most studies have investigated separately echocardiographic variables and biomarkers to identify patients at risk for later cardiotoxicity. There is little information about the ability of both techniques in the same cohort of patients. At present, it is not clear enough which of the investigated parametes - biomarkers or echocardiographic may detect earlier subtle changes in cardiac function.

Measurement of troponins and natriuretic peptides is easy of access in clinical practice. Elevation of troponin may be reliable in prediction of cardiotoxicity but different laboratories use different assays and cut-off values. Elevated troponin I (positive) was defined as any value exceeding the cut-off level of 0.4 ng/ml (Krastev et al., 2010) or 0.08 ng/ml (Cardinale et al., 2010) in different studies. For troponin T was used 0.1 ng/ml as the upper limit of the normal range and in this study elevation of troponon T levels were associated with left ventricular diastolic dysfunction, registered through prolongation of post-treatment isovolumic relaxation time (Kilickap et al., 2005). For BNP and pro-BNP are valid the same conditions in measurement.

Myocardial deformational imaging seems to have increased sensitivity compared to conventional echocardiography in detection of early cardiac changes. This may be related to the possibility of regional character of the cardiotoxicity at the beginning when global function, measured by ejection fraction is preserved. Several questions remain opened. It is not clear enough if regional dysfunction, diagnosed by strain, is clinically essential. If it is important - what are the cut-off values of these parameters for prediction of cardiotoxicity. Larger studies with long-term follow-up of children and adults after chemotherapy, with multivariable approach, are needed to clarify these issues.

5. Conclusions

Biomarkers as Troponin I and natriuretic peptides, measured before starting chemotherapy and after each cure, may be used to predict cardiotoxicity. Large prospective and multicenter studies are needed to define the potential role of new circulating biomarkers in the assessment of chemotherapy-related cardiotoxicity.

In addition to conventional 2D- and Doppler echocardiography, pulsed-wave tissue Doppler echocardiography is a reliable, simple and reproducible method, which may be included in serial echocardiographic evaluation routinely in all patients during chemotherapy. Measurement of mitral annular velocities provides information not only for left ventricular global diastolic function and filling pressures, but detects subtle changes in systolic function through measurement of systolic velocity. Myocardial deformation imaging may be used in selected patients for more detailed regional and global analysis. Further studies will establish the role of 2D-strain for prediction of cardiotoxicity. 3D-echocardiography overcomes the limits of 2D-echocardiography in measuring ejection fraction which depends on left ventricular geometry.

6. References

Abraham, T.; Dimaano, V. & Liang, HY. (2007). Role of tissue Doppler and Strain echocardiography in current clinical practice. *Circulation*, Vol. 116, No. 22, (Nov 2007), pp. 2597-2609, ISSN 1524-4539.

Aleman, B.; van den Belt-Dusebout, A.; De Bruin, M.; van 'tVeer, M.; Baaijens, M.; de Boer, J.; Hart, A.; Klokman, W.; Kuenen, M.; Quwens, G.; Bartelink, H. & van Leeuwen, F. (2007). Late cardiotoxicity after treatment for Hodgkin lymphoma. *Blood*, Vol. 109, No. 5, (Mar 2007), pp. 1878-1886, ISSN 0006-4971.

Amundsen, B.; Helle-Valle, T.; Edvardsen, T.; torp, H. ; Crosby, J. ; Lyseggen, E. ; Støylen, A. ; Ihlen, H. ; Lima, J. ; Smiseth, O. & Slørdahl, S. (2006). Noninvasive myocardial strain measurement by speckle tracking echocardiography: validation against sonomicrometry and tagged magnetic resonance imaging. *Journal of the American College of Cardiology*, Vol. 47, No. 4, (Feb 2006), pp. 789–793, ISSN 0735-1097.

Anand, I.; Latini, R.; Florea, V.; Kuskowski, M.; Rector, T.; Masson, S.; Signorini, S.; Mocarelli, P.; Hester, A.; Glazer, R.; Cohn, J. & ValHeFT Investigators. (2008). C-reactive protein in heart failure: prognostic value and the effect of valsartan. *Circulation*, Vol. 112, No. 10, (Sep 2005), pp. 1428-1434, ISSN 0009-7322.

Anker, S. & von Haehling, S. (2004). Inflammatory mediators in chronic heart failure: an overview. *Heart*, Vol. 90, No. 4, (Apr 2004), pp. 464-470, ISSN 1355-6037.

Arab, S.; Gramolini, A.; Ping, P.; Kislinger, T.; Stanley, B.; van Eyk, J.; Ouzounian, M.; MacLennan, D.; Emili, A. & Liu, P. (2006). Cardiovascular proteomics: tools to develop novel biomarkers and potential applications. *Journal of the American College of Cardiology*, Vol. 48, No. 9, (Nov 2006), pp. 1733-1741, ISSN 0735-1097.

Ayash, L.; Wright, J.; Tretyakov, O.; Gonin, R.; Elias, A.; Wheeler, C.; Eder, J.; Rosowsky, A.; Antman, K. & Frei 3d, E. (1992). Cyclophosphamide pharmacokinetics: correlation with cardiac toxicity and tumor response. *Journal of Clinical Oncology*, Vol. 10, No. 6, (June 1992), pp. 995-1000, ISSN 0732-183X.

Batist, G.; Ramakriskan, G.; Rao, C.; Chandrasekharan, A.; Gutheil, J.; Guthrie, T.; Shah, P.; Khojasteh, A.; Nair, M.; Hoelzer, K.; Tkaczuk, K.; Park, Y. & Lee, L. (2001). Reduced cardiotoxicity and preserved antitumor efficacy of liposome-encapsulated doxorubicin and cyclophosphamide compared with conventional doxorubicin and cyclophosphamide in a randomized multicenter trial of metastatic breast cancer. *Journal of Clinical Oncology*, Vol. 19, No. 5, (Mar 2001), pp. 1444-1454, ISSN 0732-183X.

Belham, M.; Kruger, A.; Mepham, S.; Faganello, G. & Pritchard, C. (2007). Monitoring left ventricular function in adults receiving anthracycline-containing chemotherapy. *European Journal of Heart failure*, Vol. 9, No. 4, (Apr 2007), pp. 409-414, ISSN 1388-9842.

Binder, T. (2002). Tridimensional echocardiography – principles and promises. *Journal of Clinical and Basic Cardiology*, Vol. 5, no. 2, (2002), pp. 149-152.

Border, W.; Michelfelder, E.; Glascock, B.; Witt, S.; Spicer, R.; Beekman, R. & Kimball, T. (2003). Color M-mode and Doppler Tissue evaluation of diastolic function in children: simultaneous correlation with invasive indices. *Journal of the American Society of Echocardiography*, Vol. 16, No. 9, (Sep 2003), pp. 988-994, ISSN 0894-7317.

Bovelli, D.; Plataniotis, G. & Roilia, F. on behalf of the ESMO Guidelines Working Group. (2010). Cardiotoxicity of chemotherapeutic agents and radiotheraphy-related heart disease: ESMO Clinical Practice Guidelines. *Annals of Oncology*, Vol. 21, No. 5, (May 2010), pp. v272-v281, ISSN 0923-7534.

Braunwald E. (2008). Biomarkers in heart failure. *The New England Journal of Medicine*, Vol. 358, No. 20, (May 2008), pp. 2148-2159, ISSN 0028-4793.

Broeyer, F.; Osanto, S.; Ritsema van Eck, H.; van Steijn, A.; Ballieux, B.; Schoemaker, R.; Cohen, A. & Burggraaf, J. (2008). *Journal of Cancer Research and Clinical Oncology*, Vol. 134, No. 9, (Sep 2008), pp. 961-968, ISSN 0171-5216.

Bu'lock, F.; Mott, M.; Oakhill, A. & Martin, R. (1995). Left ventricular diastolic function after anthracycline chemotherapy in childhood: relation with systolic function, symptoms, and pathophysiology. *British Heart Journal*, Vol. 73, No. 4, (Apr 1995), pp. 340-350, ISSN 0007-0769.

Bu'lock, F.; Mott, M.; Oakhill, A. & Martin, R. (1996). Early identification of antracycline cardiomyopathy: possibilities and implications. *Archives of disease in childhood*, Vol. 75, No. 5, (1996), pp. 416-422, doi:10.1136/adc.75.5.416, ISSN 14682044.

Cardinale, D. & Sandri, MT. (2010). Role of biomarkers in chemotherapy-induced cardiotoxicity. *Progress in Cardiovascular Diseases*, Vol. 53, No. 2, (Sep 2010), pp. 121-129, ISSN 1532-8643.

Cardinale, D.; Colombo, A.; Sandri, MT.; Lamantia, G.; Colombo, N.; Civelli, M.; Martinelli, G.; Veglia, F.; Fiorentini, C. & Cipolla, C. (2006). Prevention of high-dose chemotherapy-induced cardiotoxicity in high-risk patients by angiotensin-converting enzyme inhibition. *Circulation*, Vol. 114, No. 23, (Dec 2006), pp. 2474-2481, ISSN 0009-7322.

Cardinale, D.; Colombo, A.; Torrisi, R.; Sandri, M.; Civelli, M.; Salvatici, M.; Lamantia, G.; Colombo, N.; Cortinovis, S.; Dessanai, M.; Nolè, F.; Veglia, F. & Cipolla, C. (2010). Trastuzumab-induced cardiotoxicity: clinical and prognostic implications of Troponin I evaluation. *Journal of Clinical Oncology*, Vol. 28, No. 25, (September 2010), pp. 3910-3916, doi: 10.1200/JCO.2009.27.3615

Carver, J. (2010). Management of trastuzumab-related cardiac dysfunction. *Progress in Cardiovascular Diseases*, Vol. 53, No. 2, (Sep 2010), pp. 130-139, ISSN 1532-8643.

Centers for Disease Control and Prevention (CDC). (2011). Cancer survivors – United States, 2007. *Morbidity and mortality Weekly Report*, Vol. 60, No. 9, (Mar 2011), pp. 269-272, http://www.cdc.gov/cancer/survivorship/what_cdc_is_doing/research/survivors_article.htm

Ciocca, D. & Calderwood, S. (2005). Heat shock proteins in cancer: diagnostic, prognostic, predictive, and treatment implications. *Cell Stress Chaperones*, Vol. 10, No. 2, (June 2005), pp. 86-103, doi: 10.1379/CSC-99r.1

Cohn, J.; Levine, T.; Olivari, M.; Garberg, V.; Lura, D.; Francis, G.; Simon, A. & Rector, T. (1984). Plasma norepinephrine as a guide to prognosis in patients with chronic congestive heart failure. *The New England Journal of Medicine*, Vol. 311, No. 13, (Sep 1984), pp. 819-823, ISSN 0028-4793.

Coleman, M.; Gatta, G.; Verdecchia, A.; Estéve, J.; Sant, M.; Storm, H.; Allemani, C.; Ciccolallo, L.; Santaquilani, M.; Berrino, F. & the EUROCARE Working Group. (2003). *Annals of Oncology*, Vol. 14, Suppl. 5, (2003), pp. v128-v149, doi: 10.1093/annons/mdg756

Di Lisi, D.; Bonura, F.; Macaione, F.; Cuttitta, F.; Peritore, A.; Meschisi, M.; Novo, G.; DÁlessandro, N. & Novo, S. (2011). Chemotherapy-induced cardiotoxicity: role of the conventional echocardiography and the Tissue Doppler. *Minerva Cardioangiologica*, Vol. 59, No. 4, (Aug 2011), pp. 301-308, ISSN 0026-4725.

Dolci, A.; Dominici, R.; Cardinale, D.; Sandri, M. & Panteghini, M. (2008). Biochemical markers for prediction of chemotherapy-induced cardiotoxicity. Systematic review of the literature and recommendations for use. *American Journal of Clinical Pathology*, Vol. 130, No. 5, (Nov 2008), pp. 688-695, ISSN 0002-9173.

Ewer, M. & Ewer, S. (2010). Troponin I provides insight into cardiotoxicity and the antracycline-trastuzumab interactions. *Journal of Clinical Oncology*, Vol. 28, No. 25, (September 2010), pp. 3901-3909, ISSN 1527-7755.

Fadillioglu, E.; Oztas, E.; Erdogan, H.; Yagmurca, M.; Sogut, S.; Ucar, M. & Irmak, M. (2004). Protective effects on caffeic acid phenethyl ester on doxorubicin-induced cardiotoxicity in rats. *Journal of Applied Toxology*, Vol. 24, No. 1, (Jan-Feb 2004), pp. 47-52, ISSN 0260-437X.

Fallah-Rad, N.; Walker, J.; Wassef, A.; Lytwyn, M.; Bohonis, S.; Fang, T.; Tian, G.; Kirkpatrick, I.; Singal, P.; Krahn, M.; Grenier, D. & Jassal, D. (2011). The utility of cardiac biomarkers, tissue velocity and Strain imaging, and cardiac magnetic resonance imaging in predicting early left ventricular dysfunction in patients with human epidermal growth factor receptor II-positive breast cancer treated with adjuvant trastuzumab therapy. *Journal of the American College of Cardiology*, Vol. 57, No. 22, (May 2011), pp. 2263-2270, ISSN 0735-1097.

Fan, GC.; Zhou, X.; Wang, X.; Song, G.; Qiuan, J.; Nicolaou, P.; Chen, G.; Ren, X. & Kranias, E. (2008). Heat shock protein 20 interacting with phosphorylated akt reduces doxorubicin-triggered oxidative stress and cardiotoxicity. *Circulation Research*, Vol. 103, No. 11, (Oct 2008), pp. 1270-1279, ISSN 0009-7330.

Friedman, M.; Bozdech, M.; Billingham, M. & Rider, A. (1978). Doxorubicin cardiotoxicity. Serial endomyocardial biopsies and systolic time intervals. *JAMA*, Vol. 240, No. 15, (Oct 1978), pp. 1603-1606, ISSN 0098-7484.

Gabrielson, K.; Bedja, D.; Pin, S.; Tsao, A.; Gama, L.; Yuan, B. & Muratore, N. (2007). Heat shock protein 90 and ErbB2 in the cardiac response to doxorubicin injury. *Cancer Research*, Vol. 67, No 4, (February 2007), pp. 1436-1441, ISSN 0008-5472.

Galderisi, M.; Marra, F.; Esposito, R.; Lomoriello, V.; Pardo, M. & de Divitiis, O. (2007). Cancer therapy and cardiotoxicity: the need of serial Doppler echocardiography. *Cardiovascular ultrasound*, Vol. 5, No. 4, (Jan 2007), doi: 10.1186/1476-7120-5-4, ISSN 1476-7120.

Galiuto, L. Ignone, G. & De Maria, AN. (1998). Contraction and relaxation velocities of the normal left ventricle using pulsed-wave tissue Doppler echocardiography. *The American Journal of Cardiology*, Vol. 81, No. 5, (Mar 1998), pp. 609-614, ISSN 0002-9149.

Ganame, J.; Claus, P.; Eyskens, B.; Uyttebroeck, A.; Renard, M.; D'hooge, J.; Gewillig, M.; Bijnens, B.; Sutherland, G. & Mertens, L. (2007). Acute cardiac functional and morphological changes after anthracycline infusions in children. *American Journal of Cardiology*, Vol. 99, No. 7, (Apr 2007), pp. 974–977, ISSN 0002-9149.

Ganame, J.; Claus, P.; Uyttebroeck, A.; Renard, M.; D'hooge, J.; Bijnens, B.; Sutherland, G.;Eyskens, B. & Mertens, L. (2007). Myocardial dysfunction late after low dose anthracycline treatment in asymptomatic pediatric patients. *Journal of the American Society of Echocardiography*, Vol. 20, No. 12, (Dec 2007), pp. 1351–1358, ISSN 0894-7317.

Garcia, M.; Ares, M.; Asher, C.; Rodriguez, L.; Vandervoort, P. & Thomas, J. (1997). An index of early left ventricular filling that combined with pulsed Doppler peak E velocity may estimate capillary wedge pressure. *Journal of American College of Cardiology*, Vol. 29, No. 2, (Feb 1997), pp. 448-454, ISSN 0735-1097.

Garcia, M.; Smedira, N.; Greenberg, N.; Main, M.; Firstenberg, M.; Odabashian, J. & Thomas, J. (2000). Color M-mode Doppler flow propagation velocity is a preload insensitive index of left ventricular relaxation: animal and human validation. *Journal of American College of Cardiology*, Vol. 35, No. 1, (Jan 2000), pp. 201-208, ISSN 0735-1097.

Goffinet, C. & Vanoverschelde, JL. (2007). Speckle Tracking echocardiography, In: *European Cardiovascular Disease*, Available from: www.touchcardiology.com

Gorcsan, J. & Tanaka, H. (2011). Echocardiography assessment of myocardial strain. *Journal of the American College of Cardiology*, Vol. 58, No. 14, (Sep 2011), pp. 1401-1413, ISSN 0735-1097.

Hare, J.; Brown, J.; Leano, R.; Jenkins, C.; Woodward, N. & Marwick, T. (2009). Use of myocardial deformation imaging to detect preclinical myocardial dysfunction before conventional measures in patients undergoing breast cancer treatment with trastuzumab. *American Heart Journal*, Vol. 158, No. 2, (Aug 2009), pp. 294-301, ISSN 0002-8703.

Hashimoto, I.; Li, X.; Hejmadi, B.; Jones, M.; Zetts, A. & Sahn, D. (2003). Myocardial strain rate is a superior method for evaluation of left ventricular subendocardial function compared with tissue Doppler imaging. *Journal of the American College of Cardiology*, Vol. 42, No. 9, (Nov 2003), pp. 1574–1583, ISSN 0735-1097.

Hausdorf, G.; More, G.; Beron, G.; Erttmann, R.; Winkler, K.; Landbeck, G. & Keck, E. (1988). Long term doxorubicin cardiotoxicity in childhood: non-invasive evaluation of the contractile state and diastolic filling. *British Heart Journal*, Vol. 60, No. 4, (Oct 1988), pp. 309-315, ISSN 0007-0769.

Herman, E.; Lipshultz, S.; Rifai, N.; Zhang, J.; Papoian, T.; Yu, ZX.; Takeda, K. & Ferrans, V. (1998). Use of cardiac Troponin T levels as an indicator of doxorubicin-induced cardiotoxicity. *Cancer research*, Vol. 58, No. 2, (Jan 1998), pp. 195-197, ISSN 0008-5472.

Ho, C. & Solomon, S. (2006). A clinician's guide to tissue Doppler imaging. *Circulation*, Vol. 113, No. 10, (March 2006), pp. e396-e398, ISSN 0009-7322.

Horacek, J.; Pudil, R.; Tichy, M.; Jebavy, L.; Zak, P.; Slovacek, L. & Maly, J. (2007). Biochemical markers and assessment of cardiotoxicity during preparative regimen and hematopoetic cell transplantation in acute leukemia. *Experimental Oncology*, Vol. 29, No. 3, (Sep 2007), pp. 243-247, ISSN 1812-9269.

Horacek, J.; Vasatova, M.; Tichy, M.; Pudil, R.; Jebavy, L. & Maly, J. (2010). The use of cardiac biomarkers in detection of cardiotoxicity associated with conventional and high-dose chemotherapy for acute leukemia. *Experimental Oncology*, Vol. 32, No. 2, (June 2010), pp. 97-99, ISSN 1812-9269.

Horwich, T.; Patel, J.; MacLellan, W. & Fonarow, G. (2003). Cardiac troponin I is associated with impaired hemodynamics, progressive left ventricular dysfunction, and increased mortality rates in advanced heart failure. *Circulation*, Vol. 108, No. 7, (Aug 2003), pp. 833-838, ISSN 0009-7322.

Hudson, M.; O'Connor, C.; Gattis, W.; Tasissa, G.; Hasselblad, V.; Holleman, C.; Gaulden, L.; Sedor, F. & Ohman, E. (2004). Implications of elevated cardiac troponin T in ambulatory patients with heart failure: a prospective analysis. *American Heart Journal*, Vol. 147, No. 3, (Mar 2004), pp. 546-552, ISSN 0002-8703.

Hung, J.; Lang, R.; Flachskampf, F.; Shernan, S.; McCulloch, M.; Adams, D.; Thomas, J.; Vannan, M.; Ryan T. & ASE. (2007). 3d echocardiography: a review of the current status and future directions. *Journal of the American Society of Echocardiography*, Vol. 20, no. 3, (Mar 2007), pp. 213-233, ISSN 0894-7317.

Iwaki, K.; Chi, SH.; Dillmann, W. & Mestril, R. (1993). Induction of HSP70 in cultured rat neonatal cardiomyocytes by hypoxia and metabolic stress. *Circulation*, Vol. 87, No. 6, (June 1993), pp. 2023-2032, ISSN 0009-7322.

Jensen, B.; Skovsgaard, T. & Nielsen, L. (2002). Functional monitoring of anthracycline cardiotoxicity: a prospective, blinded, long-term observational study of outcome in 120 patients. *Annals of Oncology*, Vol. 13, No. 5, (May 2002), pp. 699-709, ISSN 0923-7534.

Jevon, M.; Dorling, A. & Hornick, I. (2008). *Progenitor cells and vascular disease*, Vol. 41, Suppl. s1, (Feb 2008), pp. 146-164.

Jurcut, R.; Wildiers, H.; Ganame, J.; D'hooge, J.; De Backer, J.; Denys, H.; Paridaens, R.; Rademakers, F. & Voigt, J. (2008). Strain rate imaging detects early cardiac effects of pegylated liposomal Doxorubicin as adjuvant therapy in elderly patients with breast cancer. *Journal of the American Society of Echocardiography*, Vol. 21, No. 12, (Dec 2008), pp. 1283-1289, ISSN 0894-7317.

Jurcut, R.; Wildiers, H.; Ganame, J.; D'hooge, J.; Paridaens, R. & Voigt, J. (2008). Detection and monitoring of cardiotoxicity - what does modern cardiology offer? *Supportive Care in Cancer*, Vol. 16, No. 5, (May 2008), pp. 437–445, ISSN 0941-4355.

Kampinga, H. & Craig, E. (2010). The Hsp70 chaperone machinery: J-proteins as drivers of functional specificity. *Nature Reviews Molecular Cell Biology*, Vol. 11, No. 8, (Aug 2010), pp. 579-592, ISSN 1471-0072.

Kilickap, S.; Barista, I.; Akgul, E.; Aytemir, K.; Aksoyek, S.; Aksoy, S.; Celik, I.; Kes, S. & Tekuzman, G. (2005). cTnT can be a useful marker for early detection of antracycline cardiotoxicity. *Annals of Oncology*, Vol. 16, No. 5, (March 2005), pp. 798-804, ISSN 0923-7534.

Kinova, E. & Kozhuharov, H. (2004). Left ventricular diastolic filling patterns as predictors of heart failure after myocardial infarction: a colour M-mode Doppler study. *Hellenic Journal of Cardiology*, Vol. 45, No. 1, (Feb 2004), pp. 23-31, ISSN 1109-9666

Krastev, B.; Kinova, E.; Pencheva, B.; Mihailov, R.; Kyurkchiev, S.; Kehayov, I.; Ivanova, E.; Zlatareva, N. & Goudev, A. (2010). The role of biomarkers in early diagnosis of chemotherapy-induced cardiotoxicity. *Cardiovascular diseases*, Vol. 41, No. 1, (2010), pp. 3-8, ISSN 0204-6865. (article in Bulgarian)

Krastev, B.; Kinova, E.; Zlatareva, N. & Goudev, A. (2010). Early detection of chemotherapy-related cardiotoxicity. *European Journal of Echocardiography*, Vol. 11, Suppl. 2, pp. ii29, ISSN 1525-2167. (Abstract)

Krastev, B.; Kinova, E.; Zlatareva, N. & Goudev, A. (2010). Echocardiographic Doppler predictors of cardiotoxicity in cancer patients during chemotherapy. *Bulgarian Cardiology*, Vol. 16, No. 1, (2010), pp. 34-41, ISSN 1310-7488. (Article in Bulgarian)

Lakoumentas, J.; Panou, F.; Kotseroglou, V.; Aggeli, K. & Harbis, P. (2005). The Tei-index of myocardial performance: applications in cardiology. *Hellenic Journal of Cardiology*, Vol. 46, No. 1, (Jan-Feb 2005), pp. 52-58, ISSN 1109-9666.

Lang, R.; Bierig, M.; Devereux, R.; Flachskampf, F.; Pellikka, P.; Picard, M.; Roman, M.; Seward, J.; Shanewise, J.l Solomon, S.; Spencer, K.; Sutton, M.; Stewart, W.; ASE nomenclature and standarts committee; Task force on chamber quatification; ACC echocardiography committee; AHA; EAE; ESC. (2006). Recommendations for chamber quantification. *European Journal of Echocardiography*, Vol. 7, No. 2, (March 2006), pp. 79-108, ISSN 1525-2167.

Lee, D. & Vasan, R. (2005). Novel markers for heart failure diagnosis and prognosis. *Current Opinion in Cardiology*, Vol. 20, No. 3, (May 2005), pp. 201-210, ISSN 1531-7080.

Lorionte, M.; Palazzoni, G.; Natali, R.; Comerci, G.; Abbate, A.; Di Persio, S. & Biondi-Zoccai, G. (2009). Apprasing cardiotoxicity associated with liposomal doxorubicin by means of tissue Doppler echocardiography end-points: rationale and design of the LITE (Liposomal doxorubicin-Investigational chemotherapy – Tissue Doppler imaging Evaluation) randomized pilot study. *International Journal of Cardiology*, Vol. 135, No. 1, (Jun 2009), pp. 72-77, ISSN 0167-5273.

Marber, M.; Mestril, R.; Chi, S.; Sayen, M.; Yellon, D. & Dillmann, W. (1995). Overexpression of the rat inducible 70-kD heat stress protein in a transgenic mouse increases the resistance of the heart to ischemic injury. *The Journal of Clinical Investigation*, Vol. 95, No. 4, (Apr 1995), pp. 1446-1456, ISSN 0021-9738.

Marwick, T. (2006). Measurement of strain and strain rate by echocardiography. Ready for prime time? *Journal of the American College of cardiology*, Vol. 47, No. 7, (Apr 2006), pp. 1313-1327, ISSN 0735-1097.

Masson, S.; Latini, R.; Anand, I.; Vago, T.; Angelici, L.; Barlera, S.; Missov, E.; Clerico, A.; Tognoni, G.; Cohn J. & Val-HeFT investigators. (2006). Direct comparison of B-type natriuretic peptide (BNP) and amino-terminal proBNP in a large population of patients with chronic and symptomatic heart failure: the Valsartan Heart Failure

(Val-HeFT) data. *Clinical Chemistry*, Vol. 52, No. 8, (Aug 2006), pp. 1528-1538, ISSN 0009-9147.

Milroy, R.; Shapiro, D.; Shenkin, A. & Banham, S. (1989). Acute phase reaction during chemotherapy in small cell lung cancer. *British Journal of Cancer*, Vol. 59, No. 6, (June 1989), pp. 933-935, ISSN 0007-0920.

Mitani, I.; Jain, D.; Joska, T.; Burthess, B. & Zaret, B. (2003). Doxorubicin cardiotoxicity: prevention of congestive heart failure with serial cardiac function monitoring with equilibrium radionuclide angiocardiography in the current era. *Journal of Nuclear Cardiology*, Vol. 10, No. 2, (Mar-Apr 2003), pp. 132-139, ISSN 1071-3581.

Møller, J.; Søndergaard, E.; Seward, J.; Appleton, C. & Egstrup, K. (2000). Ratio of left ventricular peak E-wave velocity to flow propagation velocity assessed by color M-mode Doppler echocardiography in first myocardial infarction: prognostic and clinical implications. *Journal of the American College of Cardiology*, Vol. 35, No. 2, (Feb 2000), pp. 363-370, ISSN 0735-1097.

Morris, P. Chen, C.; Steingart, R.; Fleisher, M.; Lin, N.; Moy, B.; Come, S.; Sugarman, S.; Abbruzzi, A.; Legman, R.; Patil, S.; Dickler, M.; McArthur, H.; Winer, E.; Norton, L.; Hudis, C. & Dang, C. (2010). Troponin I and C-reactive protein are commonly detected in patients with breast cancer treated with dose-dense chemotherapy incorporating trastuzumab and lapatinib. *Clinical Cancer Research*, Vol. 17, No. 10, (May 2011), pp. 3490-3499, ISSN 1078-0432.

Nagi, A.; Cserép, Z.; Tolnay, E.; Nagykálnai, T. & Forster, T. (2008). Early diagnosis of chemotherapy-induced cardiomyopathy: a prospective tissue Doppler imaging study. *Pathology and Oncology Research*, Vol. 14, No. 1, (Mar 2008), pp. 69-77, ISSN 1219-4956.

Nagi, L.; Szabo, F.; Ivanyl, J.; Nemeth, L.; Kovács, G.; Palatka, J.; Tarján, J.; Tóth K. & Rőth E. (2001). A method for detection of doxorubicin-induced cardiotoxicity: flow-mediated vasodilation of the brachial artery. *Experimental and Clinical Cardiology*, Vol. 6, No. 2, (Summer 2001), pp. 87-92, ISSN 1918-1515.

Nagueh, S.; Middleton, K.; Kopelen, H.; Zoghbi, W. & Quinones M. (1997). Doppler tissue imaging: a noninvasive technique for evaluation of left ventricular relaxation and estimation of filling pressures. *Journal of the American College of Cardiology*, Vol. 30, No. 6, (Nov 1997), pp. 1527-1533, ISSN 0735-1097.

Notomi, I.; Lysyansky, P.; Setser, R.; Shiota, T.; Popović, Z.; Martin-Miklovic, M.; Weaver, J.; Oryszak, S.; Greenberg, N.; White, R.; Thomas, J. (2005). Measurement of ventricular torsion by two-dimensional ultrasound speckle tracking imaging. *Journal of the American College of Cardiology*, Vol. 45, No 12, (Jun 2005), pp. 2034-2041, ISSN 0735-1097.

Paulus, W.; Tschöpe, C.; Sanderson, J.; Rusconi, C.; Flachskampf, F.; Rademakers, F.; Marino, P.; Smiseth, O.; De Keulenaer, G.; Leite-Moreira A.; Borbély, A.; Edes, I.; Handoko, M.;Heymans, S.; Pezzali, N.; Pieske, B.; Dickstein, K.; Fraser, A. & Brutsaert, D. (2007). How to diagnose diastolic heart failure: a consensus statement on the diagnosis of heart failure with normal left ventricular ejection fraction by the Heart failure and Echocardiography Associations of the European Society of

Cardiology. *European Heart Journal,*vol. 28, No. 20, (Oct 2007), pp. 2539-2550, ISSN 0195-668x.

Perik, P.; Vries, E.; Boomsma, F.; Messerschmidt, J.; Van Veldhuisen, D.; Sleijfer, D.; Gietema, J. & Van der Graaf, W. (2006). The relation between soluble apoptotic proteins and subclinical cardiotoxicity in adjuvant-treated breast cancer patients. *Anticancer Research,* vol. 26, No. 5B, (Sep 2006), pp. 3803-3811, ISSN 1791-7530.

Rezzani, R.; Rodella, L.; Dessy, C.; Daneau, G.; Bianchi, R. & Feron, O. (2003). Changes in Hsp90 expression determine the effects of cyclosporine A on the NO pathway in rat myocardium. *FEBS Letters,* Vol. 552, No. 2, (Sep 2003), pp. 125-129, ISSN 0014-5793.

Rodriquez-Losada, N.; Garcia-Pinilla, J.; Jimenez-Navarro, M. & Gonzalez, F. (2008). Endothelial progenitor cells in cell-based therapy for cardiovascular disease. *Cellular and Molecular Biology (Noisy-le-Grand, France),* Vol. 54, No. 1, (Oct 2008), pp. 11-23, ISSN 1165-158X.

Rohde, L.; Baldi, A.; Weber, C.; Geib, G.; Mazzotti, N.; Fiorentini, M.; Roggia, M.; Pereira, R. & Clausell, N. (2007). Tei index in adult patients submitted to adriamycin chemotherapy: failure to predict early systolic dysfunction. Diagnosis of adriamycin cardiotoxicity. *The International Journal of Cardiovascular Imaging,* Vol. 23, No. 2, (Apr 2007), pp. 185-191, ISSN 1569-5794.

Sandri, MT.; Savatici, M.; Cardinale, M.; Zorzino, L.; Passerini, R.; Lentati, P.; Leon, M.; Civelli, M.; Martinelli, G. & Cipolla, C. (2005). N-terminal pro-B-type natriuretic peptide after high-dose chemotherapy: a marker predictive of cardiac dysfunction? *Clinical Chemistry,* vol. 51, No. 8, (Aug 2005), pp. 1405-1410, ISSN 0009-9147.

Schmitt, K.; Tulzer, G.; Meri, M.; Aichhorn, G.; Grillenberger, A.; Wiesinger, G. & Hofstadler, G. (1995). Early detection of doxorubicin and daunorubicin cardiotoxicity by echocardiography: diastolic versus systolic parameters. *European Journal of Pediatrics,* Vol. 154, No. 3, (Mar 1995), pp. 201-204, ISSN 0340-6199.

Scully, R. & Lipshultz, E. (2007). Anthracycline cardiotoxicity in long-term survivors of childhood cancer. *Cardiovascular Toxicology,* Vol. 7, No. 2, (Apr 2007), pp. 122-128, doi: 10.1007/s12012-007-0006-4

Seidman, A.; Hudis, C.; Pierri, MK.; Shak, S.; Ashby, M.; Murphy, M.; Stewart, S. & Keefe D. (2002). Cardiac dysfunction in the trastuzumab clinical trials experience. *Journal of Clinical Oncology,* Vol. 20, No. 5, (Mar 2002), pp. 1215-1221, ISSN 0732-183X.

Sengupta, P.;northfelt, D.; Gentile, F.; Zamorano, J. & Kandheria, B. (2008). Trastuzumab-induced cardiotoxicity: heart failure at the crossroads. *Mayo Clinic Proceedings,* Vol. 83, No. 2, (Feb 2008), pp. 197-203, ISSN 0025-6196.

Senju, N.; Ikeda, S.; Koga, S.; Miyahara, Y.; Tsukasaki, K.; Tomonaga, M. & Kohno, S. (2007). The echocardiographic Tei-index reflects early myocardial damage induced by anthracyclines in patients with hematological malignancies. *Heart and Vessels,* Vol. 22, No. 6, (Nov 2007), pp. 393-397, ISSN 1615-2573.

Shi, Y.; Moon, M.; Dawood, S.; McManus, B. & Liu, P. (2011). Mechanisms and management of doxorubicin cardiotoxicity. *Herz,* Vol. 36, No. 4, (Jun 2011), pp. 296-305, ISSN 0340-9937.

Šimončiková, P.; Ravingerová, T. & Barančik, M. (2008). The effect of chronic doxorubicin treatment on mitogen-activated protein kinases and heart stress proteins in rat hearts. *Physiological Research*, Vol. 57, Suppl. 2, (Mar 2008), pp. S97-S102, ISSN 0862-8408.

Singal, P. & Iliskovic, N. (1998). Doxorubicin-induced cardiomyopathy. *The New England Journal of Medicine*, Vol. 339, No. , (Sep 1998), pp. 900-905, ISSN 0028-4793.

Skuta, G.; Fischer, G.; Janaky, T.; Kele, Z.; Szabo, P.; Tozser, J. & Sumegi, B. (1999). Molecular mechanism of the short-term cardiotoxicity caused by 2′,3′-dideoxycytidine (ddC): modulation of reactive oxygen species levels and ADP-ribosylation reactions. *Biochemical Pharmacology*, Vol. 58, No. 12, (Dec 1999), pp. 1915-1925, ISSN 0006-2952.

Slamon, D.; Leyland-Jones, B.; Shak, S.; Fush, H.; Paton, V.; Bajamonde, A.; Fleming, T.; Eiermann, W.; Wolter, J.; Pegram, M.; Baselga, J. & Norton, L. (2001). Use of chemotherapy plus a monoclonal antibody against HER2 for metastatic breast cancer that overexpress HER2. *The New England Journal of Medicine*, Vol. 233, No. 11, (Mar 2001), pp. 783-792, ISSN 0028-4793.

Sohn, D.; Chai, I.; Lee, D.; Kim, H.C.; Kim, H.S.; Oh, B.; Lee, M.; Park, Y.; Seo, J. & Lee Y. (1997). Assessment of mitral annulus velocity by Doppler tissue imaging in the evaluation of left ventricular diastolic function. *Journal of the American College of Cardiology*, Vol. 30, No. 2, (Aug 1997), pp. 474-480, ISSN 0735-1097.

Sugiura, T.; Takase, H.; Toriyama, T.; Goto, T.; Ueda, R. & Dohi, Y. (2005). Circulating levels of myocardial proteins predict future deterioration of congestive heart failure. *Journal of Cardiac Failure*, Vol. 11, No. 7, (Sep 2005), pp. 504-509, ISSN 1071-9164.

Suzuki, T.; Hayashi, D.; Yamazaki, T.; Mizuno, T.; Kanda, Y.; Komuro, I.; Kurabayashi, M.; Yamaoki, K.; Mitani, K.; Hirai, H.; Nagai, R. & Yazaki, Y. (1998). Elevated B-type natriuretic peptide levels after anthracycline administration. *American Heart Journal*, Vol. 136, No. 2, (Aug 1998), pp. 362-363, ISSN 0002-8703.

Tanindi, A.; Demirci, U.; Tacoy, G.; Buyukberber, S.; Alsancak, Y.; Coskun, U.; Yalcin, R. & Benekli, M. (2011). Assessment of right ventricular functions during cancer chemotherapy, In: *European Journal of Echocardiography*, Aug 30, 2011, Available from: doi: 10.1093/ejechocard/jer142

Tassan-Mangina, S.; Codorean, D.; Metivier, M.; Costa, B.; Himberlin, C.; Jouannaud, C.; Blaise, AM.; Elaerts, J. & Nazeyrollas, P. (2006). Tissue Doppler imaging and conventional echocardiography after anthracycline treatment in adults: early and late alterations of left ventricular function during a prospective study. *European Journal of Echocardiography*, Vol. 7, No. 2, (Mar 2006), pp. 141-146, ISSN 1525-2167.

Tei, C.; Ling, L.; Hodge, D.; Bailey K.; Oh, J.; Rodeheffer, R.; Tajik A. & Seward, J. (1995). *Journal of Cardiology*, vol. 26, No. 6, (Dec 1995), pp. 357-366, ISSN 1876-4738.

Torti, F.; Bristow, M.; Lum, B.; Carter, S.; Howes, A.; Aston, D.; Brown, B.; Hannigan, J.; Meyers, F.; Mitchell, E. & Billingham, M. (1986). Cardiotoxicity of epirubicin and doxorubicin: assessment by endomyocardial biopsy. *Cancer Research*, Vol. 46, No. 7, (Jul 1986), pp. 3722-3727, ISSN 0008-5472.

University Hospital, Bordeaux. (Apr 15, 2011). Early detection of anthracycline cardiotoxicity by echocardiographic analysis of myocardial deformation in 2D strain (CA2D). Available at: http://clinicaltrials.gov/ct2/show/NCT01212926

Van Dalen, E.; van der Pal, H.; Kok, W.; Caron, H. & Kremer, L. (2006). *European Journal of Cancer*, Vol. 42, No. 18, (Dec 2006), pp. 3191-3198, ISSN 0014-2964.

Venugopal, S.; Deveraj, S. & Jialal, I. (2005). Effect of C-reactive protein on vascular cells: evidence for a proinflammatory, proatherogenic role. *Current Opinion in Nephrology and Hypertension*, Vol. 14, No. 1, (Jan 2005), pp. 33-37, ISSN 1062-4821.

Yamada, H.; Oki, T.; Tabata, T. & Ito, S. (1998). Assessment of left ventricular systolic wall motion velocity with tissue Doppler imaging: comparison with peak dP/dt of the left ventricular pressure curve. *Journal of the American Society of Echocardiography*, Vol. 11, No. 5, (May 1998), pp. 442-449, ISSN 0894-7317.

Yasue, H.; Oshimura, M.; Sumida, H.; Kikuta, K.; Kugiyama, K.; Jougasaki, M.; Ogawa, H.; Okumura, K.; Mukoyama, M. & Nakao, K. (1994). Localization and mechanism of secretion of B-type natriuretic peptide in comparison with those of A-type natriuretic peptide in normal subjects and patients with heart failure. *Circulation*, vol. 90, No. 1, (Jul 1994), pp. 195-203, ISSN 1524-4539.

Zannad, F.; Alla F.; Dousset, B.; Perez, A. & Pitt, B. (2000). Limitation of excessive extracellular matrix turnover may contribute to survival benefit of spironolactone therapy in patients with congestive heart failure: insights from the Randomized Aldactone Evaluation Study (RALES). *Circulation*, Vol. 102, No. 22, (Nov 2000), pp. 2700-2706, ISSN 0009-7322.

Zethelius, B.; Berglund, L.; Sundström, J.; Ingelsson, E.; Basu, S.; Larsson, A.; Venge P. & Arnlöv, J. (2008). Use of multiple biomarkers to improve the prediction of death from cardiovascular causes. *The New England Journal of Medicine*, Vol. 358, No. 20, (May 2008), pp. 2107-2116, ISSN 0028-4793.